Spatial and Spatio-temporal Bayesian Models with R-INLA

Spatial and Spatio-temporal Bayesian Models with R-INLA

Marta Blangiardo

MRC-PHE Centre for Environment and Health, Department of Epidemiology and Biostatistics, Imperial College London, UK

Michela Cameletti

Department of Management, Economics and Quantitative Methods, University of Bergamo, Italy

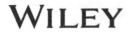

This edition first published 2015
© 2015 John Wiley & Sons, Ltd

Registered office
John Wiley & Sons Ltd, The Atrium, Southern Gate, Chichester, West Sussex, PO19 8SQ, United Kingdom

For details of our global editorial offices, for customer services and for information about how to apply for permission to reuse the copyright material in this book please see our website at www.wiley.com.

Library of Congress Cataloging-in-Publication Data

Blangiardo, Marta.
  Spatial and spatio-temporal Bayesian models with R-INLA / by Marta Blangiardo and Michela Cameletti.
    pages cm
  Includes bibliographical references and index.
  ISBN 978-1-118-32655-8 (cloth)
  1. Bayesian statistical decision theory. 2. Spatial analysis (Statistics) 3. Asymptotic distribution
(Probability theory) 4. R (Computer program language) I. Cameletti, Michela. II. Title.
  QA279.5.B63 2015
  519.5'42—dc23

2015000696

A catalogue record for this book is available from the British Library.

ISBN: 9781118326558

Set in 10/12pt TimesRoman by Laserwords Private Limited, Chennai, India.

1   2015

To MM, Gianluca, Kobi and Clarissa:
now we can enjoy life again!

Contents

Preface

This book presents the principles of Bayesian theory for spatial and spatio-temporal modeling, combining three aspects: (1) an introduction to Bayesian thinking and theoretical aspects of the Bayesian approach, (2) a focus on the spatial and spatio-temporal models used within the Bayesian framework, (3) a series of practical examples which allow the reader to link the statistical theory presented to real data problems. All the examples are coded in the R package R-INLA, and based on the recently developed integrated nested Laplace approximation (INLA) method, which has proven to be a valid alternative to the commonly used Markov Chain Monte Carlo (MCMC) simulations.

The book starts with an introduction in Chapter 1, providing the reader with the importance of spatial and spatio-temporal modeling in several fields, such as social science, environmental epidemiology, and infectious diseases epidemiology. We then show why Bayesian models are commonly used in these fields and why we focus on the INLA approach. We also describe the datasets which will be used in the rest of the book, providing information on the topics that will be used as illustration.

As all the examples are run in R, in Chapter 2 we introduce the basic concepts of the R language. Chapter 3 describes the Bayesian methods: first we introduce the paradigms of this approach (i.e., the concepts of prior and posterior distributions, Bayes theorem, conjugacy, how to obtain the posterior distribution, the computational issues around Bayesian statistics for conjugated and non conjugated models). We also include a small section on the differences between the frequentist and the Bayesian approach, focusing on the different interpretation of confidence intervals, parameters, and hypothesis testing.

Chapter 4 discusses the computational issues regarding Bayesian inference. After the Monte Carlo method is introduced, we consider MCMC algorithms, providing some examples in R for the case of conjugated and non conjugated distributions. The focus of the chapter is the INLA method, which is a computationally powerful alternative to MCMC algorithms. In particular, the R-INLA library is described by means of a small tutorial and of a step-by-step example.

Then in Chapter 5 we present the Bayesian modeling framework which is used in the fields introduced in Chapter 1 and focuses on regression models (linear and generalized linear models). In this context, we introduce the concept of exchangeability and explain how this is used to predict values from variables of interest, a topic which will be expanded later in the chapters on spatial and spatio-temporal modeling. The last section of this part is devoted to introducing hierarchical models.

Chapter 6 focuses on models for two types of spatial processes: (1) area level—introducing disease mapping models and small area ecological regressions (including risk factors and covariates) and then presenting zero inflated models for Poisson and Binomial data; (2) point level—presenting Bayesian kriging through the stochastic partial differential equations (SPDE) approach and showing how to model observed data and also to predict for new spatial locations. Chapter 7 extends the topics treated in Chapter 6 adding a temporal dimension, where we also include the time dimension in the models.

Finally, Chapter 8 introduces new developments within INLA and focuses on the following advanced applications: when data are modeled using different likelihoods, when missing data are present in covariates, a spatio-temporal model with dynamic evolution for the regression coefficients, and a spatio-temporal model for high-frequency data on time where a temporal resolution reduction is needed.

We would like to thank many people who helped with this book: Håvard Rue for his precious contribution, his endless encouragement and for introducing us to Elias Krainski, who became involved in the book; Finn Lindgren, Aurelie Cosandey Godin and Gianluca Baio for reading drafts of the manuscript and providing useful comments; Philip Li, Ravi Maheswaran, Birgit Schrödle, Virgilio Gómez-Rubio, and Paola Berchialla, who provided some of the datasets; finally, a huge thank to our families who have supported us during all this time.

We hope that this book can be helpful for readers at any level, wanting to familiarize or increase their practice and knowledge of the INLA method. Those who are approaching the Bayesian way of thinking for the first time could follow it from the beginning, while those who are already familiar with R and Bayesian inference can easily skip the first chapters and focus on spatial and spatio-temporal theory and applications.

Marta Blangiardo and Michela Cameletti

1

Introduction

1.1 Why spatial and spatio-temporal statistics?

In the last few decades, the availability of spatial and spatio-temporal data has increased substantially, mainly due to the advances in computational tools which allow us to collect real-time data coming from GPS, satellites, etc. This means that nowadays in a wide range of fields, from epidemiology to ecology, to climatology and social science, researchers have to deal with geo-referenced data, i.e., including information about space (and possibly also time).

As an example, we consider a typical epidemiological study, where the interest is to evaluate the incidence of a particular disease such as lung cancer across a given country. The data will usually be available as counts of diseases for small areas (e.g., administrative units) for several years. What types of models allow the researchers to take into account all the information available from the data? It is important to consider the potential geographical pattern of the disease: areas close to each others are more likely to share some geographical characteristics which are related to the disease, thus to have similar incidence. Also how is the incidence changing in time? Again it is reasonable to expect that if there is a temporal pattern, this is stronger for subsequent years than for years further apart.

As a different example, let us assume that we are now in the climatology field and observe daily amount of precipitation at particular locations of a sparse network: we want to predict the rain amount at unobserved locations and we need to take into account spatial correlation and temporal dependency.

Spatial and spatio-temporal models are now widely used: typing "statistical models for spatial data" in ™Google Scholar returns more than 3 million hits and "statistical models for spatio-temporal data" gives about 159,000. There are countless scientific papers in peer review journals which use more or less complex and

Spatial and Spatio-temporal Bayesian Models with R-INLA, First Edition.
Marta Blangiardo and Michela Cameletti.
© 2015 John Wiley & Sons, Ltd. Published 2015 by John Wiley & Sons, Ltd.

innovative statistical models to deal with the spatial and/or the temporal structure of the data in hand, covering a wide range of applications; the following list only aims at providing a flavor of the main areas where these types of models are used: Haslett and Raftery (1989), Handcock and Wallis (1994) and Jonhansson and Glass (2008) work in the meteorology field; Shoesmith (2013) presents a model for crime rates and burglaries, while Pavia *et al.* (2008) used spatial models for predicting election results; in epidemiology Knorr-Held and Richardson (2003) worked on infectious disease, while Waller *et al.* (1997) and Elliott *et al.* (2001) presented models for chronic diseases. Finally, Szpiro *et al.* (2010) focused on air pollution estimates and prediction.

1.2   Why do we use Bayesian methods for modeling spatial and spatio-temporal structures?

Several types of models are used with spatial and spatio-temporal data, depending on the aim of the study. If we are interested in summarizing spatial and spatio-temporal variation between areas using risks or probabilities then we could use statistical methods like disease mapping to compare maps and identify clusters. Moran Index is extensively used to check for spatial autocorrelation (Moran, 1950), while the scan statistics, implemented in SaTScan (Killdorf, 1997), has been used for cluster detection and to perform geographical surveillance in a non-Bayesian approach. The same types of models can also be used in studies where there is an aetiological aim to assess the potential effect of risk factors on outcomes.

A different type of study considers the quantification of the risk of experiencing an outcome as the distance from a certain source increases. This is typically framed in an environmental context, so that the source could be a point (e.g., waste site, radio transmitter) or a line (e.g., power line, road). In this case, the methods typically used vary from nonparametric tests proposed by Stone (1988) to the parametric approach introduced by Diggle *et al.* (1998).

In a different context, when the interest lies in mapping continuous spatial (or spatio-temporal) variables, which are measured only at a finite set of specific points in a given region, and in predicting their values at unobserved locations, geostatistical methods – such as kriging – are employed (Cressie, 1991; Stein, 1991). This may play a significant role in environmental risk assessment in order to identify areas where the risk of exceeding potentially harmful thresholds is higher.

Bayesian methods to deal with spatial and spatio-temporal data started to appear around year 2000, with the development of Markov chain Monte Carlo (MCMC) simulative methods (Casella and George, 1992; Gilks *et al.*, 1996). Before that the Bayesian approach was almost only used for theoretical models and found little applications in real case studies due to the lack of numerical/analytical or simulative tools to compute posterior distributions. The advent of MCMC has triggered the possibility for researchers to develop complex models on large datasets without the need of imposing simplified structures. Probably the main contribution to spatial and spatio-temporal statistics is the one of Besag *et al.* (1991), who developed the Besag–York–Mollié (BYM) method (see Chapter 6) which is commonly used for disease mapping, while Banerjee *et al.* (2004), Diggle and Ribeiro (2007) and Cressie and Wikle (2011) have concentrated on Bayesian geostatistical models. The main advantage of the Bayesian approach resides in its taking into account uncertainty in the estimates/predictions, and its flexibility and capability of dealing with issues like missing data. In the book, we follow this paradigm and introduce the Bayesian philosophy and inference in Chapter 3, while in Chapter 4 we review Bayesian computation tools, but the reader could also find interesting the following: Knorr-Held (2000) and Best *et al.* (2005) for disease mapping and Diggle *et al.* (1998) for a modeling approach for continuous spatial data and for prediction.

1.3   Why INLA?

MCMC methods are extensively used for Bayesian inference, but their limitation resides in their computational burden. This has become an important issue, considering the advances in data collection, leading to availability of *big datasets*, characterized by high spatial and temporal resolution as well as data from different sources. The model complexity of taking into account spatial and spatio-temporal structures with large datasets could lead to several days of computing time to perform Bayesian inference via MCMC.

To overcome this issue, here comes the integrated nested Laplace approximations (INLA), a deterministic algorithm proposed by Rue *et al.* (2009) which has proven capable of providing accurate and fast results. It started as a stand-alone program but was then embedded into R (as a package called R-INLA), and since then it has become very popular amongst statisticians and applied researchers in a wide range of fields, with spatial and spatio-temporal models being possibly one of the main applications for it. The website www.r-inla.org provides a great resource of papers and tutorials and it contains a forum where users can post queries and requests of help. In this book we provide a detailed documentation of the INLA functions and options for modeling spatial and spatio-temporal data and use a series of examples drawn from epidemiology, social and environmental science.

1.4   Datasets

In this section, we briefly describe the datasets that we will use throughout the book. They are available for download from R packages or from the INLA website (https://sites.google.com/a/r-inla.org/stbook/), where we also provide the R code used to run all the examples.[1]

---

[1] From now onward, we use the typewriter font for computer code.

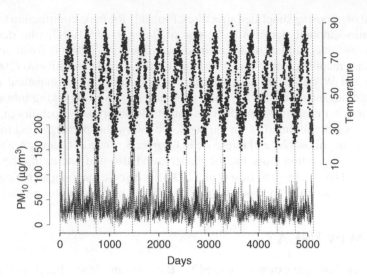

Figure 1.1   Daily temperature (points) and PM$_{10}$ concentration (line) in Salt Lake City (1987–2000).

1.4.1   National Morbidity, Mortality, and Air Pollution Study

The National Morbidity, Mortality and Air Pollution Study (NMMAPS) is a large time series study to estimate the effect of air pollution on the health of individuals living in 108 US cities during the period 1987–2000. Several papers have been published on the data, methods, and results from this study (see, for instance, Samet *et al.* 2000). Detailed information about the database can be found on the Internet-based Health and Air Pollution Surveillance System (iHAPSS) website (http://www.ihapss.jhsph.edu/). Data on the daily concentration of particulates with an aerodynamic diameter of less than 10 (PM$_{10}$) and nitrogen dioxide (NO$_2$), both measured in µg/m^3, as well as daily temperature for Salt Lake City are contained in the file NMMAPSraw.csv.

We use this dataset to study the relationship between PM$_{10}$ and temperature as an illustration of a linear regression model (Chapter 5). A plot which shows the trend of PM$_{10}$ and temperature for the 14 years of available data is presented in Figure 1.1.

1.4.2   Average income in Swedish municipalities

Statistics Sweden (http://www.scb.se/) has created a population registry of Sweden, with detailed socioeconomic information at the individual and household level for all Swedish municipalities. This dataset was used by the EURAREA Consortium (EURAREA Consortium, 2004), a European research project funded by EUROSTAT, to investigate methods for small area estimation and their application. Gómez-Rubio *et al.* (unpublished) also used this dataset to illustrate how

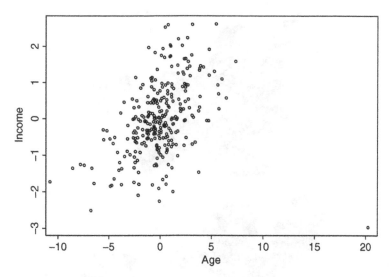

Figure 1.2   Relationship between the average age of the household and the average household income for 284 Swedish municipalities.

Bayesian hierarchical models can be implemented to provide good quality small area estimates and focused on the relationship between the average household income and the average age of the household heads. We are using a simulated version of the dataset[2] to show how to implement the Student t likelihood to deal with outliers in a linear regression model in Chapter 5.

The data are available in the file income.csv and contains the simulated average household income (income) and the average age for the head of the household (age) for 284 Swedish municipalities. Both variables are standardized. Figure 1.2 shows the relationship between the two variables.

1.4.3   Stroke in Sheffield

Maheswaran *et al.* (2006) analyzed the effect of outdoor modeled nitrogen oxide (NOx) levels, classified into quintiles, on stroke mortality in Sheffield (UK) between 1994 and 1998, using a Bayesian hierarchical model with spatial random effects. An association was observed between higher levels of NOx (in $\mu g/m^3$) and stroke mortality at the small area level (1030 enumeration districts, including on average 150 households). We use this dataset as an illustration of the Binomial generalized linear model in Chapter 5 and then of the hierarchical models in the same chapter.

The numbers of observed and expected stroke cases in each enumeration district, together with the NOx exposure and a measure of social deprivation (Townsend

---

[2] It was not possible to use the real data for privacy issues.

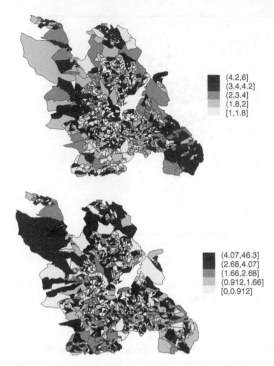

Figure 1.3   NOx concentration (top) and proportion of strokes registered per 1000 individuals (bottom) for enumeration districts in Sheffield (UK).

index), are available in the file Stroke.csv. Both variables are available in quintiles. Figure 1.3 shows the maps of NOx concentration (top) and the proportion of observed (O) strokes registered per 1000 individuals obtained as $\frac{O_i}{Pop_i} \times 1000$ (bottom) at the enumeration district level.

1.4.4   Ship accidents

McCullagh and Nelder (1989) used this dataset to study the rate of incidents in ships. The data are provided in the file Ships.csv. They include identification number (id), ship type (type), construction period (built), operation period (oper), and number of incidents (y). The natural logarithm of the number of months in operation is specified as the offset (months).

We use this dataset to illustrate the Poisson regression presented in Chapter 5. Figure 1.4 shows boxplots of the relationship between each predictor and the number of incidents (outcome).

1.4.5   CD4 in HIV patients

We consider simulated data from a clinical trial comparing two alternative treatments for HIV-infected individuals. 80 patients with HIV infection were randomly

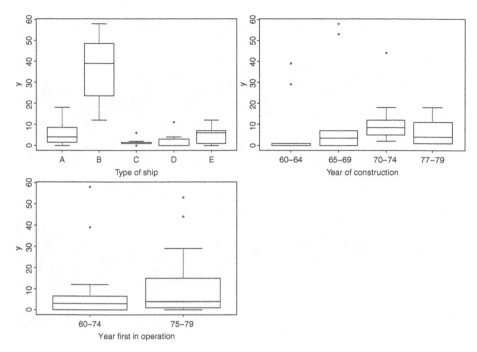

Figure 1.4   Boxplots of the relationship between each predictor and the number of accidents: type of ship (top left), year of construction (top right), and year when first in operation (bottom left).

assigned to one of two treatment groups: drug = 0 (didanosine, ddI) and drug = 1 (zalcitabine, ddC). Counts of CD4, cells commonly used in HIV positive patients as they are part of the immune system, were recorded at study entry (time $t = 0$) and again at 2, 6, and 12 months. An indicator of whether the patient had already been diagnosed with AIDS at study entry was also recorded (AIDS = 1 if patient diagnosed with AIDS, and 0 otherwise). The data can be found in the file CD4.csv.

We use this dataset to illustrate the hierarchical structure in regression models in Chapter 5. Figure 1.5 shows the distribution of CD4 for each patient, stratified by the use of drugs and the AIDS diagnosis.

1.4.6   Lip cancer in Scotland

Clayton and Kaldor (1987) analyzed the lip cancer rates in Scotland in the years 1975–1980 at the county level in order to evaluate the presence of an association between sun exposure and lip cancer. The example is part of the GeoBUGS Manual (Spiegelhalter *et al.* 1996; see http://mathstat.helsinki.fi /openbugs/Manuals/GeoBUGS/Manual.html) and is used here to illustrate hierarchical models (Chapter 5). The dataset is available as an R workspace (see Section 3.3), named LipCancer.RData, containing the number of counties

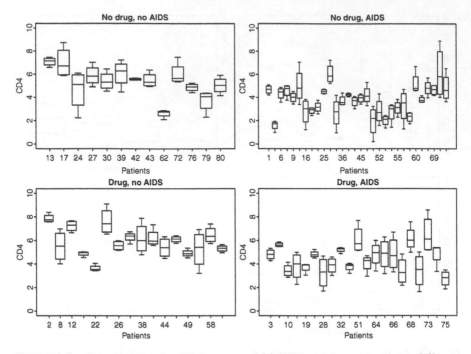

Figure 1.5   Boxplots for the CD4 counts of 80 HIV positive patients (at different time points), stratified by the drug use and the AIDS diagnosis.

($N = 56$), the observed cases of lip cancer in each county (O), the expected number of cases adjusted by the age and sex distribution of the population in the county (E), and the exposure variable (X), which measures the percentage of the population working in an outdoor environment (agriculture, fishing, or forestry), thus highly exposed to the sun. Figure 1.6 shows the map of the exposure variable (top) and of the standardized morbidity ratio ($SMR_i = O_i/E_i$, bottom) for the 56 counties.

1.4.7   Suicides in London

Congdon (2007) studied suicide mortality in 32 London boroughs (excluding the City of London) in the period 1989–1993 for male and female combined, using a disease mapping model and an ecological regression model.

We use this example to illustrate the intrinsic conditional autoregressive (iCAR) structure described in Chapter 6. The dataset is available as an R workspace, named LondonSuicides.RData, which contains the number of boroughs (N), the number of observed suicides in the period under study (O), the number of expected cases of suicides (E), an index of social deprivation (X1), and an index of social fragmentation (X2), which represents the lack of social connections and of sense of community.

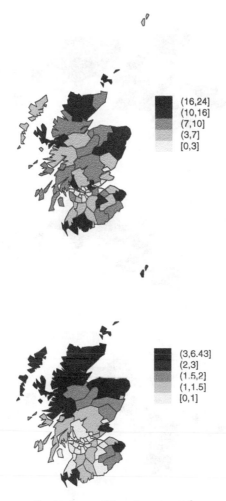

Figure 1.6   Percentage of people working in an outdoor environment (top) and SMR for lip cancer (bottom) in the 56 Scottish counties.

Figure 1.7 shows the distribution of the social deprivation index (top), the social fragmentation index (center) and the SMR for suicides (bottom) in the 32 London boroughs.

1.4.8   Brain cancer in Navarra, Spain

Gómez-Rubio and Lopez-Quilez (2010) developed a statistical method to perform cluster detection on rare diseases and applied it to the study of the brain cancer incidence in Navarra (Spain), following the previous work of Ugarte *et al.* (2006). The data are available as an R workspace named Navarre.RData: the object brainnav contains the observed cases (OBSERVED), expected (EXPECTED)

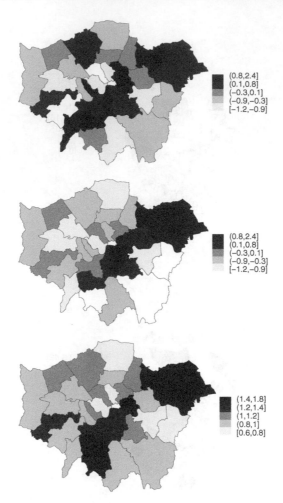

Figure 1.7   Distribution of social deprivation index (top), social fragmentation index (center), and SMR of suicide (bottom) in the 32 London boroughs.

ones, and SMR (SMR) of brain cancer in 1988–1994 for the 40 health districts in the Navarra region of Spain.

As the data contains a large proportion of zeros (32.5%), the standard Poisson model used for disease mapping is not appropriate, so we use this example to illustrate the zero inflated Poisson models (ZIP) in Chapter 6.

Figure 1.8 shows the SMR for brain cancer in the 40 health districts.

1.4.9   Respiratory hospital admission in Turin province

Atmospheric pollution is known to be associated with respiratory hospital admissions and mortality in small area studies (see, for instance, Sunyer *et al.*, 1997, 2003). We use an example on data for PM_{10} and hospital admissions for respiratory

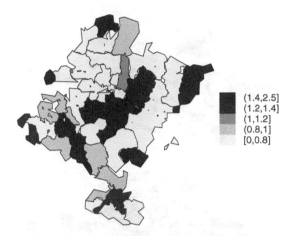

Figure 1.8   SMR of brain cancer for the 40 health districts in Navarra (Spain).

causes in the Turin province (Italy) in 2004 to introduce a zero inflated binomial regression model (ZIB) in Chapter 6, as the outcome variable is very sparse and the risk factor is spatially structured. The number of observed hospitalizations for respiratory causes at municipality level, the population for the same spatial units, and the average annual concentration of PM_{10} are available in the file dataResp.csv.

The map in Figure 1.9 (top) shows the distribution of the percentage of respiratory hospital admissions (over the total population) in the 315 municipalities considered in this example. The map in Figure 1.9 (bottom) shows the distribution of the average PM_{10} for the same period and the same areas.

1.4.10   Malaria in the Gambia

Diggle *et al.* (2002) studied the prevalence of malaria in children sampled from a village in the Gambia using generalized linear models. The dataset gambia (available as dataframe in the geoR package) contains data on eight variables and 2035 children living in 65 villages. The response variable (pos) is a binary indicator of the presence of malarial parasites in a blood sample. Other child level covariates are: age (age, in days), usage of bed nets (netuse), and information about whether the bed nets are treated with insecticide (treated). Village level covariates regard the vegetation index (green) and the inclusion or not of the village in the primary health care system (phc).

We use this example to illustrate the Bayesian kriging in Chapter 6 through the stochastic partial differential equation (SPDE) approach of Lindgren *et al.* (2011). The map in Figure 1.10 shows the Gambia region with the location of the villages.

1.4.11   Swiss rainfall data

In 1997 a statistical exercise named *The Spatial Interpolation Comparison 97 project* was organized by the Radioactivity Environmental Monitoring (Joint

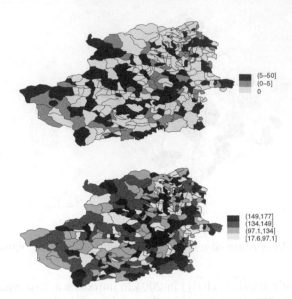

Figure 1.9   Distribution of the percentage of hospital admissions for respiratory causes in 2004 (over the total population) in the 315 municipalities in the Turin province, Italy (top). Map of the average PM$_{10}$ concentration in 2004 for the 315 municipalities (bottom).

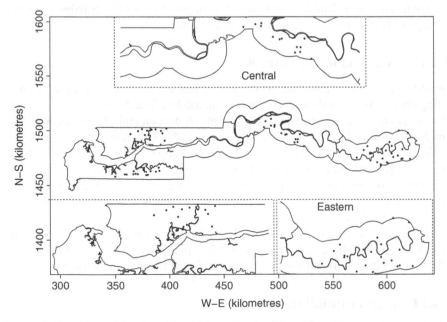

Figure 1.10   Map of the Gambia, Africa: the dots identifies villages where malaria prevalence has been recorded in children.

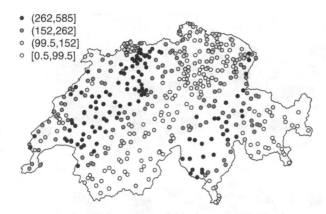

Figure 1.11   Rainfall data (in 10th of mm) collected on May 8, 1986, at 467 locations in Switzerland.

Research Centre, European Commission) to explore the impact of human factors in selecting and using spatial interpolation algorithms for mapping purposes (Dubois, 1998). The participants were asked to estimate daily rainfall values at 367 sites in Switzerland using 100 observed measurements (in 10th of mm) taken on May 8, 1986.

The data are included in the geoR library as an object named SIC which is formed by four geodata objects (a geodata object is a list with two obligatory arguments given by coords and data) denoted by sic.all, sic.100, sic.367, and sic.some, which differ in the number of spatial locations. Each object contains the following variables: location coordinates (coords), rainfall measurements (data), and elevation values (altitude). Additionally, a matrix named sic.borders with Switzerland borders is included.

The spatial distribution of the rainfall data measured at the 467 spatial locations is displayed in Figure 1.11. In Chapter 6, we use the rainfall data to illustrate spatial prediction (i.e., kriging) for a continuous spatial process.

1.4.12   Lung cancer mortality in Ohio

Lawson (2009) presented a space–time disease mapping model on lung cancer mortality in the Ohio counties (USA) for the years 1968–1988. We use the same dataset here to illustrate the parametric spatio-temporal disease mapping approach in Chapter 7.

The data are stored in the OhioRespMort.csv file, which consists of a matrix of (88×21) rows (counties × years) and six columns with the name and the ID of the county (NAME and county), the year (year), the number of deaths (y), the number of exposed individuals (n), and the expected number of deaths (E).

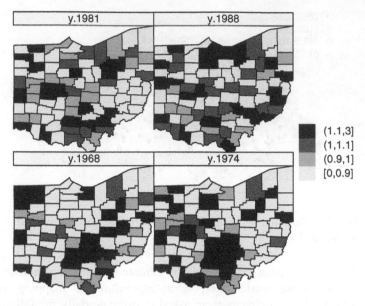

Figure 1.12   Distribution of standardized mortality rates of lung cancer in 88 counties in Ohio (USA) during 1968, 1974, 1981, and 1988.

Figure 1.12 displays the distribution of standardized mortality ratios ($SMR_i = y_{it}/E_{it}$) of respiratory cancer deaths for four years.

1.4.13   Low birth weight births in Georgia

Lawson (2009) considered counts of very low birth weight (<1500 g) in the counties of Georgia (USA) for the years 1994–2004 to perform spatio-temporal disease mapping. Here we consider counts of low birth weight (<2500 g) for the 159 counties of Georgia during 2000–2010 in order to illustrate the spatio-temporal Poisson nonparametric approach in Chapter 7.

The data were obtained from the Georgia Department of Public Health website through the OASIS web query system (http://oasis.state.ga.us/) and are stored in the Lowbirthweight_births.csv and Total_births.csv files, which contain for each county and year the number of low birth weight births and the total number of births, respectively.

Figure 1.13 displays the distribution of standardized incidence ratios of low birth weight for the 11 considered years.

1.4.14   Air pollution in Piemonte

Cameletti *et al.* (2011) analyzed PM_{10} concentration measured in the Piemonte region (Northern Italy) during October 2005–March 2006. The data come from a monitoring network composed of 24 stations.

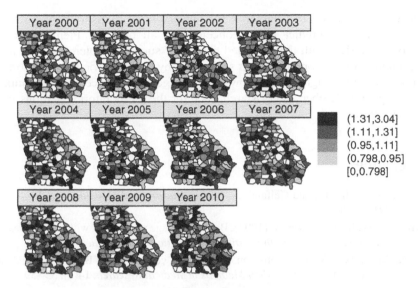

Figure 1.13   Distribution of standardized incidence rate of low birth weight births in 159 counties in Georgia (USA) during 2000–2010.

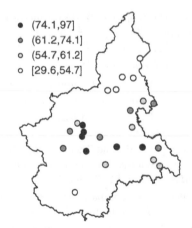

Figure 1.14   Average PM$_{10}$ (μg/m^3) concentration during October 2005–March 2006 for the 24 monitoring stations in the Piemonte region (Northern Italy).

The data are stored in the `Piemonte_data_byday.csv` file which contains daily PM$_{10}$ concentration (`PM10`, in μg/m^3) and some covariates: daily maximum mixing height (`HMIX`, in m), daily total precipitation (`PREC`, in mm), daily mean wind speed (`WS`, in m/s), daily mean temperature (`TEMP`, in K), daily emission rates of primary aerosols (`EMI`, in g/s), altitude (`A`, in m), and spatial coordinates (`UTMX` and `UTMY`, in km).

We use this dataset in Chapter 7 for implementing a spatio-temporal model with covariates to predict PM_{10} concentration all over the Piemonte region. Moreover, we deal with the so-called change of support problem in order to get concentration predictions at a lower scale given by health districts where mortality data are available. Figure 1.14 shows the average PM_{10} concentration computed over the period October 2005–March 2006 for the 24 monitoring stations in the Piemonte region.

References

Banerjee, S., Carlin, B., and Gelfand, A. (2004). *Hierarchical Modeling and Analysis for Spatial Data*. CRC.

Besag, J., York, J., and Mollie, A. (1991). Bayesian image restoration, with two applications in spatial statistics. *Annals of the Institute of Statistical Mathematics*, **43**, 1–59.

Best, N., Richardson, S., and Thompson, A. (2005). A comparison of Bayesian spatial models for disease mapping. *Statistical Methods in Medical Research*, **14**(1), 35–59.

Cameletti, M., Ignaccolo, R., and Bande, S. (2011). Comparing spatio-temporal models for particulate matter in Piemonte. *Environmetrics*, **22**, 985–996.

Casella, G. and George, E. (1992). Explaining the Gibbs sampler. *American Statistician*, **46**, 167–174.

Clayton, D. and Kaldor, J. (1987). Empirical Bayes estimates of age-standardized relative risks for use in disease mapping. *Biometrics*, **43**, 671–681.

Congdon, P. (2007). *Bayesian Statistical Modelling*. John Wiley and Sons, Ltd.

Cressie, N. (1991). *Statistics for Spatial Data*. Wiley.

Cressie, N. and Wikle, C. (2011). *Statistics for Spatio-Temporal Data*. Wiley.

Diggle, P. and Ribeiro, J. P. (2007). *Model-based Geostatistics*. Springer.

Diggle, P., Moyeed, R., and Tawn, J. (1998). Model-based geostatistics. *Journal of the Royal Statistical Society, Series C*, **47**, 299–350.

Diggle, P., Moyeed, R., Rowlingson, B., and Thomson, M. (2002). Childhood Malaria in the Gambia: A case-study in model-based geostatistics. *Journal of the Royal Statistical Society, Series C (Applied Statistics)*, **51**(4), 493–506.

Dubois, G. (1998). Spatial interpolation comparison 97: Foreword and introduction. *Journal of Geographic Information and Decision Analysis*, **2**, 1–10.

Elliott, N., Wakefield, J., Best, N., and Briggs, D., editors (2001). *Spatial Epidemiology*. Oxford University Press.

EURAREA Consortium (2004). *Project reference volume*. EURAREA Consortium. http://www.ons.gov.uk/ons/guide-method/method-quality /general-methodology/spatial-analysis-and-modelling /eurarea/index.html.

Gilks, W., Richardson, S., and Spiegelhalter, D. (1996). *Markov Chain Monte Carlo in Practice*. Chapman & Hall/CRC.

Gómez-Rubio, V. and Lopez-Quilez, A. (2010). Statistical methods for the geographical analysis of rare diseases. *Advances in Experimental Medicine and Biology*, **686**, 151–171.

Handcock, M. and Wallis, J. (1994). An approach to statistical spatial-temporal modelling of meteorological fields. *Journal of the American Statistical Association*, **86**, 368–390.

Haslett, J. and Raftery, A. (1989). Space time modelling with long memory dependence: Assessing Ireland's wind power resource. *Journal of Applied Statistics*, **38**(1), 1–50.

Jonhansson, M. and Glass, G. (2008). High-resolution spatio-temporal weather models for climate studies. *International Journal of Health Geographics*, **7**(52), 1–8.

Killdorf, M. (1997). A spatial scan statistics. *Communications in Statistics: Theory and Methods*, **26**, 1481–1496.

Knorr-Held, L. (2000). Bayesian modelling of inseparable space-time variation in disease risk. *Statistics in Medicine*, **19** (17–18), 2555–2567.

Knorr-Held, L. and Richardson, S. (2003). A hierarchical model for space-time surveillance data on meningococcal disease incidence. *Journal of the Royal Statistical Society, Series C*, **52**(2), 169–183.

Lawson, A. (2009). *Bayesian Disease Mapping. Hierarchical Modeling in Spatial Epidemiology*. CRC Press.

Lindgren, F., Rue, H., and Lindström, J. (2011). An explicit link between Gaussian fields and Gaussian Markov random fields: The stochastic partial differential equation approach (with discussion). *Journal of Royal Statistical Society, Series B*, **73**(4), 423–498.

Maheswaran, R., Haining, R., Pearson, T., Law, J., Brindley, P., and Best, N. (2006). Outdoor NOx and stroke mortality: Adjusting for small area level smoking prevalence using a Bayesian approach. *Statistical Methods in Medical Research*, **15**(5), 499–516.

McCullagh, P. and Nelder, J. (1989). *Generalized Linear Models, Second Edition*. Chapman & Hall.

Moran, P. (1950). Notes on continuous stochastic phenomena. *Biometrika*, **37**(1), 17–23.

Pavia, J., Larraz, B., and Montero, J. (2008). Election forecasts using spatio-temporal models. *Journal of the American Statistical Association*, **103**(483), 1050–1059.

Rue, H., Martino, S., and Chopin, N. (2009). Approximate Bayesian inference for latent Gaussian model by using integrated nested Laplace approximations (with discussion). *Journal of Royal Statistical Society, Series B*, **71**, 319–392.

Samet, J., Dominici, F., Zeger, S., Schwartz, J., and Dockery, D. (2000). The National Morbidity, Mortality, and Air Pollution Study, Part I: Methods and Methodologic Issues. *Research Report of the Health Effects Institute*, **94**.

Shoesmith, G. (2013). Space time autoregressive models and forecasting national, regional and state crime rates. *International Journal of Forecasting*, **29**(1), 191–201.

Spiegelhalter, D., Thomas, A., Best, N., and Gilks, W. (1996). BUGS: Bayesian Inference Using Gibbs Sampling, Version 0.5, (version ii). MRC Biostatistics Unit.

Stein, M. (1991). *Interpolation of Spatial Data: Some Theory of Kriging*. Springer.

Stone, R. (1988). Investigations of excess environmental risks around putative sources: Statistical problems and a proposed test. *Statistics in Medicine*, **7**, 649–660.

Sunyer, J., Spix, C., Quenel, P., Ponce-de Leon, A., Ponka, A., Barumandzadeh, T., Touloumi, G., Bacharova, L., Wojtyniak, B., Vonk, J., Bisanti, L., Schwartz, J., and Katsouyanni, K. (1997). Urban air pollution and emergency admissions for asthma in four European cities: the APHEA Project. *Thorax*, **52**(9), 760–765.

Sunyer, J. Atkinson, R., Ballester, F., Le Tertre, A., Ayres, J. G., Forastiere, F., Forsberg, B., Vonk, J. M., Bisanti, L., Anderson, R. H., Schwartz, J., Katsouyanni, K. (2003). Respiratory effects of sulphur dioxide: a hierarchical multicity analysis in the APHEA 2 study. *Occupation Environmental Medicine*, **60**(8), e2.

Szpiro, A., Sampson, P., Sheppard, L., Lumley, T., Adar, S., and Kaufman, J. (2010). Predicting intra-urban variation in air pollution concentrations with complex spatio-temporal dependencies. *Environmetrics*, **21**(6), 606–631.

Ugarte, M., Ibanez, B., and Militino, F. (2006). Modelling risks in disease mapping. *Statistical Methods in Medical Research*, **15**, 21–35.

Waller, L., Carlin, B., Xia, H., and Gelfand, A. (1997). Hierarchical spatio-temporal mapping of disease rates. *Journal of the American Statistical Association*, **92**(438), 607–617.

2

Introduction to R

2.1 The R language

R is a statistical computer program which provides a rich environment for data analysis and graphics. It can be freely downloaded from the website http://www.r-project.org/ under the GNU General Public License. Its installation is straightforward and at this stage we assume that R is installed on your machine. This section attempts at introducing R for beginners focusing only on the items which are useful to know for this book. For more details about R basics and its use for statistical analysis, we refer the reader to Crawley (2007), Chambers (2008), Dalgaard (2008), Everitt and Hothorn (2009) and Zuur *et al.* (2012). Moreover, the literature is rich of books devoted to applications with R such as, for example, time series analysis and econometrics (Kleiber and Zeileis, 2008; Cowpertwait and Metcalfe, 2009; Shumway and Stoffer, 2011), ecology (Stevens, 2009; Zuur *et al.*, 2009), Bayesian inference (Albert, 2009), geostatistics (Bivand *et al.*, 2008), as well as epidemiology and biostatistics (Peng and Dominici, 2008; Logan, 2010).

After launching R, the user can type commands in the console, for instance, starting with some simple arithmetic expressions

```
> 3 * 2
[1] 6
```

and getting the corresponding result, where > and [1] denote the cursor and the response, respectively. The elementary arithmetic operators are the usual +, -, *, /, and ^. Moreover, all the common arithmetic functions are available, such as log, exp, sin, sqrt. For instance,

---

Spatial and Spatio-temporal Bayesian Models with R-INLA, First Edition.
Marta Blangiardo and Michela Cameletti.
© 2015 John Wiley & Sons, Ltd. Published 2015 by John Wiley & Sons, Ltd.

```
> exp(2)
[1] 7.389056
> log(10) #Comment: base = e
[1] 2.302585
> sqrt(4)
[1] 2
```

Note that it is possible to include comments in the code using the # symbol.

To store a value or the result of an arithmetic operation in a variable, we use the assignment operator <- as follows[1]:

```
> x <- 3   #Comment: this is an assignment.
> x
[1] 3
> y <- sqrt(4)
> y
[1] 2
```

It is worth noting that R is case sensitive, so that y is different from Y.

To perform statistical analysis, we need a collection of values which can be stored in more complex objects, like vectors, matrices, lists and dataframes, all described in the following section.

2.2 R objects

Vectors

To create a vector named x, the function c (that stands for concatenate or collect) is used, as in

```
> x <- c(2, 4, 6, 8)
```

Then if we type

```
> x
[1] 2 4 6 8
```

R will return all the values stored in x. In certain cases, it may be useful to check the number of elements in the vector, which can be done typing

```
> length(x)
[1] 4
```

Arithmetic operations on vectors are carried out element by element. So, for instance, if we want to multiply x by a constant or to compute its square root we type the following commands:

```
> x2 <- x * 2
> x2
[1]  4  8 12 16
```

---

[1] For assignment it is also possible to use the = operator.

```
> x3 <- sqrt(x)
> x3
[1] 1.414214 2.000000 2.449490 2.828427
```

Calculations can also involve two or more vectors at a time, as in

```
> x4 <- x2 + x3
> x4
[1]  5.414214 10.000000 14.449490 18.828427
> x5 <- x3^2 * log(x4)
> x5
[1]  3.378055  9.210340 16.023955 23.482942
```

R can do operations also when the vector lengths differ; in this case the elements of the shorter vector are recycled as often as necessary to create a vector with the same length of the longer term, as in the following example:

```
> z <- c(10,20)
> x + z
[1] 12 24 16 28
```

Note that R provides a warning message when the longer object length is not a multiple of the shorter object length.

It is possible to summarize the values of vectors using functions like sum, min, max, range, mean, var. For example, the mean of x5 is given by

```
> mean(x5)
[1] 13.02382
```

that is equivalent to

```
> sum(x5)/length(x5)
[1] 13.02382
```

In the same way, the sample variance can be computed typing

```
> var(x5)
[1] 75.32582
```

or

```
> sum((x5 - mean(x5))^2) / (length(x5) - 1)
[1] 75.32582
```

A regular sequence is a particular type of vector which can be set up calling the seq or rep function. Before using it, it is worth having a look at the help page of seq that can be invoked with help(seq) or ?seq. The help page provides the following definition:

```
seq(from = 1, to = 1, by = ((to - from)/(length.out - 1)),
                    length.out = NULL, along.with = NULL, ...)
```

where from, to, by, length.out, and along.with are the arguments of the function whose description is given in the help page. For example, from and to define the starting and ending value of the sequence, that are set by default to 1. Not all the arguments of the function need to be specified when the function is called; R will assign to these their default values if not told otherwise. For example, if we enter

```
> seq(from = 1, to = 10)
[1]  1  2  3  4  5  6  7  8  9 10
```

we get the sequence of integer values from 1 to 10. On the contrary, with the command

```
> seq(from = 1, to = 5, by = 0.5)
[1] 1.0 1.5 2.0 2.5 3.0 3.5 4.0 4.5 5.0
```

we obtain the sequence of values from 1 to 10 with step equal to 0.5. Again, if we just fix the starting (or ending) value of the sequence and its length, we get

```
> seq(from = 1, length.out = 10)
 [1]  1  2  3  4  5  6  7  8  9 10
> seq(to = 1, length.out = 10)
 [1] -8 -7 -6 -5 -4 -3 -2 -1  0  1
```

R employs the so-called positional matching. Thus, if we call a function specifying the arguments in the same order they appear in the function definition (as given in the help page), it is not necessary to specify the name of the arguments. For example, the command

```
> seq(from = 1, to = 5, by = 0.5)
[1] 1.0 1.5 2.0 2.5 3.0 3.5 4.0 4.5 5.0
```

gives the same output of

```
> seq(1, 5, 0.5)
[1] 1.0 1.5 2.0 2.5 3.0 3.5 4.0 4.5 5.0
```

But attention is needed because, for instance,

```
> seq(from = 1, to = 10, length.out = 3)
[1]  1.0  5.5 10.0
```

is not equal to

```
> seq(1, 10, 3)
[1]  1  4  7 10
```

as 3 in this case refers to the step of the sequence (by) and not to its length. Instead, if we specify the argument names we can change their order as we like, and they can also be truncated provided they are not ambiguous. So, for example, the following commands are equivalent:

```
> seq(to = 10, from = 1, length.out = 3)
[1]  1.0  5.5 10.0
> seq(f = 1, t = 10, l= 3)
[1]  1.0  5.5 10.0
```

Another useful function is rep, which creates vectors with repeated elements, as in

```
> rep(x = 2, times = 4)
[1] 2 2 2 2
```

The same function also allows us to repeat a whole vector or the elements of a vector for a fixed number of times:

```
> rep(x2, times = 3)
 [1]  4  8 12 16  4  8 12 16  4  8 12 16
> rep(x2, each = 3)
 [1]  4  4  4  8  8  8 12 12 12 16 16 16
```

A particular type of vectors is the logical one, which consists of the sequence of TRUE and FALSE values. Usually a logical vector is created by checking if a condition is met. For example, if we enter the following command on x2 (recall that x2<-c(4,8,12,16)):

```
> x6 <- x2 > 8
> x6
[1] FALSE FALSE  TRUE  TRUE
```

we get the vector named x6 whose length is the same as of x2 and with elements equal to TRUE if the condition is met (x2 >8) and FALSE otherwise. The logical operators are: <, <=, >, >= for relational operations, == for exact equality and != for inequality. Moreover, the classical operators *AND*, *OR*, and *NOT* are reproduced using &, | and !. Some examples are given below[2]:

```
> x7 <- c(seq(1, 5), rep(6,3))
> x7
[1] 1 2 3 4 5 6 6 6
> x7 == 4
[1] FALSE FALSE FALSE  TRUE FALSE FALSE FALSE FALSE
> x7 != 4
[1]  TRUE  TRUE  TRUE FALSE  TRUE  TRUE  TRUE  TRUE
> x7 == 4 | x7 == 6
[1] FALSE FALSE FALSE  TRUE FALSE  TRUE  TRUE  TRUE
> x7%%2 == 0 & x7 > 4 #even values > 4; %% is the modulo operation
[1] FALSE FALSE FALSE FALSE FALSE  TRUE  TRUE  TRUE
> !(x7%%2 == 0) #odd values
[1]  TRUE FALSE  TRUE FALSE  TRUE FALSE FALSE FALSE
```

A vector can also contain missing values which are denoted by NA (not available). The function is.na indices the missing values in a vector, returning a TRUE for each missing value:

```
> x7 <- c(2, NA, 3, 4, NA, 1, 2, NA)
> is.na(x7)
[1] FALSE  TRUE FALSE FALSE  TRUE FALSE FALSE  TRUE
```

If we are interested in counting the number of missing values in a vector, we just type

---

[2] In one of the example, we use the modulo operation, reproduced in R by %%, that computes the remainder of the division. For example, the R commands 4%%2 and 5%%2 give 0 and 1 as output, respectively.

```
> sum(is.na(x7))
[1] 3
```

In this case, R transforms the logical values TRUE and FALSE to numeric values (1 and 0, respectively) so that the sum of ones is equal to the number of missing values.

It is also possible to create vectors containing strings given by a sequence of characters delimited by double quotes (also single quotes can be used), as in

```
> x8 <- c("a", "b", "hello2", "z")
> x8
[1] "a"      "b"      "hello2" "z"
```

Obviously in this case, no numerical operations can be performed, but the logical ones are still valid.

The selection of subsets of values in a vector (also known as *indexing*) is performed using square brackets. For example, the command

```
> x7[7]
[1] 2
```

yields the value that occupies the 7th position in vector x7. Brackets are also used for changing the value of a vector element as in the following example where 0 is assigned to the 7th value of x7:

```
> x7[7] <- 0
> x7
[1]  2 NA  3  4 NA  1  0 NA
```

To select more than one value at a time, we need to use a vector inside the square brackets. For instance, with the following syntax we select the first, third, and seventh elements of x7:

```
> x7[c(1, 3, 7)]
[1] 2 3 0
```

A way to select the nonmissing values in a vector is to use the following code:

```
> x8 <- c(0, 2, NA, 3, 4, 9, NA, 12)
> na_indices <- is.na(x8) #a logical vector
> x8_new <- x8[! na_indices]
> x8_new
[1]  0  2  3  4  9 12
```

It is also possible to use negative indices to remove terms from a vector:

```
> x8_new[- c(1,length(x8_new))] #remove the first and the last values
[1] 2 3 4 9
```

Matrices

Matrices are generalizations of vectors defined by two indices (one for the rows and one for the columns). A first way to create a matrix from a given vector is to use the function `matrix`:

```
> z <- seq(from = 0, to = 21, by =3)  #length(z)=8
> z
[1]   0   3   6   9 12 15 18 21
> Z <- matrix(z, nrow=4, ncol=2)
> Z
     [,1] [,2]
[1,]    0   12
[2,]    3   15
[3,]    6   18
[4,]    9   21
```

It is worth noting that the matrix is filled by columns (so the first four elements of z are stored in column 1 of Z and the remaining in column 2); nevertheless, it is possible to set the argument `byrow` equal to `TRUE`, so that R will first fill the first row, then the second one and so on. The commands `nrow(Z)` and `ncol(Z)` are used to retrieve the number of rows and columns of matrix Z, respectively. With `dim(Z)`, we retrieve both dimensions stored in a vector.

Another possibility to create a matrix is to employ the functions `cbind` and `rbind` which combine elements of given vectors by column or by row, respectively. The following example illustrates their use:

```
> y1 <- c(1, 2, 3, 4, 5)
> y2 <- c(5, 10, 15, 20, 25)
> Y1 <- cbind(y1, y2)     #by column
> Y1
     y1 y2
[1,]  1  5
[2,]  2 10
[3,]  3 15
[4,]  4 20
[5,]  5 25
> dim(Y1)
[1] 5 2
> Y2 <- rbind(y1, y2)     #by row
> Y2
   [,1] [,2] [,3] [,4] [,5]
y1    1    2    3    4    5
y2    5   10   15   20   25
> dim(Y2)
[1] 2 5
```

For extracting elements from a matrix, we need to specify two indices inside square brackets separated by a comma, i.e., `[ , ]`:

```
> Y2[1,1]   #value in 1st row and 1st column
y1
 1


> Y2[1, c(1,3)]   #values in 1st row, 1st and 3rd columns
[1] 1 3
```

One of the indices can be omitted if we want to select an entire row or column, as in

```
> Y2[2,]    #2nd row
[1]  5 10 15 20 25

> Y2[,1]  #1st column
y1 y2
 1  5
```

Matrix multiplication is performed by means of the * and %*% operators, that perform element-by-element and matrix product, respectively. The following examples illustrate how to use them:

```
> A <- matrix(c(1, 2, 3, 4), nrow=2, ncol=2)
> A
     [,1] [,2]
[1,]    1    3
[2,]    2    4
> B <- matrix(c(1, 1, 0, 1), nrow=2, ncol=2)
> B
     [,1] [,2]
[1,]    1    0
[2,]    1    1
> C <- matrix(c(0, 2, 4, 6, 8, 10), nrow=2, ncol=3)
> C
     [,1] [,2] [,3]
[1,]    0    4    8
[2,]    2    6   10
> A * B #element by element product: only for
        #matrices of the same size
     [,1] [,2]
[1,]    1    0
[2,]    2    4
> A %*% C    #matrix product
     [,1] [,2] [,3]
[1,]    6   22   38
[2,]    8   32   56

> C %*% A   #matrix product

Error in C %*% A : non-conformable arguments
```

In the last example, we get an error because C and A are nonconformable matrices, as the number of columns of C is three while the number of rows of A is two.

A matrix can also be transposed (with the function t) or its determinant computed (with the function det) as follows:

```
> t(A)
     [,1] [,2]
[1,]    1    2
[2,]    3    4
> det(A)  #A must be a square matrix
[1] -2
```

The function diag is used to extract the diagonal of an existing matrix or to create a new identity matrix:

```
> diag(A) #extract the diagonal of A
[1] 1 4
> diag(2) #create a new identity matrix of size 2
     [,1] [,2]
[1,]    1    0
[2,]    0    1
```

With the same function, it is possible to construct a diagonal matrix, as in

```
> diag(x=2,nrow=3,ncol=3)
     [,1] [,2] [,3]
[1,]    2    0    0
[2,]    0    2    0
[3,]    0    0    2
```

where the first value defines the diagonal. If ncol is not given, R creates a square matrix, so diag(x=2,nrow=3,ncol=3) can be shorten to diag(2,3). Sometimes it may be useful to set column and row names using vectors of strings:

```
> colnames(A) <- c("First col.", "Second col.")
> rownames(A) <- c("First row", "Second row")
> A
            First col. Second col.
First row            1           3
Second row           2           4
```

In this case, it is possible to extract elements from the matrix using names with single or double quotes instead of indices, like in the following case:

```
> A[, "First col."] #equivalent to A[, 1]
 First row Second row
         1          2
```

Factors

A factor in R is equivalent to a categorical variable: each entry is not just a simple string of text but one of the levels of the variable. We create a factor typing for example,

```
> factor(c(1, 2, 3))
[1] 1 2 3
Levels: 1 2 3
```

Note that the levels of the factor could be different from the ones that the data have taken. So we could have five levels but only three of them observed, as in

```
> factor(c(1, 2, 3), levels = seq(from=1, to=5))
[1] 1 2 3
Levels: 1 2 3 4 5
```

Another option of the factor function is labels which allows us to specify possible labels for each level, as follows:

```
> factor(c(1, 2, 3), levels = seq(from=1, to=5),
          labels = c("a", "b", "c", "d", "e"))
[1] a b c
Levels: a b c d e
```

We now illustrate with a short example how to create a factor starting from a vector of $n = 100$ random number simulated from a standard Normal distribution using the function rnorm (see Section 4.3 for more details about random number generation in R):

```
> set.seed(8584) #set the seed
> sim_data <- rnorm(n=100)
```

The command set.seed is used to specify the random number seed in order to ensure result reproducibility (once the seed is set, R will always produce the same random numbers). Then, by using the cut function we divide the simulated data into four classes defined as $(-3, -1]$, $(-1, 0]$, $(0, +1]$, $(+1, +3]$ and get the corresponding frequency distribution using table:

```
> sim_data_class <- cut(sim_data, breaks = c(-3, -1, 0, 1, +3))
> table(sim_data_class)
sim_data_class
(-3,-1]   (-1,0]    (0,1]    (1,3]
     15       34       36       15
```

The output stored in sim_data_class is a factor with four levels and length equal to 100. To check this, we extract the first four elements of sim_data_class:

```
> sim_data_class[seq(1,4)]
[1] (-1,0]   (-1,0]   (-1,0]    (-3,-1]
Levels: (-3,-1] (-1,0] (0,1] (1,3]
```

If required, the level labels can be changed as follows:

```
> sim_data_class2 <- factor(sim_data_class,
                    labels=c("VeryLow","Low","High","VeryHigh"))
> sim_data_class2[seq(from=1,to=4)]
[1] Low      Low      Low      VeryLow
Levels: VeryLow Low High VeryHigh
```

Lists

A list is an ordered collection of objects, which could be of different types or dimensions, and provides a convenient way to return the results of statistical analysis. The following code creates a list, named w, composed by vectors of strings, logical, and numerical values:

```
> names <- c("Maria", "John", "Sam")
> gender <- c("F", "M", "M")
> married <- c(TRUE, FALSE, TRUE)
> age <- c(33, 38, 34)
```

```
> size <- 3
> w <- list(Names = names, Gender = gender, Age = age,
          Married = married, Size=size)
```

Important attributes regard the component names and the length of the list; the information are retrieved typing the following commands:

```
> names(w)
[1] "Names"    "Gender"  "Age"      "Married" "Size"
> length(w)
[1] 5
```

Note that if names are omitted when the list is created, then the components are only numbered.

The components of a list are accessed using indices in double square brackets (i.e., [[ ]]) or using the names after the sign $:

```
> w[[1]] #first component in the list
[1] "Maria" "John"  "Sam"
> w$Names
[1] "Maria" "John"  "Sam"
> w[[2]][1] #first element inside the second component of the list
[1] "F"
> w$Gender[1]
[1] "F"
```

The names of the components may be abbreviated down to the minimum number of letters needed to identify them uniquely. Thus, w$G returns the same output of w$Gender. With $ it is also possible to add a new component to an existing list, as in

```
> w$Height = c(168, 180, 178)
> names(w)
[1] "Names"    "Gender"  "Age"      "Married" "Size"     "Height"
```

Dataframes

A dataframe is an important and versatile data structure in R. It is a table of data in which each column refers to a variable and each row to a case. The creation of a new dataframe is performed by means of the function data.frame, collecting together existing variables of the same length:

```
> df <- data.frame(Gender = gender, Married = married, Age = age)
> rownames(df) <- names
> df
      Gender Married Age
Maria      F    TRUE  33
John       M   FALSE  38
Sam        M    TRUE  34
```

The object df is a dataframe containing information about three cases (in the rows) and three variables (in the columns). The dimension of the dataframe can be easily checked typing dim(df). Note that the type of the variables can be different (but of the same length), so we can combine numeric variables with logical values and factors. A useful command is str that displays in a compact way the content of the dataframe:

```
> str(df)
'data.frame': 3 obs. of  3 variables:
 $ Gender : Factor w/ 2 levels "F","M": 1 2 2
 $ Married: logi   TRUE FALSE TRUE
 $ Age    : num   33 38 34
```

Typing the command data(), it is possible to list all the dataframes supplied with R and that are accessible by name. We consider here the dataframe named iris, which gives the measurements (in cm) of petal and sepal length and width for 50 flowers from each of three iris species (setosa, versicolor, and virginica). See help(iris) for more information. The dataframe is loaded with

```
> data(iris)
```

and the head command is used to access only the top of the dataframe

```
> head(iris)
  Sepal.Length Sepal.Width Petal.Length Petal.Width Species
1          5.1         3.5          1.4         0.2  setosa
2          4.9         3.0          1.4         0.2  setosa
3          4.7         3.2          1.3         0.2  setosa
4          4.6         3.1          1.5         0.2  setosa
5          5.0         3.6          1.4         0.2  setosa
6          5.4         3.9          1.7         0.4  setosa

> str(iris)

'data.frame': 150 obs. of  5 variables:
 $ Sepal.Length: num  5.1 4.9 ...
 $ Sepal.Width : num  3.5 3 ...
 $ Petal.Length: num  1.4 1.4 ...
 $ Petal.Width : num  0.2 0.2 ...
 $ Species     : Factor w/ 3 levels "setosa","versicolor",..: 1 1 ...
```

To extract subsets of a dataframe we can use, like for matrices, two indices between square brackets. So, for example, iris[1,2] returns the sepal width of the first flower. As an alternative, it is possible to use name after the $ sign, as for lists:

```
> iris$Sepal.Width[seq(1,3)] #this is equivalent to iris[seq(1,3), 2]
[1] 3.5 3.0 3.2
```

If the dataframe contains a factor (as Species in the iris dataframe), it can be used to select subsets of data. The following code creates a new dataframe, named iris2, which contains data regarding only virginica species flowers:

```
> indices <- iris$Species == "virginica"
> iris2 <- iris[indices, ]
```

```
> dim(iris2)
[1] 50   5
> head(iris2)
    Sepal.Length Sepal.Width Petal.Length Petal.Width   Species
101          6.3         3.3          6.0         2.5 virginica
102          5.8         2.7          5.1         1.9 virginica
103          7.1         3.0          5.9         2.1 virginica
104          6.3         2.9          5.6         1.8 virginica
105          6.5         3.0          5.8         2.2 virginica
106          7.6         3.0          6.6         2.1 virginica
```

2.3   Data and session management

In this book, we will often use data available in comma-separated values (*csv*)
format. In this case, it is possible to import the data into R and store them into
a dataframe using the function `read.table`. As an example, we consider the
data described in Section 1.4.3 about strokes in Sheffield and saved in the file
`Stroke.csv`:

```
> df2 <- read.table(file="Stroke.csv", header =TRUE, sep=",", dec=".")
```

```
> dim(df2)
[1] 1030      9
> colnames(df2)
[1] "SP_ID"          "wbID"           "stroke_exp"     "pop"
[5] "y"              "Townsend.class" "NOx.class"      "Townsend"
[9] "NOx"
```

The argument `header` of the command `read.table` takes a logical value indicating whether the file contains the names of the variables as its first row. Moreover, the option `sep` allows us to specify the character of the separator between
columns while `dec` refers to the character used for decimal points. If necessary,
we can provide which column contains the row names by means of the argument
`row.names`; see `help(read.table)` for the complete definition of the function. If not specified, the row names are given by the sequence of number from 1
to the number of rows of the dataframe.

A simplified version of `read.table` is `read.csv` that uses by default
`header = TRUE`, `sep = ","` and `dec = "."`:

```
> df2 <- read.csv("Stroke.csv")
```

All the objects created in R are stored in a common workspace whose content is
listed typing `ls()`. To remove all the objects and clear the workspace type

```
> remove(list=ls())
```

On the contrary, to remove a single object we specify its name between double
quotes, as in

```
> remove("NameOfTheObjectToBeRemoved")
```

At any time, it is possible to save the workspace objects (but not the used commands or the output) in a file using the command:

```
> save.image("NameOfTheWorkspace.RData")
```

R creates a file called `NameOfTheWorkspace.RData` in the working directory (to get or set your current working directory type `getwd()` or `setwd("yourPath")`). Then, if we close R (with `q()`) and start a new session again, the saved workspace is loaded by typing

```
> load("NameOfTheWorkspace.Rdata")
```

Use `ls()` to check that all the saved objects are available.

2.4   Packages

Packages are collections of R functions, data and compiled code in a well-defined format. The basic installation of R includes some packages but many others are available from the CRAN repository (see `http://cran.r-project.org/web/packages/`). Type `help(install.packages)` for information about how to install new packages.

Throughout this book, we will use the following packages: `geoR` (a package for geostatistical data analysis), `sp` (a package providing classes and methods for spatial data), `INLA` (a package to perform full Bayesian analysis on generalized additive mixed models using integrated nested Laplace approximations), `maptools` (tools for manipulating and reading geographic data), `rgdal` (projection/transformation operations from the PROJ.4 library), `fields` (for curve, surface and function fitting), `arm` (data analysis using regression and multilevel/hierarchical models), `splancs` (spatial and spate-time point pattern analysis), `lattice` (lattice graphics), `gstat` (spatial and spatio-temporal geostatistical modeling, prediction and simulation), `spdep` (spatial dependence, weighting schemes, statistics and models), and `abind` (combine multidimensional arrays).

The command

```
> library()
```

returns the list of the installed packages. Before it can be accessed by the user, an installed package needs to be loaded into R. For example, we can load the `geoR` package with

```
> library(geoR)
```

This makes its datasets and functions available. Note that the loaded packages are not included in the workspace and when we close R and start a new session with a saved workspace, the packages have to be loaded again.

2.5   Programming in R

R has a huge collection of built-in functions but new functions (and packages) can be created by the users (see, for example, Chambers, 2008). This may be useful if the user needs to run a specific operation which cannot be executed using a R function. Moreover, when a relevant number of instructions are run many times (with different data or parameter setting), it is worth collecting all of them in a new function to be called iteratively.

A new function is defined in R using the following syntax:

```
> funct.name <- function(arg1, arg2, ...) {
  #Body of the function
  expression
  expression
  ...
  value
  }
```

where funct.name is the name of the function, arg1, arg2, . . . are the input arguments and expression denotes the operations to be executed by R using some of the inputs. Finally, value is the output of the function (note that when multiple objects are required as output – instead of a single value – it is necessary to collect them in a list). Once the function is defined, it can be called by typing

```
funct.name(arg1 = value1, arg2 = value2, ...)
```

As an example, we define a function that takes two vectors as input and computes their weighted average[3], with weights given by the vector lengths:

```
> w.average <- function(vect1, vect2) {
    n1 <- length(vect1)
    n2 <- length(vect2)
    x <- (mean(vect1) * n1 + mean(vect2) * n2) / (n1+n2)
    x
  }
```

In the following, we define two vectors (x and y) and compute their weighted average with the w.average function:

```
> x <- seq(0, 10, by = 0.2)
> x
 [1]  0.0  0.2  0.4  0.6  0.8  1.0  1.2  1.4  1.6  1.8  2.0  2.2  2.4  2.6
[15]  2.8  3.0  3.2  3.4  3.6  3.8  4.0  4.2  4.4  4.6  4.8  5.0  5.2  5.4
[29]  5.6  5.8  6.0  6.2  6.4  6.6  6.8  7.0  7.2  7.4  7.6  7.8  8.0  8.2
[43]  8.4  8.6  8.8  9.0  9.2  9.4  9.6  9.8 10.0
> y <- seq(0, 10, by = 0.5)
> y
 [1]  0.0  0.5  1.0  1.5  2.0  2.5  3.0  3.5  4.0  4.5  5.0  5.5  6.0  6.5
[15]  7.0  7.5  8.0  8.5  9.0  9.5 10.0
```

---

[3] This function already exists in R; see ?weighted.mean.

```
> w.average(vect1 = x, vect2 = y)
[1] 5
```

When one or some operations need to be executed repeatedly, it may be necessary to use *loop* constructions. One of these is the for loop[4] which is reproduced in R using the following syntax:

```
for(i in index){
    expression
    expression
    ...
}
```

where i is the loop variable and index is a vector of values often generated by the seq function. All the expressions enclosed in braces are repeatedly evaluated as i ranges through the values in the index vector. To illustrate how the for loop works, we repeat five times the simulation of 10 values from the standard Normal distribution (using the rnorm function that will be discussed in details in Section 4.3) and the calculation of the sample mean, which is printed in the output after being rounded to two decimal places (with the round function):

```
> set.seed(123)
> for(i in 1:5){
    x <- rnorm(10) #simulate 10 values from the std Normal distr.
    print(round(mean(x),2)) #print the rounded mean
  }
[1]  0.07
[1]  0.21
[1] -0.42
[1]  0.32
[1] -0.01
```

Another possibility for specifying the loop variable i, which ranges from 1 to 5, is given by for(i in seq(1,5)). It may be useful to store the 5 averages in a vector instead of printing them. In this case, we first use the numeric function to create a vector of length 5 with elements equal to 0:

```
> aver.vect <- numeric(5)
> aver.vect
[1] 0 0 0 0 0
```

and then we change the for loop code in order to store the ith average in the corresponding position of the aver.vect vector, as follows:

```
> set.seed(123)
> for(i in 1:5){
    x <- rnorm(10)
    aver.vect[i] <- round(mean(x),2) #store the mean
  }
> aver.vect
[1]  0.07  0.21 -0.42  0.32 -0.01
```

---

[4] Other loop constructions available in R are while and repeat.

In R it is also possible to define a conditional construction using a `if` statement which is defined as follows:

```
if (condition) {
  expression 1a
  expression 1b
  ...
} else {
  expression 2a
  expression 2b
  ...
}
```

where `condition` is a logical value or an expression that leads to a single logical value. If `condition` is TRUE, the first block of operations (`expression 1a`, `expression 1b`, ...) will be executed; otherwise R will run the expressions in the second block. Note that the `else` statement can be omitted if it is not required. As an example, we modify the code used previously to illustrate the `for` loop. In particular, if the sample average is positive we compute and save its square root (rounded to two decimals), otherwise we return a NA value.

```
> set.seed(123)
> for(i in 1:5){
    x <- rnorm(10)
    if(mean(x) > 0){ #check if the mean is positive
    aver.vect[i] <- round(sqrt(mean(x)),2)
    } else {
    aver.vect[i] <- NA
    }
  }
> aver.vect
[1] 0.27 0.46   NA 0.57   NA
```

2.6   Basic statistical analysis with R

In this section, we illustrate some basic statistical analysis that can be carried out on a dataframe. First of all, we can compute some synthetic indices using the `summary` function. With reference to the `iris` dataset, if we type

```
> summary(iris)
  Sepal.Length    Sepal.Width     Petal.Length    Petal.Width
 Min.   :4.300   Min.   :2.000   Min.   :1.000   Min.   :0.100
 1st Qu.:5.100   1st Qu.:2.800   1st Qu.:1.600   1st Qu.:0.300
 Median :5.800   Median :3.000   Median :4.350   Median :1.300
 Mean   :5.843   Mean   :3.057   Mean   :3.758   Mean   :1.199
 3rd Qu.:6.400   3rd Qu.:3.300   3rd Qu.:5.100   3rd Qu.:1.800
 Max.   :7.900   Max.   :4.400   Max.   :6.900   Max.   :2.500
       Species
 setosa    :50
 versicolor:50
 virginica :50
```

we obtain for each numeric variable the minimum, the maximum, the quartiles and the mean. For factor variables – like `Species` – the frequency distribution is returned. We may also be interested in computing the synthetic indices for each level of the factor variable. The `aggregate` function splits the data into subsets, defined usually by factor levels, and computes summary statistics for each of them. For example, if we want to calculate the mean petal length for each species we enter

```
> aggregate(Petal.Length ~ Species, data=iris, FUN=mean)
      Species Petal.Length
1      setosa        1.462
2  versicolor        4.260
3   virginica        5.552
```

Other options for the `FUN` argument are `median`, `min`, `max`, `range`, `quantile`, `var`, `sd` (see `?aggregate`). The ~ syntax denotes a formula object that is used especially as a symbolic description of a model to be fitted by R. A typical model takes the form `response ~ predictors`, where response is the dependent variable and predictors consist of a series of explanatory variables. In the code above, we use the formula notation for specifying the aggregated and grouping variables (`Petal.Length` and `Species`, respectively).

A `.` (dot) in the formula is used to select all the remaining variables contained in `data`, as in

```
> aggregate( . ~ Species, data = iris, FUN = mean)
      Species Sepal.Length Sepal.Width Petal.Length Petal.Width
1      setosa        5.006       3.428        1.462       0.246
2  versicolor        5.936       2.770        4.260       1.326
3   virginica        6.588       2.974        5.552       2.026
```

When performing statistical analysis, graphical representations are extremely useful. For example, the boxplots reported in Figure 2.1 display the distribution of the petal length by species and are obtained by using the following code:

```
> boxplot(Petal.Length ~ Species, data = iris,
          ylab ="Petal length", xlab = "Species", col="gray")
```

where we use the options `ylab` and `xlab` for specifying the axis labels and `col` for setting the boxplot color. For more information on the `boxplot` function, see `help(boxplot)`.

When we consider two numeric variables jointly, it may be interesting to compute the Pearson correlation coefficient or to plot one variable against the other to investigate the presence of a linear relationship. For example, with reference to the `iris` dataframe, the correlation coefficient between `Petal.Width` and `Petal.Length` is simply calculated by typing

```
> cor(iris$Petal.Width, iris$Petal.Length)
[1] 0.9628654
```

The corresponding dispersion plot is displayed in Figure 2.2 (top) and is obtained using the `plot` function with the `Petal.Length ~ Petal.Width` formula:

```
> plot(Petal.Length ~ Petal.Width, data=iris)
```

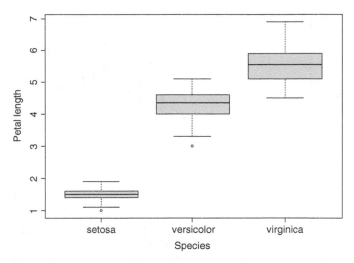

Figure 2.1   Boxplots of `Petal.Length ~ Species` *for the* `iris` *dataframe.*

or alternatively

```
> plot(iris$Petal.Length, iris$Petal.Width)
```

The `plot` function is a generic function for plotting R objects and many options can be specified. See `help(plot)` for the function options and `demo(graphics)` for a gallery of some plots that can be obtained with R. The dispersion plot can be improved by plotting points with different symbols according to the level of the `Species` factor. This can be easily obtained with

```
> plot(Petal.Length ~ Petal.Width, data = iris,
      pch = c(21, 8, 19)[as.numeric(iris$Species)])
> legend("topleft", pch = c(21, 8, 19),
       legend = levels(iris$Species), box.lty = 0)
```

and the output is reported in the bottom frame of Figure 2.2. With `pch`, we specify the type of points as explained in `help(points)`; here we create a vector of three symbols (21 = filled circle, 8 = asterisk, and 19 = solid circle) according to the values (1, 2, and 3) obtained transforming the factor `Species` into a numeric vector (using `as.numeric`). The plot legend is placed in the top-left part of the plot using the `legend` function.

To assess the presence of a linear relationship between `Petal.Length` and `Petal.Width`, a linear model can be specified. This is implemented in R using the `lm` function (linear model), as follows:

```
> lm1 <- lm(Petal.Length ~ Petal.Width, data=iris)
> abline(lm1) #add the fitted line in the dispersion plot
> summary(lm1)

Call:
lm(formula = Petal.Length ~ Petal.Width, data = iris)
```

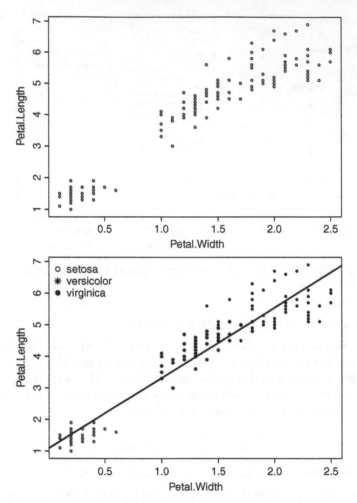

Figure 2.2   Dispersion plots of Petal.Length ~ Petal.Width *for the* iris *dataframe. In the bottom plot, the point symbol is given by the levels of the* Species *factor, as specified in the legend. The straight line is added after fitting a linear model to the data.*

```
Residuals:
    Min       1Q    Median       3Q      Max
-1.33542 -0.30347 -0.02955  0.25776  1.39453

Coefficients:
            Estimate Std. Error t value Pr(>|t|)
(Intercept)  1.08356    0.07297   14.85   <2e-16 ***
Petal.Width  2.22994    0.05140   43.39   <2e-16 ***
—
Signif. codes:  0 '***' 0.001 '**' 0.01 '*' 0.05 '.' 0.1 ' ' 1
```

```
Residual standard error: 0.4782 on 148 degrees of freedom
Multiple R-squared:  0.9271, Adjusted R-squared:  0.9266
F-statistic:  1882 on 1 and 148 DF,  p-value: < 2.2e-16
```

If we apply the summary function to the lm1 object, we obtain a table containing parameter estimates, standard errors and significance as well as residual statistics, and the R-squared index for goodness of fit. The abline command adds the fitted straight line to the plot displayed in Figure 2.2 (bottom). Note that lm includes the intercept by default; if we want to omit it we need to use the formula Petal.Length ~ Petal.Width -1.

There are some specialized functions that allow us to extract elements from a linear model object. For example, fitted(lm1) and residuals(lm1) return the fitted values and the residuals, respectively, while

```
> coefficients(lm1)
(Intercept) Petal.Width
   1.083558    2.229940
```

provides the estimated coefficients. To list all the objects produced by the lm function type

```
> names(lm1)
 [1] "coefficients"  "residuals"      "effects"      "rank"
 [5] "fitted.values" "assign"         "qr"           "df.residual"
 [9] "xlevels"       "call"           "terms"        "model"
```

In R, there are also functions for regression diagnostics that are used to evaluate the model assumptions and investigate whether or not there are observations with a large influence on the regression output. We do not cover this or other advanced regression issues here and we refer the reader to more specialized book such as Faraway (2004), Dalgaard (2008), Sheather (2008) and Fox and Weisberg (2011).

It is worth noting that in a linear model it is also possible to include a categorical variable (i.e., a factor object in R) as a predictor. In this case, R represents the factor as a set of *dummy* (or indicator) variables. In particular, if the factor has k levels, besides the intercept we will have $k - 1$ dummy variables taking values 1 or 0 when the corresponding factor level occurs or not. For example, if we intend to fit the model that considers the sepal length as a function of the species, we type

```
> lm2 <- lm(Sepal.Length ~ Species, data=iris)
> summary(lm2)
Call:
lm(formula = Sepal.Length ~ Species, data = iris)

Residuals:
    Min      1Q  Median      3Q     Max
-1.6880 -0.3285 -0.0060  0.3120  1.3120

Coefficients:
                  Estimate Std. Error t value Pr(>|t|)
(Intercept)         5.0060     0.0728  68.762  < 2e-16 ***
Speciesversicolor   0.9300     0.1030   9.033 8.77e-16 ***
Speciesvirginica    1.5820     0.1030  15.366  < 2e-16 ***
```

—

```
Signif. codes:  0 '***' 0.001 '**' 0.01 '*' 0.05 '.' 0.1 ' ' 1

Residual standard error: 0.5148 on 147 degrees of freedom
Multiple R-squared:  0.6187, Adjusted R-squared:  0.6135
F-statistic: 119.3 on 2 and 147 DF,  p-value: < 2.2e-16
```

This model corresponds to the following symbolic representation:

$$\texttt{Sepal.Length} \sim \beta_0 + \beta_1 I_{\text{versicolor}} + \beta_2 I_{\text{virginica}}$$

where β_0 is the intercept. Moreover, $I_{\text{versicolor}}$ and $I_{\text{virginica}}$ are the dummy variables that are equal to 1 for Species==versicolor and Species==virginica, respectively, and 0 elsewhere (in this case the setosa species is considered as base level). If we omit the intercept using the formula Sepal.Length ~ Species -1, R will include one additional dummy variable for the setosa species but the model output will not change. The lm2 model output with the three fitted straight lines (one for each level) is displayed in Figure 2.3 (top).

Numerical and categorical variables can be included jointly in the linear model formula (using +) and interactions can be considered as well (specified using : or *).[5] As an example, we may be interested in a more complex model for sepal length without intercept and which includes as regressors the Species factor and its interaction with the numeric variable Sepal.Width. This kind of model corresponds to the following symbolic representation:

$$\texttt{Sepal.Length} \sim \beta_1 I_{\text{setosa}} + \beta_2 I_{\text{versicolor}} + \beta_3 I_{\text{virginica}}$$

$$+ \beta_4 I_{\text{setosa}} \times \texttt{Sepal.Width} + \beta_5 I_{\text{versicolor}}$$

$$\times \texttt{Sepal.Width}$$

$$+ \beta_6 I_{\text{virginica}} \times \texttt{Sepal.Width}$$

In R, we fit this model using the following code where the intercept is omitted specifying -1 in the formula:

```
> lm3 <- lm(Sepal.Length ~ Species + Sepal.Width:Species -1, data=iris)
> summary(lm3)
Call:
lm(formula = Sepal.Length ~ Species + Sepal.Width:Species - 1,
    data = iris)

Residuals:
     Min       1Q   Median       3Q      Max
-1.26067 -0.25861 -0.03305  0.18929  1.44917

Coefficients:
```

---

    [5] The specification of the form a : b indicates the set of terms obtained by taking the interactions of all terms in a with all terms in b. The specification a*b corresponds to a + b + a:b and includes single effects and interactions.

	Estimate	Std. Error	t value	Pr(>|t|)	
Speciessetosa	2.6390	0.5715	4.618	8.53e-06	***
Speciesversicolor	3.5397	0.5580	6.343	2.74e-09	***
Speciesvirginica	3.9068	0.5827	6.705	4.25e-10	***
Speciessetosa:Sepal.Width	0.6905	0.1657	4.166	5.31e-05	***
Speciesversicolor:Sepal.Width	0.8651	0.2002	4.321	2.88e-05	***
Speciesvirginica:Sepal.Width	0.9015	0.1948	4.628	8.16e-06	***

```
-
Signif. codes:  0 '***' 0.001 '**' 0.01 '*' 0.05 '.' 0.1 ' ' 1

Residual standard error: 0.4397 on 144 degrees of freedom
Multiple R-squared:  0.9947, Adjusted R-squared:  0.9944
F-statistic:  4478 on 6 and 144 DF,  p-value: < 2.2e-16
```

The model output shows that all the parameters are significative and the corresponding three fitted lines are displayed in Figure 2.3 (bottom).

A natural extension of the linear regression framework is the class of generalized linear models (GLM) that are employed when the outcome variable is measured on a binary scale or represents the count of events (i.e., the outcome is characterized by a Binomial or Poisson distribution). A key point of GLM is the *link function* which specifies the mean of the response variable as a linear function of the regressors (see Agresti, 2002; McCullagh and Nelder, 1989 for the general GLM theory). The R function for fitting a GLM is glm which is very similar to the lm function except that it requires to specify the family argument (the distribution of the outcome) and the link function. See help(glm) and help(family) for more details. By default R adopts the logit and the log link function for the Binomial and the Poisson case, respectively.

To illustrate the glm function, we first consider a simple example regarding a Binomial GLM for the proportions of female children who have reached menarche. This example refers to the dataframe named menarche, which is included in the library MASS:

```
> library(MASS)
> data(menarche)
> str(menarche)
'data.frame': 25 obs. of  three variables:
 $ Age     : num  9.21 10.21 10.58 10.83 11.08 ...
 $ Total   : num  376 200 93 120 90 88 105 111 100 93 ...
 $ Menarche: num  0 0 0 2 2 5 10 17 16 29 ...
```

As we can see from the output of the str function, the dataframe consists of 25 rows (representing groups) and three variables: Age (the average group age), Total (the number of female children in each group) and Menarche (the number of girls who has reached menarche). To fit in R the Binomial GLM with age as regressor we use the following code, where the argument weight is used to specify the total number of trials:

```
> glm1 <- glm(Menarche/Total ~ Age, weight = Total,
            data=menarche, family=binomial)
```

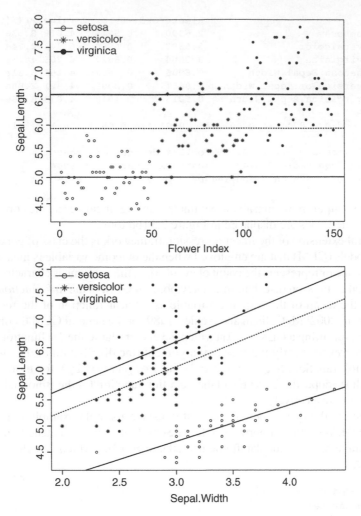

Figure 2.3   Plot of Sepal.Length *of the* iris *dataframe with point symbol according to* Species *(top). Plot of* Sepal.Length *vs* Sepal.Width *of the* iris *dataframe with point symbol according to* Species *(bottom). For both the plots, the straight lines are added after fitting linear models including dummy variables.*

```
> summary(glm1)
Call:
glm(formula = Menarche/Total ~ Age, family = binomial,
    data = menarche, weights = Total)

Deviance Residuals:
    Min       1Q    Median       3Q       Max
-2.0363  -0.9953  -0.4900   0.7780   1.3675
```

```
Coefficients:
             Estimate Std. Error z value Pr(>|z|)
(Intercept) -21.22639    0.77068  -27.54   <2e-16 ***
Age           1.63197    0.05895   27.68   <2e-16 ***
-
Signif. codes:  0 '***' 0.001 '**' 0.01 '*' 0.05 '.' 0.1 ' ' 1

(Dispersion parameter for binomial family taken to be 1)

    Null deviance: 3693.884  on 24  degrees of freedom
Residual deviance:   26.703  on 23  degrees of freedom
AIC: 114.76

Number of Fisher Scoring iterations: 4
```

Both the intercept and the age parameter are significative. The `glm` function produces a set of objects which can be listed typing `names(glm1)`. For example, the
object `glm1$fitted.values` contains the fitted mean values obtained using
the inverse of the link function. The fitted values can be used to graphically check
the goodness of fit of the model in a plot where age is on the *x*-axis and the proportion of girls who reached menarche is on the *y*-axis, as in Figure 2.4 (top) which is
obtained using the following code:

```
> plot(Menarche/Total ~ Age, data=menarche)
> lines(menarche$Age, glm1$fitted.values)
```

Another simple example about GLM considers the case when the outcome
follows a Poisson distribution. In particular, we analyze the `warpbreaks` data
about the number of warp breaks per loom. The data, which are stored in the
dataframe named `warpbreaks`, refers to 54 observations and three variables:
`breaks` (number of breaks), `wool` (the type of wool, A or B), and `tension`
(the tension level, L, M or H). The following output describes the structure of the
dataframe:

```
> data(warpbreaks)
> str(warpbreaks)


'data.frame': 54 obs. of  3 variables:
 $ breaks : num  26 30 ...
 $ wool    : Factor w/ 2 levels "A","B": 1 1 ...
 $ tension: Factor w/ 3 levels "L","M","H": 1 1 ...
```

Using the `xtabs` function, it is possible to obtain the contingency table for the
`warpbreaks` data with the total number of breaks for each type of wool and
tension level:

```
> xtabs(warpbreaks)
    tension
wool   L   M   H
```

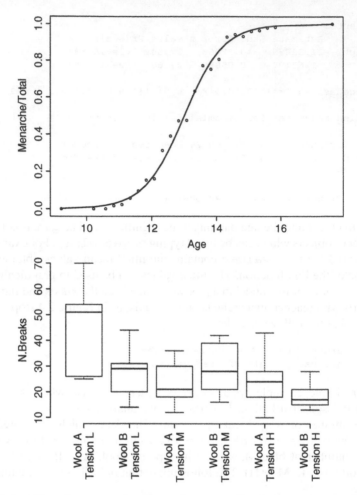

Figure 2.4   Plot of Menarche/Total ~ Age *for the* menarche *dataframe (top). The line is added after fitting a Binomial GLM to the data. Boxplots of* breaks ~ wool:tension *for the warpbreaks dataframe (bottom).*

```
A 401 216 221
B 254 259 169
```

The data distribution can also be summarized using the boxplots displayed in Figure 2.4 (bottom) and obtained using the following code (note that the syntax wool:tension is used for considering the interactions between the two factors):

```
> boxplot(breaks ~ wool:tension,data = warpbreaks,
        ylab="N.Breaks", xlab="", axes=F)
> axis(side=2, at=seq(10,70,10), labels=seq(10,70,10))
> axis(side=1, at= seq(1,6),
      labels=c("Wool A\nTension L", "Wool B\n Tension L",
      "Wool A\nTension M",
```

```
"Wool B\nTension M", "Wool A\nTension H", "Wool B\nTension H"),
las=2, cex.axis=0.7)
```

Note that the option `axes=F` is used to omit the plot axes which are then added through the `axis` function (see `help(axis)`).

To implement the Poisson GLM model, we employ the `glm` function with `family=poisson`:

```
> glm2 <- glm(breaks ~ wool + tension,
 data=warpbreaks, family=poisson)
> summary(glm2)
Call:
glm(formula = breaks ~ wool + tension, family = poisson,
    data = warpbreaks)

Deviance Residuals:
    Min       1Q   Median       3Q      Max
-3.6871  -1.6503  -0.4269   1.1902   4.2616

Coefficients:
            Estimate Std. Error z value Pr(>|z|)
(Intercept)  3.69196    0.04541  81.302  < 2e-16 ***
woolB       -0.20599    0.05157  -3.994 6.49e-05 ***
tensionM    -0.32132    0.06027  -5.332 9.73e-08 ***
tensionH    -0.51849    0.06396  -8.107 5.21e-16 ***
—
Signif. codes:  0 '***' 0.001 '**' 0.01 '*' 0.05 '.' 0.1 ' ' 1

(Dispersion parameter for poisson family taken to be 1)

    Null deviance: 297.37  on 53  degrees of freedom
Residual deviance: 210.39  on 50  degrees of freedom
AIC: 493.06

Number of Fisher Scoring iterations: 4
```

Note that, as in the case of linear regression, R introduces the factors in the GLM as *dummy* variables. All the parameter estimates appear to be statistically significative.

References

Agresti, A. (2002). *Categorical Data Analysis*. Second edition. John Wiley and Sons, Ltd.

Albert, J. (2009). *Bayesian Computation with R*. Springer.

Bivand, R., Pebesma, E., and Gómez-Rubio (2008). *Applied Spatial Data Analysis with R*. Springer.

Chambers, J. (2008). *Software for Data Analysis. Programming with R*. Springer.

Cowpertwait, P. and Metcalfe, A. (2009). *Introductory Time Series with R*. Springer.

Crawley, M. (2007). *The R Book*. John Wiley and Sons, Ltd.

Dalgaard, P. (2008). *Introductory Statistics with R*. Springer.

Everitt, B. and Hothorn, T. (2009). *A Handbook of Statistical Analyses Using R*, Second Edition. CRC Press.

Faraway, J. (2004). *Linear Models with R*. Chapman & Hall/CRC.

Fox, J. and Weisberg, S. (2011). *An R Companion to Applied Regression. Second Edition*. SAGE Publications, Inc.

Kleiber, C. and Zeileis, A. (2008). *Applied Econometrics with R*. Springer.

Logan, M. (2010). *Biostatistical Design and Analysis Using R: A Practical Guide*. Wiley–Blackwell.

McCullagh, P. and Nelder, J. (1989). *Generalized Linear Models*. John Wiley and Sons, Ltd.

Peng, R. and Dominici, F. (2008). *Statistical Methods for Environmental Epidemiology with R. A Case Study in Air Pollution and Health*. Springer.

Sheather, S. (2008). *A Modern Approach to Regression with R*. Springer.

Shumway, R. and Stoffer, D. (2011). *Time Series Analysis and Its Applications, with R Examples*. Third Edition. Springer.

Stevens, M. (2009). *A Primer of Ecology with R*. Springer.

Zuur, A., Ieno, E., Walker, N., Saveliev, A., and Smith, G. (2009). *Mixed Effects Models and Extensions in Ecology with R*. Springer.

Zuur, A., Ieno, E., and Meesters, E. (2012). *A Beginner's Guide to R*. Springer.

3

Introduction to Bayesian methods

3.1 Bayesian philosophy

The popularity of Bayesian methods has constantly increased since the 1950s, and is now at its peaks, with Bayesian models used in virtually every research area, from social science (Jackman, 2009) to medicine and public health (Berry and Stangl, 1999), from finance (Rachev *et al.*, 2008) to ecology (McCarthy, 2007) to health economics (Baio, 2012), and econometrics (Gómez-Rubio *et al.*, 2014). Nevertheless, the history of Bayesian thinking dates back to the eighteen century; in this section we are going to follow the steps of the great scientists who have invented and developed the theory which is the core of this book, but for an extensive and complete history of Bayesian theory, we encourage the reader to refer to the following publications: Howie (2002), Fienberg (2006), and Bertsch Mcgrayne (2011).

3.1.1 Thomas Bayes and Simon Pierre Laplace

All started with the work of two men: the reverend Thomas Bayes and the scientist Simon Pierre Laplace. Thomas Bayes, born in 1701 in Hertfordshire (England), was a presbyterian minister and mathematician. He started thinking about probability as a way to explain cause–effect relationships in a mathematical way. He was inspired by the work of the Scottish philosopher David Hume who in 1748 published an essay where he attacked some of the pillars of Christianity based on traditional belief and affirmed that we can only base our knowledge on our experience. Without knowing it, he was introducing a cornerstone of Bayesian theory, that experience plays an essential role in informing about cause–effect mechanism. He did not

Spatial and Spatio-temporal Bayesian Models with R-INLA, First Edition.
Marta Blangiardo and Michela Cameletti.
© 2015 John Wiley & Sons, Ltd. Published 2015 by John Wiley & Sons, Ltd.

provide any mathematical detail, but concluded that "we can only find probable causes from probable effects" (Bertsch Mcgrayne, 2011).

Bayes' interest laid on demonstrating that knowing an effect it was possible to obtain the probability of the causes that might have generated it, essentially giving the foundations for the so-called inverse probability theory which is embraced by the Bayesian philosophy. In "An Essay Towards Solving a Problem in the Doctrine of Chances" (Bayes, 1763), published posthumously by Richard Price in 1763, he wrote: *Given the number of times in which an unknown event has happened and failed: required the chance that the probability of its happening in a single trial lies somewhere between any two degrees of probability that can be named.* This sentence might seem a little obscure, but can be rephrased using the simple following example: an event which occurs n times (e.g., tossing a coin and getting head) is governed by a probability of occurrence π, which is characterized by a suitable probability distribution; in other words, Bayes proposes a direct elicitation of the cause which rules the occurrence of the effect, that is the probability of the occurrence for the particular event.

Independently from Bayes, Simon Pierre Laplace, a French scientist, presented in 1774 the fundamental principle of Bayesianism and inverse probability theory, simply stating that the probability of a cause is proportional to the probability of an event (given the cause) and providing with the first version of what we call today Bayes theorem (Laplace, 1774; Stigler, 1986). In his "Mémoire sur la probabilité des causes par les évènemens" he presented his principle as follows: *If an event can be produced by a number n of different causes, then the probabilities of these causes given the event are to each other as the probabilities of the event given the causes, and the probability of the existence of each of these is equal to the probability of the event given the cause, divided by the sum of all the probabilities of the event given each of these causes.* He first assumed that the probability of the causes must be equal and worked on applications of his principle, first on gambling, which was the only field at that time where probability was used (even though the notion of inverse probability was not). Later he wanted to test how this worked with large amount of data. To do so, demography was the natural field where to look; parishes had a large collection of data from births to marriages and deaths. He concentrated on births by gender and concluded that based on the evidence the probability that a baby boy was born was slightly higher than a baby girl. He started with equal probabilities for the two events (being born as a boy or as a girl) and then applying the inverse probability theory he included the evidence from the data to update his probabilities, using the very same idea that is at the basis of Bayesian inference and which will be introduced in Section 3.4.1.

Laplace worked extensively on demography and in 1781 he estimated the size of the French population, using data from parishes and also additional information about the size of the population available for the eastern regions of the country; in the same year he also generalized his inverse probability principle, allowing for the causes to have different probabilities and proposing the final form of Bayes theorem (which will be introduced in Section 3.3). Subjectivism is a natural characteristic of inverse probability theory: different people will have a different view of what cause is more probable for a particular event, based on their experience; in case of no information, the individual is allowed to consider all the causes as equally probable.

After Laplace died in 1827, the concept of probability used to quantify uncertainty due to unknown was despised for almost a century and so was subjectivism. Francis Ysidro Edgeworth and Karl Pearson returned on the idea of inverse probability at the end of the nineteenth/early twentieth century (Edgeworth, 1887; Pearson, 1920) and after that the subjectivism became the central topic in the work of Bruno de Finetti.

3.1.2   Bruno de Finetti and colleagues

Bruno de Finetti, an Italian actuary (1906–1985) worked all his life on the subjective concept of probability. He wrote 17 papers by the 1930 (according to Lindley, 1986), but the most famous are two: one published in 1931 where he put the basis for his subjective probability theory and the other "Theory of Probability," written in Italian in 1970 and translated in English (de Finetti, 1974) where he wrote: *My thesis, paradoxically, and a little provocatively, but nonetheless genuinely, is simply this: Probability does not exist. The abandonment of superstitious beliefs about the existence of the Phlogiston, the Cosmic Ether, Absolute Space and Time, ... or Fairies and Witches was an essential step along the road to scientific thinking. Probability, too, if regarded as something endowed with some kind of objective existence, is no less a misleading misconception, an illusory attempt to exteriorize or materialize our true probabilistic beliefs.* What he means by this statement is that the concept of objective probability is nonexistent and each individual is entitled to their own *degree of belief* in the causes which govern the occurrence of events.

Independently from de Finetti, Frank Ramsey, an English mathematician and philosopher, arrived to the same conclusions and in his "Studies in Subjective Probability" (Ramsey, 1931), he introduced the idea of subjective belief comparing it to the lowest odds, which a person will accept in a bet. On the other hand, Harold Jeffrey, an English mathematician, while maintaining a Bayesian framework, focused his theory on the concept of objective probability, which assumes ignorance on all the probabilities of occurrence for the events. In his "Theory of Probability" (Jeffrey, 1939), he insisted on the importance of learning from experience.

During the Second World War, many scientists contributed to the development of Bayesian methods, mostly in an applied perspective: amongst the others, Alan Turing, an English mathematician and computer scientist, who is mostly known for the invention of the modern computers, pioneered sequential data analysis using a Bayesian framework.

3.1.3   After the Second World War

It is after the Second World War that the so-called neo-Bayesianism revival started (Fienberg, 2006), focusing mainly on decision theory: the father of this philosophy is Leonard Savage, an American mathematician and statistician, who in his book "The Foundations of Statistics", published in 1954 (Savage, 1954), synthesized the subjectivism theory of de Finetti and Ramsey, introducing the basis for the maximization of subjective expected utility. At the same time, universities like Chicago (where Savage worked) and Harvard experienced a large affluence of Bayesian scholars. Dennis Lindley, a British statistician, was visiting Chicago University when Savage's book was published and was strongly influenced by his subjective view of probability. In a paper in 1957, he discussed how the Frequentist and Bayesian approach can be in disagreement regarding hypothesis testing in certain situations, something which is now known as Lindley's paradox (Lindley, 1957). His work was always centered on the concept of subjective uncertainty and in his latest book "Understanding uncertainty", he wrote *Uncertainty is a personal matter; it is not the uncertainty but your uncertainty* (Lindley, 2006).

Such great advances in Bayesian theory did not correspond to the same advances in empirical applications of the theories due to the computational issues arising when dealing with large datasets. It is finally in 1962 that we see the first use of Bayesian framework for solving a practical problem: John Tukey, an American statistician, and colleagues proposed a Bayesian methodology to predict the results of the 1962 US election which were presented at the NBC television during that night. They used various data on previous elections and expert opinion from leading social scientists and included a hierarchical structure (in his paper on Bayesianism, Fienberg (2006) refers that Tukey spoke extensively about borrowing strength, the main feature of hierarchical models, which will be central in Chapter 5).

3.1.4   The 1990s and beyond

The advent of computational algorithms to perform Bayesian inference and modeling started in the 1990s with the development of Gibbs sampling, and then generalized to Markov chain Monte Carlo (MCMC) methods (Gelfand and Smith, 1990; Casella and George, 1992). The availability of such computational methods allowed statisticians to perform Bayesian computation on large datasets and to specify complex models. In 1989, the project "Bayesian inference Using Gibbs Sampling" developed a user friendly software (BUGS, Spiegelhalter *et al.*, 1995) to perform Gibbs sampling simulations, later extended to include different MCMC methods, such as Metropolis–Hastings and slice sampling. Toward the end of the 1990s, the first version of WinBUGS (BUGS operating under Windows, Spiegelhalter *et al.*, 1999) was launched and in less than a decade has made it possible for applied researchers like social scientists, epidemiologists, geographers, etc., to perform Bayesian modeling on large datasets.

A more recent alternative to MCMC, based on integrated nested Laplace approximations (INLA) was developed by Rue *et al.* (2009). This method ensures faster computation than MCMC for a particular class of models, the so-called latent Gaussian models. The methodology behind INLA will be extensively treated in Chapter 4 and Chapters 5–8 will provide several examples of how INLA can be used in real data problems.

Having looked back at the essential steps taken by Bayesianism and how it has affirmed itself during more than three centuries, in the rest of the chapter we are going to present the fundamental principles of Bayesian methods, starting with the concept of conditional and inverse probability. We will then focus on the three components of Bayesian inference: likelihood, prior, and posterior, and how the posterior can be obtained through Bayes theorem. The families of conjugate models will follow, particular types of models which are easy to treat analytically, but that are limited in their flexibility. We then conclude the chapter with a section presenting different choices for prior distribution.

3.2 Basic probability elements

3.2.1 What is an event?

Given a random experiment, Ω is the sample space, that is the collection of all its possible outcomes. For example, if we roll a six faces dice once, the sample space will be $\Omega = \{1, 2, 3, 4, 5, 6\}$ or if we toss a coin twice it will be $\Omega = \{$Tail–Tail, Tail–Head, Head–Tail, Head–Head$\}$. An event can be defined as the outcome(s) from the experiment that we are interested in. Events always belong to Ω. For instance an event A could be "Tossing a coin twice will give me two tails", which can also be written as $A = \{$Tail–Tail$\}$. For each event A there is a *complement* event A^C which can only happen if A does not occur. For instance, A^C will be "Tossing a coin twice will NOT give me two tails", which can also be written as $A^C = \{$Head–Head, Tail–Head, Head–Tail$\}$.

Considering two simple events A and B, the *intersection* event, which can be written as $A \cap B$, occurs when both happen at the same time, while the *union* event, which can be written as $A \cup B$, occurs when at least one of the two events happens. Because the entire sample space is the collection of all the possible events (and therefore one of them will occur), Ω is said to be the *certain* (*or sure*) event. Conversely, an empty set $\emptyset$ (i.e., a set containing no events) is called the *impossible* event. If $A \cap B = \emptyset$ the two events are called *incompatible* or *mutually exclusive*. The union of each event with its complement gives the certain event, while the intersection of each event with its complement gives the empty set. For instance going back to the coin example, $A = \{$Tail–Tail$\}, A^C = \{$Head–Head, Tail–Head, Head–Tail$\}$, we can write the union and the intersection between these two events as follows:

$$A \cup A^C = \{\text{Tail–Tail, Tail–Head, Head–Tail, Head–Head}\} = \Omega$$

$$A \cap A^C = \{\} = \emptyset.$$

3.2.2 Probability of events

Having defined sample space and events in an experiment, the next step is that of assigning these a probability measure, which represents the chance each event will occur. Such probability can vary between 0 and 1, representing, at its extremes, complete certainty that the event is occurring (probability $= 1$) or is not occurring (probability $= 0$); anything between these two values provides the degree of uncertainty on the event being true.

There are different formulations of probability (see Dawid, 1991 for an exhaustive description); as this book focuses on the Bayesian framework, we will introduce here the subjective approach, which is its foundation. Nevertheless, we will also briefly present the classical or frequentist approach, commonly used in introductory statistical courses, and generally used as a benchmark.

Classical probability

In the frequentist approach the concept of probability is the limit of a long-run relative frequency. This means that for an event A the uncertainty on its occurrence is calculated as the ratio of the number of times the event occurred to the number of trials. For instance, applying this formulation to the dice example described above, considering $A = \{2\}$ and assuming that the dice is fair, if we roll it for a large M number of times, A will occur approximately $M/6$ of the times; thus, its probability (frequency) will be $Pr(A) = 1/6$. From this definition it follows that the probability is objective, it is a characteristic of objects (e.g., of the dice) and cannot differ for different subjects.

In this framework, a probability must satisfy the three Kolmogorov axioms:

(I) for an event A in Ω, the probability $Pr(A) \geq 0$;

(II) the probability for the certain event Ω is equal to 1;

(III) the probability of the union of n incompatible events is equal to the sum of the probabilities of each of them $Pr(\cup_{i=1}^{n} A_i) = \sum_{i=1}^{n} Pr(A_i)$. This is also called axiom of total probabilities, which we will see in Section 3.3 is linked to Bayes theorem.

From these axioms it also follows that

1. the probability of the empty set is 0. As the intersection between the certain event and the impossible event is empty ($\Omega \cap \emptyset = \emptyset$) and the union between the certain event and the impossible event is the sure event ($\Omega \cup \emptyset = \Omega$), then Ω and $\emptyset$ are incompatible and for the axiom of total probabilities it follows that $Pr(\Omega) = Pr(\Omega) + Pr(\emptyset)$ from which $Pr(\emptyset) = Pr(\Omega) - Pr(\Omega) = 0$;

2. given the event A, the probability of its contrary event A^C is $1 - Pr(A)$. As $A \cup A^C = \Omega$, then $Pr(A \cup A^C) = Pr(\Omega) = 1$; also as A and A^C are incompatible, from the axiom of total probabilities $Pr(A \cup A^C) = Pr(A) + Pr(A^C) = 1$ from which $Pr(A^C) = 1 - Pr(A)$;

3. given the two events A and B, if A is included in B ($A \subseteq B$), then B can be written as the union of the event A and of the difference between B and A ($A \cup (B - A) = A \cup (B \cap A^C)$), which are incompatible; then from the law of total probabilities it follows that $Pr(B) = Pr(A) + Pr(B - A)$, from which, $Pr(B) \geq Pr(A)$, as from the first axiom of probability $Pr(B - A) \geq 0$;

4. the probability of the union of any two events A and B, $Pr(A \cup B)$ can be written as $Pr(A) + Pr(B) - Pr(A \cap B)$. Using the Venn diagram[1] in Figure 3.1, $A \cup B$ can be seen as the union of the three following incompatible events: only A occurs (left-hand side of the Venn diagram), characterized by the probability $Pr(A - (A \cap B))$; only B occurs (right-hand side of the Venn diagram), characterized by the probability $Pr(B - (A \cap B))$; A and B occur at the same time, (central part of the Venn diagram) characterized by the probability $Pr(A \cap B)$; as these three events are incompatible, applying the axiom of total probabilities, we obtain $Pr(A - (A \cap B)) = Pr(A) - Pr(A \cap B)$ (and similarly for $Pr(B - (A \cap B))$), so that $Pr(A \cup B) = Pr(A) - Pr(A \cap B) + Pr(B) - Pr(B \cap A) + Pr(B \cap A) = Pr(A) + Pr(B) - Pr(A \cap B)$. Note that if A and B are incompatible $Pr(A \cap B) = 0$, so $Pr(A \cup B)$ becomes the sum of the probabilities of the two events, as already seen in the axiom of total probabilities.

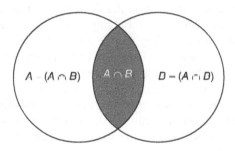

Figure 3.1   Venn diagram for two nonmutually exclusive events A and B.

There are two main concerns related to the classical (or frequentist) definition of probability: first considering the probability of an event A as a relative frequency means that we are only able to calculate it if we know the entire sample space Ω. Such condition can be satisfied in a simple example (e.g., in the dice or coin experiments previously presented), but it becomes problematic in more realistic and complex settings; for instance, if we are interested in assessing the probability of underage drinking in men living in London, or the probability of experiencing breast cancer in France, we would only be able to use the proportion if we knew the occurrence of the event of interest in the entire target population, which is in practice very unlikely. Second, this probability definition is based on the concept of repeatability, which is not necessarily a characteristic of the event of interest: for instance the events "Caesar crossed the Rubicon" or "The next US president will be a woman" do not satisfy this assumption as they can only happen once. In these cases the classical probability fails and a different approach is needed.

---

[1] The Venn diagram is formed by a collection of overlapping circles and is used to visualize logical relationships between classes (e.g., events).

Subjective probability

A substantially different definition is that of the subjective probability, which, as it has been introduced in Section 3.1, is the basis of Bayesian thinking. It was originally introduced by de Finetti (1931) in terms of betting, that is the probability is the rate at which the individual is willing to bet on the occurrence of an event. In more general terms, this probability formulation reflects a degree of belief that the individual has on the occurrence of an event. It is clear that the great difference between this and the classical approach lies on the idea that each individual is entitled to their own degree of belief. Thus, the probability is *subjective* (recall from Section 3.1 that de Finetti claimed that probability does not exist; it should be now clear that he meant the probability in the frequentist perspective). In de Finetti's definition, the only rule for a measure to be considered a probability is coherence, which he formulated in betting terms as follows: an individual will never bet on the occurrence of an event if they are certain that they will lose.

De Finetti (1931) proved that this concept of coherence is equivalent to the Kolmogorov axioms (presented in Section 3.2.2), meaning that these rules are still valid in the subjective definition of probability. An important aspect is that in the subjective interpretation a probability can be attached to any event, so that if we are interested in "Caesar crossed the Rubicon" or "The next US president will be a woman", it is always possible to indicate the degree of belief that a person has on their occurrence, making such definition more flexible and versatile than the classical one, as it does not rely on the assumption that the events should be repeatable. Nevertheless, frequentist reasoning can be used to inform the subjective probability, that is, information on the previous occurrence of the event can be used to define the degree of belief that an individual has got.

3.2.3 Conditional probability

Given the two events A and B, we can define the *conditional* event – denoted by $A|B$ – as the event A under the condition that the event B has already occurred. Then a probability measure can be associated to this event, measuring how likely the event A will occur *given that* the event B has already been observed. This probability measure is called the *conditional probability*. In other words, if we consider a conditional probability, we are interested in the subset of the sample space Ω where both A and B can occur and as basis for the comparison, we focus only on the subset where B can occur instead of considering the entire sample space Ω. Thus, the conditional probability can be specified as follows:

$$Pr(A|B) = \frac{Pr(A \cap B)}{Pr(B)}. \tag{3.1}$$

Looking at the Venn diagram in Figure 3.1, this is equivalent to divide the probability that both events happen (central part) by the sum of this probability and the one that only B occurs (right part). To fully appreciate the concept of conditional probability, we present two simple examples.

Example 3.1: Consider a standard deck of 52 cards (13 cards for each seed); we are interested in calculating the probability of drawing two aces in a row. The event B can be defined as "an ace is extracted at the first draw" and as there are four aces in the deck:

$$Pr(B) = \frac{4}{52}.$$

The event A can be defined as "an ace is extracted at the second draw". This depends on the result of the first draw: if an ace did not occur then there are still four aces in the deck (and 51 cards in total), so $Pr(A|B^C) = \frac{4}{51}$, while if an ace was extracted in the first draw it means that only 3 are still available, so $Pr(A|B) = \frac{3}{51}$. This last result can also be obtained by using Eq. (3.1) as follows:

$$Pr(A|B) = \frac{4/52 \times 3/51}{4/52} = \frac{3}{51} = 0.059$$

concluding that around 6% of the time two consecutive aces will be drawn from a deck with 52 cards.

Example 3.2: Simon (1988) studied the 13-year cycle cicada, a noisy insect similar to the grasshopper which appears periodically in some southern US states. Table 3.1 describes a sample of cicada captured in Tennesee in 1998 by weight and gender.

Suppose that we are interested in the probability that a cicada weights more than 25 g (an event that we indicate as W) given that it is female (an event that we indicate as F). The event of interest can be written as follows:

$$W|F = \{\text{Weight} > 25 \text{ g } given \text{ that } \text{Gender} = \text{Female}\}.$$

Using the formula in Eq. (3.1), the probability of interest $Pr(W|F)$ can be written as follows:

$$Pr(W|F) = \frac{Pr(W \cap F)}{Pr(F)}$$

and using the data in Table 3.1 we obtain

$$Pr(W|F) = \frac{11/104}{59/104} = 0.186.$$

Table 3.1 Number of Cicadas captured in Tennessee by weight and gender.

	Female (F)	Male (F^C)	Total
≤ 25 g (W^C)	48	43	91
> 25 g (W)	11	2	13
Total	59	45	104

Similarly it is possible to calculate the probability that the weight is above 25 g given that the gender of the cicada is male:

$$Pr(W|F^C) = \frac{2/104}{45/104} = 0.044,$$

so we can conclude that it is four times more likely that the weight of a cicada is above 25 g if it is a female than if it is a male.

3.3   Bayes theorem

Conditional probability plays an important role in Bayesian statistics (see Dawid, 1979, for a technical review on the topic) and Bayes theorem follows naturally from it: rearranging the definition given in Eq. (3.1), it is possible to write the probability of the intersection between the events A and B as follows:

$$Pr(A \cap B) = Pr(A|B) \times Pr(B). \tag{3.2}$$

If now we are interested in the probability of the event B, conditioning on A, applying again Eq. (3.1) we get

$$Pr(B|A) = \frac{Pr(A \cap B)}{Pr(A)} \tag{3.3}$$

and substituting Eq. (3.2) into Eq. (3.3), we obtain the so-called Bayes theorem

$$Pr(B|A) = \frac{Pr(A|B) \times Pr(B)}{Pr(A)}. \tag{3.4}$$

The interpretation of Bayes theorem follows from the inverse probability theory introduced by Thomas Bayes and Pierre Simon Laplace, as described in Section 3.1; the interest lies in the probability of the event B given that A occurs. $Pr(B)$ is calculated before we observe A; then the probability of observing A given B is used to update the original $Pr(B)$ so that $Pr(B|A)$ is obtained. If we frame Bayes theorem in an experimental setting, we can rephrase the abovementioned sentence saying that before running the experiment the researcher has some information about B whose level of uncertainty is expressed by $Pr(B)$, which is combined with the result of the experiment, expressed by $Pr(A|B)$, to obtain an updated probability for B, that is, $Pr(B|A)$.

Now if we extend this concept and consider a set of events $B_1, \ldots, B_K$, they are defined *mutually exclusive* if $B_i \cap B_j = \emptyset$, for $i \neq j$ and *exhaustive* if $U_{i=1}^K B_i = \Omega$. Then $Pr(U_{i=1}^K B_i) = \sum_{i=1}^K Pr(B_i) = 1$, so that the probability of A can be written as

$$Pr(A) = \sum_{i=1}^K Pr(A \cap B_i), \text{ as } A \cap B_i \text{ are mutually exclusive events}$$

or alternatively

$$Pr(A) = \sum_{i=1}^{K} Pr(A|B_i) \times Pr(B_i), \text{ applying Eq. (3.2).}$$

These two formulations are called the law of total probabilities and can be used to rewrite Bayes theorem as follows:

$$Pr(B_i|A) = \frac{Pr(A|B_i)Pr(B_i)}{\sum_{i=1}^{K} Pr(A|B_i)Pr(B_i)}. \tag{3.5}$$

Example: A new HIV test is supposed to have 95% sensitivity (defined as probability that the test is positive given that a person has HIV) and 98% specificity (defined as probability that the test is negative given that a person has not HIV). In the English population, HIV prevalence (proportion of a population with HIV) is 0.0015 and we are interested in evaluating the probability that a patient has HIV given that the test is positive.

Let A be the event that the patient is truly HIV positive and A^C be the event that they are truly HIV negative. As either A or A^C will definitively happen, but they cannot happen at the same time, we can conclude that A and A^C are exhaustive and mutually exclusive events. Let B be the event that the patient tests positive, we want to assess the probability of the event A given B: $Pr(A|B)$.

From the available information on the test, "95% sensitivity" can be translated in probability terms as $Pr(B|A) = 0.95$, while "98% specificity" can be written as $Pr(B|A^C) = 0.02$. Then applying Bayes theorem in its formulation presented in Eq. (3.5), we obtain

$$Pr(A|B) = \frac{Pr(B|A)Pr(A)}{Pr(B|A)Pr(A) + Pr(B|A^C)Pr(A^C)}$$
$$= \frac{0.95 \times 0.0015}{0.95 \times 0.0015 + 0.02 \times 0.9985} = 0.067.$$

Thus, we can conclude that about 6.7% of those testing positive will in fact have HIV.

3.4   Prior and posterior distributions

The HIV example shows that despite the high sensitivity (95%) and specificity (98%) of the test, the fact that the proportion of HIV positive in a population is very small (0.15%) has a strong impact on the final probability of being HIV positive, given that the test returns a positive result. Assuming now that the proportion of

HIV positives in the population is 20%, the probability $Pr(A|B)$ would increase as follows:

$$Pr(A|B) = \frac{0.95 \times 0.2}{0.95 \times 0.2 + 0.02 \times 0.8} = 0.92.$$

This can be explained if we think that the disease prevalence $Pr(A)$ is the information on the event of interest (being HIV positive in the example) available *a priori*, that is before carrying out any experiment (also called *prior information*). Observing a positive result through the diagnostic test updates the prior, leading to an increased *posterior* probability of having the disease. So the posterior probability will depend on the prior information as well as on the results of the experiment: when the prevalence of the disease is very low $(Pr(A) = 0.0015)$, the posterior probability after observing a positive result will increase to $Pr(A|B) = 0.067$, while when the prevalence is higher $(Pr(A) = 0.2)$, the posterior probability after observing a positive result will reach $Pr(A|B) = 0.92$.

3.4.1 Bayesian inference

Bayes theorem applied to observable events (as in diagnostic testing) is uncontroversial and well established, on the other hand more controversial is its use in general statistical analyses, where *parameters* are unknown quantities and their prior distribution needs to be specified, in order to obtain the corresponding *posterior* distribution. This process is known as *Bayesian inference* and it makes fundamental distinction between observable and unknown quantities.

Consider a random variable[2] Y; its uncertainty is modeled using a probability distribution or a density function (according to whether Y is a discrete or continuous random variable, respectively) indexed by a generic parameter θ. Let

$$L(\theta) = p(Y = y|\theta) \tag{3.6}$$

be the so-called *likelihood* function which specifies the distribution of the data y under the model defined by θ. Notice that $p(\cdot)$ is used to indicate the probability distribution or density function for a random variable, while $Pr(\cdot)$ is used for the probability of events (see Section 3.2). For instance, the random variable Y could be the number of deaths for respiratory diseases, we observe y and we are interested in studying the death rate θ in the population. From now on, for the sake of simplicity, we will refer to the likelihood as $p(y|\theta)$.

The variability on y depends only on the sampling selection (sampling variability). In other words we assume that the data are a random sample from the study population and the uncertainty originates by the fact that we only observe that sample instead of all the other possible ones. Conversely, the parameter θ is an unknown

---

[2] Given the outcomes of an experiment defined in the sample space Ω, a random variable is a variable which maps each outcome of Ω to real numbers. There are two types of random variables: discrete, if they can only assume integer values, e.g., $0, 1, \ldots, n, \ldots$; continuous if they can assume any values in a specified range, e.g., $(-\infty, +\infty)$.

quantity modeled through a suitable *prior* probability distribution $p(\theta)$ before we observe any realization y of the random variable Y and reflects our *prior* belief on θ. In the presence of a hierarchical structure or spatial (or temporal) dependence between the parameters, it would be more common to express the knowledge on θ through *hyperparameters* ψ, so that its distribution would become $p(\theta|\psi)$. The concept of hyperparameters will be treated extensively in Chapters 5–7.

Given the two components (likelihood and prior), in a Bayesian perspective the inferential problem is solved using Bayes theorem, where instead of probability of events we now include probability distributions (for the parameter θ and for the data y):

$$p(\theta|y) = \frac{p(y|\theta) \times p(\theta)}{p(y)} \tag{3.7}$$

to obtain the *posterior* distribution $p(\theta|y)$, which represents the uncertainty about the parameter of interest θ after having observed the data, thus the conditioning on y. Note that $p(y)$, in the denominator of Eq. (3.7) is the *marginal distribution* of the data and it is considered a normalization constant as it does not depend on θ, so the Bayes theorem is often reported as

$$p(\theta|y) \propto p(y|\theta) \times p(\theta),$$

where the *equal to* sign (=) is replaced by the *proportional to* sign ($\propto$).

The process to obtain the marginal distribution $p(y)$ is similar to what we showed in Eq. (3.5), where we applied the law of total probabilities for mutually exclusive and exhaustive events. To explain this point, assume that θ is a discrete parameter which can only assume values 0 and 1. We first consider the conditional probability $p(y|\theta = 0)$, weighting it by the probability that θ will assume value 0, $p(\theta = 0)$; then consider the conditional probability $p(y|\theta = 1)$, weighting it by the probability that θ will assume value 1, $p(\theta = 1)$; finally $p(y)$ will simply be the sum of the two weighted probabilities:

$$p(y) = p(y|\theta = 0) \times p(\theta = 0) + p(y|\theta = 1) \times p(\theta = 1).$$

In other words, marginalizing $p(y)$ means *integrating out* all the uncertainty on θ. This process can easily be extended to a case when θ can assume discrete values in Θ, leading to

$$p(y) = \sum_{\theta \in \Theta} p(y|\theta)p(\theta).$$

When θ is a continuous variable, the sum in the previous equation is replaced by the integral calculation

$$p(y) = \int_{\theta \in \Theta} p(y|\theta)p(\theta)d\theta.$$

Note that as the posterior distribution is a combination of prior and likelihood, it is always somewhere in between these two distributions. We will see in Section 3.6 what this means in practice with two examples based on two different prior distributions.

3.5   Working with the posterior distribution

A great advantage of working in a Bayesian framework is the availability of the entire posterior probability distribution for the parameter(s) of interest. Obviously, it is always possible and useful to summarize it through some suitable synthetic indicators. The summary statistic typically used is the posterior mean, which, for a hypothetical continuous parameter of interest θ, is

$$E(\theta|y) = \int_{\theta \in \Theta} \theta p(\theta|y) d\theta,$$

where Θ are all the possible values that the variable θ can assume. Note that if θ is discrete the integral is replaced by the sum.

In a similar way, it is also easy to calculate indicators which divide conveniently the probability distribution. For instance, the posterior median $\theta_{0.5}$ is defined as the value which divides the probability distribution in two equal halves, so that

$$p(\theta \leq \theta_{0.5}|y) = 0.5 \text{ and } p(\theta \geq \theta_{0.5}|y) = 0.5,$$

while the 95% credibility interval (CI) is defined as the pair of θ values ($\theta_{0.025}$ and $\theta_{0.975}$) so that

$$p(\theta \leq \theta_{0.025}|y) = 0.025 \text{ and } p(\theta \geq \theta_{0.975}|y) = 0.025.$$

Note that despite the apparent similarity of the credibility interval to the confidence intervals as defined in the frequentist approach, the interpretation of the two is completely different.

In the frequentist philosophy, the $(100 - \alpha)\%$ confidence interval suggests that if we could repeat the same experiment, under the same conditions, for a large number M of times, then the real value of θ would fall out of the intervals only $\alpha\%$ of the times. This convoluted statement is not equivalent to asserting that the probability of θ lying within the confidence interval is $(100 - \alpha)\%$, since the parameter is considered a fixed, unknown value, and it is not a random variable characterized by a probability distribution.

Conversely, within the Bayesian approach, a credibility interval will explicitly indicate the posterior probability that θ lies within its boundaries, $p(\theta \in CI|y)$; this is made possible by the fact that the parameter of interest is associated with a probability distribution, so that we can make probabilistic statements and take the underlying uncertainty into account. To highlight this difference, we talk about credibility (as opposed to confidence) intervals.

Following the same rationale, Bayesian inference can provide any probability statements about parameters; for instance, it is easy to calculate the posterior probability that θ is larger (or smaller) than an assigned threshold (e.g., $p(\theta > 1|y)$, see Figure 3.2). This probability is commonly computed in epidemiological studies,

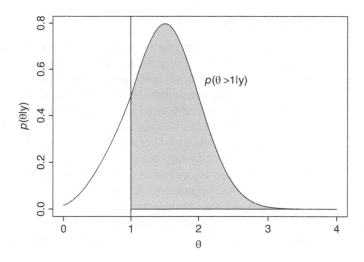

Figure 3.2   Posterior distribution for the θ parameter. The gray area corresponds to the posterior probability that θ > 1.

assuming that θ is the relative risk[3] of disease (or death), and it is particularly interesting to evaluate the probability of an increased relative risk ($\theta > 1$). In comparison, inference under the frequentist approach could only lead to the estimate of the p-value for an increased relative risk. This is not equivalent to $p(\theta > 1|y)$, as it only provides a quantification of how extreme is the estimated θ, thus giving a statement about the plausibility of the data under the hypothesis that the true value of θ is 1 (Casella and Berger, 2002).

3.6   Choosing the prior distribution

When performing Bayesian inference, the choice of prior distribution is a vital issue, as it represents the information that is available for the parameters of interest. In particular, there are two aspects which need to be taken into account: (i) the type of distribution, which should be representative of the nature of the parameters, and (ii) the hyperparameters, which would make the distribution more or less informative, thus providing the level of information (or ignorance) available for the parameters.

---

[3] The relative risk (RR) is a measure commonly used in epidemiology to determine the change in the probability of experiencing a particular outcome (e.g., disease or death) for exposed and unexposed groups. A different measure equally common in epidemiology and used throughout the book is the odds ratio (OR), which compares the odds of the outcome amongst exposed and nonexposed. In case of rare events, e.g., when the probability of disease or death is small, then RR ≈ OR.

3.6.1   Type of distribution

Based on the nature of the parameters of interest there is usually a "natural" candidate for the type of prior distribution. For instance, if the parameter under study is a proportion (e.g., the probability of death in the population or the proportion of responses for a particular drug), the uncertainty on the parameter should be represented by a distribution varying between 0 and 1; if the parameter of interest is a continuous symmetric variable (e.g., the average age in the population, the daily temperature in a year or the log transformed concentration of air pollutants), the prior distribution should be allowed to vary between 0 and $+\infty$ or between $-\infty$ and $+\infty$; if the parameter of interest is a continuous positive variable (e.g., the hospitalization or mortality rate in the population), the prior distribution should only be allowed to vary between 0 and $+\infty$. Starting from three examples, we now look at commonly used models, describing the typical choice of prior distribution and the Bayesian inferential process which leads to the posterior distribution.

Binomial-Beta model

A study is carried out to evaluate the prevalence of high blood pressure among people living within 5 miles of Heathrow airport (London, UK). For each individual, the outcomes are the following:

$$1 = \text{high blood pressure}; \quad 0 = \text{normal or low blood pressure}.$$

Defining a "success" if the ith person has high blood pressure and considering n people sampled independently from the reference population, the number of successes y represents the data in the study and can be described by a Binomial distribution

$$y|\pi \sim \text{Binomial}(\pi, n),$$

characterized by the probability function

$$p(y|\pi) = \binom{n}{y} \pi^y (1 - \pi)^{n-y} \propto \pi^y (1 - \pi)^{n-y},$$

where π corresponds to the generic parameter θ and represents the proportion (or probability) of successes; $\binom{n}{y}$ is called *binomial coefficient* and represents all the possible combinations of y successes in n trials. It can also be expressed through the factorial function: $\binom{n}{y} = \frac{n!}{y!(n-y)!}$, where $n!$ stands for "n factorial" and can be calculated as $n \times (n-1) \times (n-2) \times \cdots \times 2 \times 1$.

To complete a Bayesian model, we need to specify a suitable prior distribution for the proportion parameter π, such that it can only assume values between 0 and 1. A good candidate is the Beta distribution. This is a continuous distribution defined in $[0, 1]$, denoted by

$$\pi \sim \text{Beta}(a, b)$$

and characterized by two hyperparameters usually indicated as a and b. The density function of the Beta distribution is the following:

$$p(\pi) = \frac{\Gamma(a+b)}{\Gamma(a)\Gamma(b)} \, \pi^{a-1}(1-\pi)^{b-1} \qquad a, b > 0, \tag{3.8}$$

where $\frac{\Gamma(a+b)}{\Gamma(a)\Gamma(b)}$ is the Beta function and $\Gamma(a)$ is the Gamma function, defined as $\int_0^\infty \exp(-t)t^{a-1}\mathrm{d}t$, which, if a is an integer, can also be expressed using the factorial function: $\Gamma(a) = (a-1)!$.

We stress here that a *probability function* indicates the probability distribution for discrete random variables (e.g., the Binomial distribution of the data in this example), while *density function* is used for continuous random variables (e.g., the Beta distribution of the π parameter in this example). Nevertheless, for the sake of simplicity in the rest of the book we will refer to them interchangeably.

It can be shown that the mean and the variance for the Beta distribution are functions of the hyperparameters:

$$E(\pi) = \frac{a}{a+b} \tag{3.9}$$

$$\mathrm{Var}(\pi) = \frac{ab}{(a+b)^2(a+b+1)}. \tag{3.10}$$

Changing the value for a and b leads to different shapes and scales for the Beta distribution. This circumstance renders this distribution quite flexible and capable of handling different situations. See Figure 3.3 for an example of Beta density functions changing the hyperparameters a and b.

To obtain the posterior distribution for π, we need to apply Bayes theorem, combining the Binomial likelihood and the Beta prior:

$$p(\pi|y) \propto p(y|\pi) \times p(\pi) \tag{3.11}$$
$$\propto \pi^y(1-\pi)^{n-y} \times \pi^{a-1}(1-\pi)^{b-1}$$
$$\propto \pi^{y+a-1}(1-\pi)^{n-y+b-1},$$

which is the functional form of another Beta random variable:

$$\pi|y \propto \mathrm{Beta}(y+a, \; n-y+b),$$

where the parameters are a function of the prior (a and b) and of the observations (y and n). In particular, the mean of the posterior Beta distribution (also the so-called *posterior mean*) is

$$E(\pi|y) = \frac{y+a}{n+a+b}, \tag{3.12}$$

which indicates how the posterior average proportion of successes is a function of the prior average proportion, depending only on a and b, updated by the number of observed successes and the total number of trials (individuals).

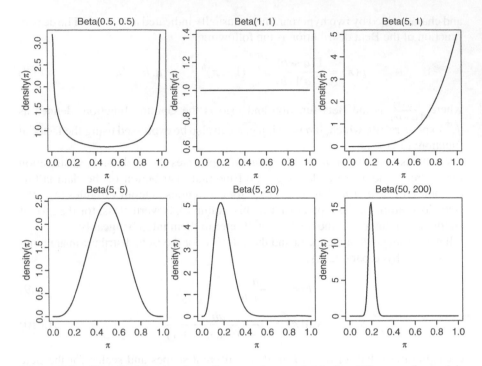

Figure 3.3   Density function for a Beta random variable for different values of the a and b hyperparameters.

Normal–Normal model

To estimate the annual mean of air pollution in Greater London (μ), daily measures of ozone (O_3) are collected in the study area using monitors for 1 year. As the values of O_3 can only be positive and generally are characterized by a long right tail, they are log transformed to resemble a Normal distribution. Note that this is typically done for skewed variables (see Gelman and Hill, 2007, Page 59). For each day ($i = 1, \ldots, n = 365$), the distribution of the log concentration (likelihood) is specified as follows:

$$y_i = \log(O_{3i})$$
$$y_i | \mu, \sigma^2 \sim \text{Normal}(\mu, \sigma^2)$$
$$p(y|\mu, \sigma^2) = \prod_{i=1}^{n} p(y_i|\mu, \sigma^2) = \left(\frac{1}{2\pi\sigma^2}\right)^{n/2} \exp\left(-\frac{1}{2\sigma^2}\sum_{i=1}^{n}(y_i - \mu)^2\right),$$

with $y = (y_1, \ldots, y_n)$, $-\infty < \mu < +\infty$. In this model, the parameter $\sigma^2 > 0$ is the sampling variability, which for the sake of simplicity we assume to know, and μ corresponds to the generic parameter θ.[4]

---

[4] Note that in the likelihood π is the mathematical constant that is the ratio of a circle's circumference to its diameter, equal to 3.14159...

As the parameter of interest μ is an average value of normally distributed observations, its prior distribution should be defined between $-\infty$ and $+\infty$. A good candidate is the Normal distribution characterized by the hyperparameters μ_0 and σ_0^2:

$$\mu \sim \text{Normal}(\mu_0, \sigma_0^2).$$

Combining the likelihood and the prior distribution leads to a posterior distribution, which is again a Normal random variable:

$$\mu|y \sim \text{Normal}\left(\frac{\sigma_0^2 n\bar{y} + \sigma^2 \mu_0}{n\sigma_0^2 + \sigma^2}, \frac{\sigma^2 \sigma_0^2}{n\sigma_0^2 + \sigma^2}\right), \tag{3.13}$$

where its mean is a weighted average between the prior mean (μ_0) and the mean of the data (sample mean $\bar{y} = \sum_{i=1}^{n} y_i/n$), with weights equal to the prior and the sampling variance:

$$E(\mu|y) = \frac{\sigma_0^2 n\bar{y} + \sigma^2 \mu_0}{n\sigma_0^2 + \sigma^2}.$$

Poisson–Gamma model

Consider a study to evaluate ρ, the average rate of leukemia in Milan (Italy) in 2010. The data are the count of cases (y), i.e., a discrete variable that can assume values between 0 and $+\infty$ and can be modeled using a Poisson distribution

$$y|\lambda \sim \text{Poisson}(\lambda),$$

where λ can be written as ρE, and E represents the expected number of leukaemia cases in the study area and period. Note that this formulation is typically used when the parameter of interest is the relative risk ρ (as in our case) as opposed to when the interest lays on the mean λ of the Poisson distribution and is the basis for small area studies which will be extensively treated in Chapter 6.

The distribution of the data (likelihood) can be specified as follows:

$$p(y|\rho) = \frac{(E\rho)^y \exp(-E\rho)}{y!} \qquad \rho > 0.$$

The parameter of interest ρ corresponds to the generic θ introduced previously. As it is a rate, its prior distribution should be a continuous variable defined on the positive axis, so that ρ can only assume values between 0 and $+\infty$. One of the most used random variables in this case is the Gamma, characterized by hyperparameters (usually identified with a and b) representing the shape and the scale of the following density function[5]:

$$\rho \sim \text{Gamma}(a, b)$$

$$p(\rho) = \frac{b^a}{\Gamma(a)} \rho^{a-1} \exp(-b\rho) \qquad a, b > 0, \tag{3.14}$$

---

[5] Alternatively, to use the specification implemented in R, the scale parameter could be replaced by the so-called *rate*, defined as $1/b$.

where $\Gamma(a)$ is the Gamma function. The mean and variance for the Gamma distribution are functions of the hyperparameters:

$$E(\rho) = \frac{a}{b} \tag{3.15}$$

$$\mathrm{Var}(\rho) = \frac{a}{b^2}. \tag{3.16}$$

Similarly to what we have seen for the Beta distribution, changing the values of a and b impacts on the shape and scale of the distribution, so that also the Gamma distribution is very flexible. Figure 3.4 shows the Gamma density function for different values of a and b.

The posterior distribution is once again obtained combining the likelihood and the prior:

$$p(\rho|y) \propto \frac{b^a}{\Gamma(a)} \rho^{a-1} \exp(-b\rho) \frac{(\rho E)^y \exp(-\rho E)}{y!}.$$

Leaving aside $\frac{b^a}{\Gamma(a)}$ and $\frac{1}{y!}$ which do not depend on ρ, thus can be seen as normalization factors, we obtain

$$p(\rho|y) \propto \rho^{a+y-1} \exp(-(b+E)\rho)$$

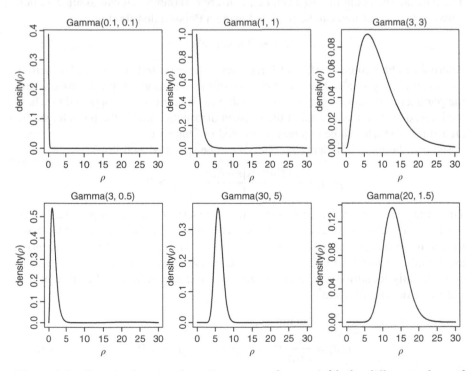

Figure 3.4   Density function for a Gamma random variable for different values of the shape and scale hyperparameters.

which is the functional form of a Gamma random variable:

$$\rho|y \sim \text{Gamma}(a + y, b + E).$$

It is characterized by a posterior mean which is a function of the hyperparameters (a and b) as well as of the data (y and E):

$$E(\rho|y) = \frac{a + y}{b + E}. \tag{3.17}$$

3.6.2   Conjugacy

The three models presented in Section 3.6.1 have one thing in common, that is the posterior distribution belongs to the same family as the prior distribution (Beta, Normal, and Gamma, respectively). This property is called *conjugacy* in Bayesian terms. Equivalently it can be said that the prior *is conjugated* to the likelihood. Conjugacy is a convenient property: as the functional form of the posterior distribution is known, as well as its hyperparameters, it is easy to extract summary statistics (like the posterior mean or median, 95% credibility intervals, etc.) or derive analytically any other quantities of interest. For instance, the posterior means for the three models described above are reported in Eq. (3.12) for the Beta distribution, Eq. (3.13) for the Normal distribution, and in Eq. (3.17) for the Gamma distribution. Table 3.2 gives a list of conjugate models and provides their prior and posterior probability distributions.

Nevertheless, it is important to notice that conjugate models are not often used in practice as they have very limited flexibility: not all the likelihoods have an associated conjugate prior or conjugacy is broken when generalized linear regression models are specified (see Chapter 5 for a detailed description of regression models in a Bayesian framework), that is the class of models typically used to assess the presence of an association between predictors (e.g., risk factors) and outcomes (e.g., health end points). In these cases, it is always possible to perform Bayesian inference, but appropriate simulative or approximation methods (MCMC, INLA) need to be applied, which will be the focus of Chapter 4.

3.6.3   Noninformative or informative prior

Once the functional form of the prior distribution has been specified, the definition of its parameters should be informed by whatever knowledge is available. This has always been a critical issue in Bayesian inference and a source of major criticism from the frequentist school. We briefly present the most used noninformative and informative priors and refer the reader to Lesaffre and Lawson 2012, Chap. 5, for a more detailed review.

Noninformative prior

The specification of a so-called *noninformative* prior has always been very appealing, particularly for applied researchers who often lack information on the

Table 3.2   Some relevant conjugate models.

	Case 1	Case 2
Likelihood	$y\|\mu, \sigma^2 \sim \text{Normal}(\mu, \sigma^2)$	$y\|\rho \sim \text{Poisson}(E\rho)$
Prior	$\mu \sim \text{Normal}(\mu_0, \sigma_0^2)$	$\rho \sim \text{Gamma}(a, b)$
Posterior	$\mu\|y \sim \text{Normal}(\mu_1, \sigma_1^2)$	$\rho\|y \sim \text{Gamma}(a_1, b_1)$
Hyperparameters	$\mu_1 = \dfrac{\sigma_0^2 n\bar{y} + \sigma^2 \mu_0}{n\sigma_0^2 + \sigma^2}$	$a_1 = a + y$
Hyperparameters	$\sigma_1^2 = \dfrac{\sigma^2 \sigma_0^2}{n\sigma_0^2 + \sigma^2}$	$b_1 = b + E$

	Case 3	Case 4
Likelihood	$y\|\pi \sim \text{Binomial}(\pi, n)$	$y\|\lambda \sim \text{Exponential}(\lambda)$
Prior	$\pi \sim \text{Beta}(a, b)$	$\lambda \sim \text{Gamma}(a, b)$
Posterior	$\pi\|y \sim \text{Beta}(a_1, b_1)$	$\lambda\|y \sim \text{Gamma}(a_1, b_1)$
Hyperparameters	$a_1 = y + a$	$a_1 = a + n$
Hyperparameters	$b_1 = n - y + b$	$b_1 = b + n\bar{y}$

parameters in their studies and want the data to *speak for themselves*. As Bayes and Laplace presented in the so-called *Bayes–Laplace postulate*, in case of ignorance the prior must be flat, i.e., assign equal probability on all the values in the possible range (if discrete) or equivalently equal density (if continuous). For instance, if the data are distributed as a Binomial, $y \sim \text{Binomial}(\pi, n)$, then a flat prior would be characterized by a density function $p(\pi) \propto 1$, with $\pi \in [0, 1]$. The major drawback of this specification is that it is not invariant for transformation of the parameters. For instance if we are interested in $\exp(\pi)$, its prior will no longer be flat, but it will show high density on small values (see Figure 3.5).

Several rules have been proposed to build a noninformative prior which is not affected by reparameterizations. Probably the most famous is the one proposed by Jeffrey (1946). His idea was to build a prior based on Fisher information, so that it would be a function of the likelihood, thus invariant to transformations:

$$p(\pi) \propto \sqrt{\Im(\pi)},$$

where $\Im = E\left[\left(\frac{\partial}{\partial \pi} \log p(y|\pi)\right)^2\right]$. For the Binomial model this becomes

$$p(\pi) \propto \frac{1}{\sqrt{\pi \times (1 - \pi)}}$$

equivalent to a $\text{Beta}(1/2, 1/2)$ prior. See Figure 3.6 for the density distribution of Jeffrey's prior compared to the flat one.

In 1979, Bernardo presented a different approach based on the maximization of the Kullback–Leibler distance between prior and posterior, defined as

$$D_{KL} = \int_{-\infty}^{\infty} \ln \left(\frac{p(\pi)}{p(\pi|y)} \right) p(\pi) d\pi,$$

called *reference* prior, and showed that for the most important cases the reference prior coincides with Jeffrey's prior.

Despite being appealing as invariant to transformation, most of Jeffrey and Bernardo's priors are improper, meaning that if we integrate them out the integral is not equal to 1. This is not necessarily a big issue, assuming that the posterior is proper, but unfortunately in some cases this prior leads to improper posterior as well. In addition, in a multiparameter model it is more controversial to get results from Jeffrey's prior (Gelman *et al.*, 2004).

Given these drawbacks, instead of building a prior which is noninformative on the entire support of the parameter(s), most of the times it is enough to assure ignorance only on a subset of the parameters where the likelihood is far from 0. This strategy leads the so-called *vague* prior, which is often used to approximate noninformative prior, encompassing the issue of impropriety. So, for instance, a Normal($0, 10^6$) could be used as prior for a mean or regression parameter (see Chapter 5). A similar reasoning can be carried out on the inverse of the variance, specifying for instance a Gamma with parameters $(0.01, 0.01)$. However, this formulation has no limiting proper posterior and puts the majority of the mass far from 0, in fact leading to a quite informative prior (Gelman, 2006; Fong *et al.*, 2009).

Informative prior

On the other extreme, if prior information is available it should be incorporated in the model via an informative prior. Typically such information derives from the results of previous experiments on the same topic, or from elicitation of experts' opinions (Ayyub, 2001; O'Hagan *et al.*, 2006; Albert *et al.*, 2012).

As an example of informative prior, let us assume to be interested in the early investigation of a new drug and to know that previous experiments with similar compounds have suggested response rates between 0.2 and 0.6. It is possible to transform this information in a prior distribution centered around 0.4 (the middle point between 0.2 and 0.6) and with a standard deviation equal to 0.1. Starting with the mean and variance formulas in Eqs. (3.9) and (3.10), and solving these equations for a and b, we obtain

$$a = E(\pi) \left(\frac{E(\pi)(1 - E(\pi))}{\text{Var}(\pi)} - 1 \right)$$

$$b = (1 - E(\pi)) \left(\frac{E(\pi)(1 - E(\pi))}{\text{Var}(\pi)} - 1 \right),$$

and plugging in the data from this example we get the prior distribution Beta(9.2, 13.8), presented in Figure 3.7(a).

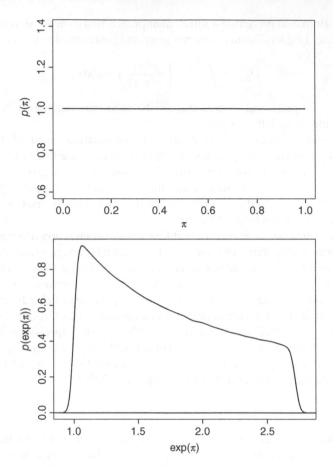

Figure 3.5   Example of how noninformative prior are not invariant to the scale.

Imagine now that we perform a trial on $n = 50$ subjects and we observe $y = 38$ successes (a success is defined as the subject responding to the drug). The likelihood is displayed in Figure 3.7(b). As the prior is conjugated to the likelihood, combining these two leads to a posterior which is Beta(47.2, 31.8), presented in Figure 3.7(c). Recalling Eq. (3.11), it can be appreciated that the parameters of the posterior distribution are influenced by the hyperparameters (a and b) and by the data (n and y); at the same time looking at the three plots in Figure 3.7 it can be seen that, as we specified a strongly informative prior, its influence on the posterior is greater than the data, thus the posterior distribution is closer to the prior than to the likelihood.

If, on the other hand, we now assume that the drug we want to investigate is the first one designed to treat a particular condition, thus does not have similarities with other compounds, we specify a noninformative prior using a Beta distribution with hyperparameters $a = 1$ and $b = 1$ and represented in Figure 3.8(a). The likelihood

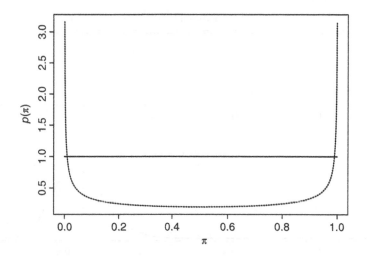

Figure 3.6 Example of Jeffrey's prior (dotted line) and Uniform prior (solid line) for a Binomial likelihood.

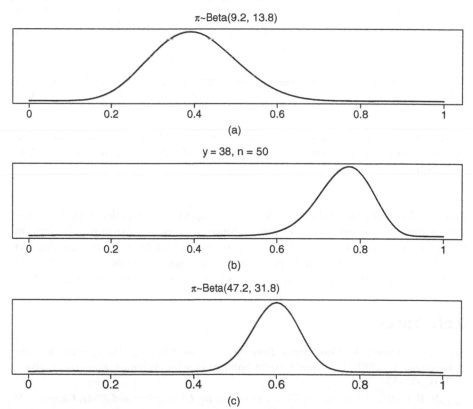

Figure 3.7 Inference on proportions using a strong informative prior. The figure shows the informative Beta prior (a), the likelihood (b) and the Beta posterior (c).

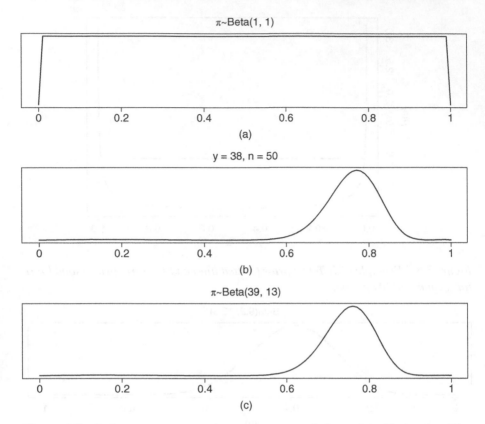

Figure 3.8   Inference on proportions using a noninformative (flat) prior. The figure shows the noninformative Beta prior (a), the likelihood (b) and the Beta posterior (c).

function does not change (Figure 3.8(b)), while applying Bayes theorem, thus combining the prior distribution and the likelihood, leads to a posterior distribution Beta(39, 13), plotted in Figure 3.8(c). It can be seen that this posterior distribution is still a compromise between the prior and the likelihood, but this time it is closer to the likelihood, as the prior is noninformative, so it has less influence than the data.

References

Albert, I., Donnet, S., Guihenneuc-Jouyaux, C., Low-Choy, S., Mengersen, K., and Rousseau, J. (2012). Combining expert opinions in prior elicitation. *Bayesian Analysis*, **7**(3), 503–532.

Ayyub, B. (2001). *Elicitation of Expert Opinions for Uncertainty and Risks*. Chapman & Hall/CRC.

Baio, G. (2012). *Bayesian Methods in Health Economics*. CRC Chapman & Hall.

Bayes, T. (1763). An essay towards solving a problem in the doctrine of chances. *Philosophical Transactions of the Royal Society of London*, **53**, 370–418.

Bernardo, J. (1979). Reference posterior distribution for bayesian inference. *Journal of the Royal Statistical Society, Series B*, **41**(2), 113–147.

Berry, D. and Stangl, D., editors (1999). *Bayesian Biostatistics*. Marcel Dekker.

Bertsch Mcgrayne, S. (2011). *The Theory That Would Not Die: How Bayes' Rule Cracked the Enigma Code, Hunted Down Russian Submarines, and Emerged Triumphant from Two Centuries of Controversy*. Yale University Press.

Casella, G. and Berger, R. (2002). *Statistical Inference*. Duxbury, Thomson Learning.

Casella, G. and George, E. (1992). Explaining the Gibbs Sampler. *The American Statistician.*, **46**(3), 167–174.

Dawid, A. (1979). Conditional independene in statistical theory. *Journal of the Royal Statistical Society, Series B*, **41**, 1–31.

Dawid, P. (1991). *Probability and Proof: some basic concepts, Appendix to "Analysis of Evidence,"* Anderson, TJ Schum, DA and Twining WL. Weidenfeld and Nicolson.

de Finetti, B. (1931). Sul significato soggettivo della probabilità. *Fundamenta Mathematicae*, **17**, 298–329.

de Finetti, B. (1974). *Theory of Probability*, volume 1. John Wiley and Sons.

Edgeworth, F. (1887). On observations related to several quantities. *Hermathena*, **6**(13), 279–285.

Fienberg, S. (2006). When did Bayesian inference become "Bayesian"? *Bayesian Analysis*, **1**, 1–40.

Fong, Y., Rue, H., and Wakefield, J. (2009). Bayesian inference for generalized linear mixed models. *Biostatistics*, **11**, 397–412.

Gelfand, A. and Smith, A. (1990). Sampling-based approaches to calculating marginal densities. *Journal of the American Statistical Association*, **85**, 398–409.

Gelman, A. (2006). Prior distributions for variance parameters in hierarchical models. *Bayesian Analysis*, **1**(3), 515–533.

Gelman, A. and Hill, J. (2007). *Data Analysis Using Regression and Multilevel/Hierarchical Models (Analytical Methods for Social Research)*. Cambridge University Press.

Gelman, A., Carlin, J., Stern, H., and Rubin, D. (2004). *Bayesian Data Analysis*. Chapman & Hall/CRC.

Gómez-Rubio, V., Bivand, R., and Rue, H. (2014). Approximate Bayesian inference for spatial econometrics models. *Spatial Statistics*, **9**, 146–165.

Howie, D. (2002). *Interpreting Probability – Controversies and Developments in the Early Twentieth Century*. Cambridge University Press.

Hume, D. (1748). *An Enquiry Concerning Human Understanding*, volume 37. Harvard Classics.

Jackman, S. (2009). *Bayesian Analysis for the Social Sciences*. John Wiley and Sons.

Jeffrey, H. (1939). *Theory of Probability*. The Clarendon Press, Oxford.

Jeffrey, H. (1946). An invariant form for the prior probability in estimation problems. *Proceedings of the Royal Society of London, Series A*, **186**, 453–461.

Laplace, P. (1774). Oeuvres complètes de laplace: Mémoire sur la probabilité des causes par les évènemens. *Mémoires de l'Academie royale des sciences de Paris*, pages 634–656.

Lesaffre, E. and Lawson, A. (2012). *Bayesian Biostatistics*. John Wiley and Sons.

Lindley, D. (1957). A statistical paradox. *Biometrika*, **44**(1–2), 187–192.

Lindley, D. (1986). Bruno de finetti, 1906-1985 (obituary). *Journal of the Royal Statistical Society, Series A*, **149**, 252.

Lindley, D. (2006). *Understanding Uncertainty*. Wiley–Blackwell.

McCarthy, M. (2007). *Bayesian Methods for Ecology*. John Wiley and Sons.

O'Hagan, A., Buck, C., Daneshkhah, A., Eiser, J., Garthwaite, P., Jenkinson, D., Oakley, J., and Rakow, T. (2006). *Uncertain Judgements: Eliciting Expert Probabilities*. John Wiley and Sons.

Pearson, K. (1920). The fundamental problem of practical statistics. *Biometrika*, **13**(1), 1–16.

Rachev, S., Hsu, J., Bagasheva, B., and Fabozzi, F. (2008). *Bayesian Methods in Finance*. John Wiley and Sons.

Ramsey, F. (1931). *Studies in Subjective Probability*. Robert Krieger.

Rue, H., Martino, S., and Chopin, N. (2009). Approximate Bayesian inference for latent Gaussian models using integrated nested Laplace approximations (with discussion). *Journal of the Royal Statistical Society, Series B*, **71**(2), 319–392.

Savage, J. (1954). *The Foundations of Statistics*. New York: John Wiley and Sons.

Simon, C. (1988). Evolution of 13- and 17-year periodical cicadas. *Bulletin of the Entomological Society of America*, **34**, 163–176.

Spiegelhalter, D., Thomas, A., Best, N., and Gilks, W. (1995). *BUGS: Bayesian Inference Using Gibbs Sampling, Version 0.5, (version ii)*. MRC Biostatistics Unit.

Spiegelhalter, D., Thomas, A., and Best, N. (1999). *WinBUGS: version 1.2 User Manual*. MRC Biostatistics Unit.

Stigler, S. (1986). *The History of Statistics: The Measurement of Uncertainty Before 1900*. Harvard University Press.

4

Bayesian computing

In Chapter 3, we introduced the foundations for Bayesian inference and provided
some examples for conjugate models, i.e., where the functional form of the posterior distribution is known. Nevertheless, conjugacy is a very stringent property,
which does not hold in most practical cases. When conjugacy is not appropriate, it
is not possible to manipulate the posterior distribution analytically and we need to
resort to simulation methods in order to explore it. Statistical simulations generate
random values from a given density function by a computer and can become a
computationally intensive procedure when the involved distributions are complex
or the amount of data is large. In this chapter, we deal with the computational
aspects of Bayesian inference, we start with simulation-based methods for generating values from posterior distributions, such as Monte Carlo (MC) and Markov
chain Monte Carlo (MCMC). Then, we focus on the integrated nested Laplace
approximations (INLA) approach. This was recently proposed by Rue *et al.* (2009)
and has become a valid and computational effective alternative to MCMC. For
each method, we alternate theory and examples providing also the R code.

4.1 Monte Carlo integration

Suppose that we are interested in calculating the following integral:

$$H = \int h(x)f(x)\mathrm{d}x, \tag{4.1}$$

where $h(\cdot)$ is a function of the random variable X with density function $f(\cdot)$. If it is
not possible to solve the integral analytically through standard calculus computations, we resort to simulations for approximating H. Note that also numerical integration methods could be used for approximating the integral (such as, for example,
Simpson's and the trapezium rules), but they are not discussed in details in this book

Spatial and Spatio-temporal Bayesian Models with R-INLA, First Edition.
Marta Blangiardo and Michela Cameletti.
© 2015 John Wiley & Sons, Ltd. Published 2015 by John Wiley & Sons, Ltd.

(see, e.g., Press *et al.*, 2007 and Lange, 2010), except for the Laplace approximation which is the core of the INLA approach and is introduced in Section 4.7.

In this section, we focus on the simulation-based MC method that approximates Eq. (4.1) using the empirical average given by

$$\hat{H} = \frac{\sum_{i=1}^{m} h(x^{(i)})}{m}, \tag{4.2}$$

where $\{x^{(1)}, \ldots, x^{(m)}\}$ is a random sample of values drawn independently from the density $f(\cdot)$. Adopting a more formal point of view, this means that the sample $\{x^{(1)}, \ldots, x^{(m)}\}$ is generated from m independent and identically distributed (*iid*) random variables $X^{(1)}, \ldots, X^{(m)}$ all distributed like X, i.e., with the density function $f(\cdot)$. By the strong law of large numbers[1] (Casella and Berger, 2002), we know that the empirical average $\mathcal{H} = \frac{\sum_{i=1}^{m} h(X^{(i)})}{m}$ converges almost surely (*as*) to the true value H when $m \to +\infty$:

$$\mathcal{H} \xrightarrow{as} H.$$

The accuracy of the MC approximation increases when the size m of the MC sample gets bigger and it can be evaluated by means of the MC standard error (*se*) of $\hat{H}$ estimated by

$$se(\hat{H}) = \sqrt{\frac{\sum_{i=1}^{m} (h(x^{(i)}) - \hat{H})^2}{m^2}}. \tag{4.3}$$

Note that the accuracy of the approximation is inversely proportional to the square root of the sample size m. Hence, for example, if we want to halve the standard error we need to quadruple m.

Moreover, the central limit theorem (Casella and Berger, 2002) states that, as long as the variance of X is finite, for $m \to +\infty$, $\mathcal{H}$ converges in distribution (*d*) to a Gaussian random variable:

$$\mathcal{H} \xrightarrow{d} \text{Normal}(H, se(\hat{H})^2).$$

Using this result, it is possible to derive an asymptotic 95% confidence interval for H given by

$$\hat{H} \pm 1.96 \times se(\hat{H}). \tag{4.4}$$

---

[1] Let $X_1, \ldots, X_n$ be iid random variables with $E(X_i) = \mu$ and $\text{Var}(X_i) = \sigma^2 < \infty$ for each $i = 1, \ldots, n$. Then $\frac{\sum_{i=1}^{n} X_i}{n}$ converges to μ almost surely for $n \to +\infty$, which means that

$$P\left(\lim_{n \to +\infty} \left|\frac{\sum_{i=1}^{n} X_i}{n} - \mu\right| < \epsilon\right) = 1$$

for every $\epsilon > 0$.

Note that this interval should be interpreted in a frequentist perspective, as described in Section 3.5, so if the simulation is repeated 100 times, we expect that 95 times H will be included in the intervals.

4.2   Monte Carlo method for Bayesian inference

Recall from Section 3.4.1 that Bayesian inference is centered around the posterior distribution of a generic (univariate) parameter θ

$$p(\theta|y) \propto p(y|\theta) \times p(\theta),$$

where y is the vector of observations. In Section 3.5, we presented how to obtain the posterior mean for θ; it is also possible to compute the posterior mean of a function $h(\cdot)$ of θ, defined as

$$E(h(\theta)|y) = \int_{\theta \in \Theta} h(\theta)p(\theta|y)d\theta. \qquad (4.5)$$

This integral has the same form of Eq. (4.1) with $f(x)$ being the posterior distribution $p(\theta|y)$. Thus, assuming that we know $p(\theta|y)$, we can resort to MC for approximating the posterior mean of $h(\theta)$. This consists of simulating a sample of m independent values of θ denoted by $\{\theta^{(1)}, \ldots, \theta^{(m)}\}$ – drawn directly from the posterior distribution $p(\theta|y)$ – and of approximating $E(h(\theta)|y)$ with the empirical average as in Eq. (4.2):

$$\frac{\sum_{i=1}^{m} h(\theta^{(i)})}{m}.$$

More generally, as the empirical distribution of the MC sample approximates the posterior distribution $p(\theta|y)$, the set $\{\theta^{(1)}, \ldots, \theta^{(m)}\}$ can be used to compute approximations to the relevant posterior summaries. For example, the posterior probability that θ takes value in a given set $\mathcal{A}$

$$p(\theta \in \mathcal{A}|y) = \int_{\theta \in \mathcal{A}} p(\theta|y)d\theta$$

is approximated by the sample proportion given by the number (#) of simulated values $\theta^{(i)}$ belonging to $\mathcal{A}$ over the sample size m:

$$\frac{\#(\theta^{(i)} \in \mathcal{A}, i = 1, \ldots, m)}{m}.$$

Another posterior summary of interest might be the qth quantile θ_q defined as

$$\int_{-\infty}^{\theta_q} p(\theta|y)d\theta = q,$$

which can be approximated by the qth empirical quantile of the MC sample $\{\theta^{(1)}, \ldots, \theta^{(m)}\}$.

To implement MC methods, we just need to be able to simulate independent values from the given posterior distribution, that is a straightforward task if $p(\theta|y)$ has a known distribution. Note that random values generated by computer are actually pseudorandom numbers in the sense that they are generated using a deterministic algorithm and can be reproduced fixing some initial conditions. Having said that, in this book we will use R functions to simulate random numbers assuming that the R algorithms produce values having the same relevant statistical properties of a sequence of random numbers. For a deeper discussion about number generators and simulations, refer to Ripley (1987) and Gentle (2009, Chapter 7).

The following section is devoted to the description of the R commands used to draw random values from a chosen random variable. We also present the functions for computing quantiles and for evaluating probabilities or density functions.

4.3   Probability distributions and random number generation in R

R provides some functions for working with discrete and continuous random variables (see ?Distributions for a list of the available probability distributions). In particular, four R functions are available for each distribution as summarized in Table 4.1.

For example, if we consider X as a Poisson random variable with parameter $\lambda = 2$ and we want to evaluate the probability $p(X = 4)$ we will type

```
> dpois(x=4, lambda=2)
[1] 0.09022352
```

Additionally, the probability $p(X \leq q)$ can be obtained using the ppois function which evaluates the cumulative probability that a Poisson random variable is smaller than or equal to q. So if $q = 4$ the probability $p(X \leq 4)$ is given by

```
> ppois(q=4, lambda=2)
[1] 0.947347
```

Table 4.1   R functions for discrete and continuous random variables. In each function, the string *name* refers to the name of the considered random variable as given in ?Distributions.

Function	Description
d*name*(parameters)	Probability or density function
p*name*(parameters)	Cumulative probability or density function
q*name*(parameters)	Quantile function
r*name*(parameters)	Random number generation

It follows that the tail probability $p(X > 4)$ can be obtained typing

```
> 1-ppois(q=4, lambda=2)
[1] 0.05265302
```

If we are interested in calculating quantiles (e.g., the median, see Section 3.5), we will use the function qpois specifying with p the required probability:

```
> qpois(p=0.5, lambda=2) #Median
[1] 2
```

Suppose now that we want to plot the density function of a continuous distribution. The following code employs the R function curve to plot the density function of the Gamma distribution[2] (see Eq. (3.14)) with the shape parameter $a = 2$ and the scale parameter $b = 2$ for values between 0 and 6. The curve is displayed in Figure 4.1 (top).

```
> a <- 2
> b <- 2
> curve(dgamma(x, shape=a, rate=b), from=0, to=6, ylab="Density")
```

Moreover, the same plot shows the median and the tail probability $p(X > 2.5)$ which are calculated as follows:

```
> qgamma(p=0.5, shape=a, rate=b) #median
[1] 0.8391735
> 1 - pgamma(q=2, shape=a, rate=b) #tail probability
[1] 0.09157819
```

If we need to simulate $m = 1000$ values from a Normal distribution with mean $\mu = 2$ and variance $\sigma^2 = 1$, we make use of the rnorm function specifying the sample size and the parameter values (we save the generated numbers in a vector named Normal.sim):

```
> mu <- 2
> variance <- 1
> m <- 1000
> set.seed(123) #for reproducibility
> Normal.sim <- rnorm(n=m, mean=mu, sd=sqrt(variance))
```

The empirical distribution of the m simulated values can be graphically represented through the histogram displayed in Figure 4.1 (bottom). The true density function of a Normal(2, 1) given as output of the dnorm function for values ranging from -2 to 6, is displayed in the same plot as a solid line.

```
> hist(Normal.sim, freq = F, xlim = c(-2, 6), main = "", xlab = "x")
> curve(dnorm(x, mean = 2, sd = 1), from = -2, to = 6, lwd = 2,
         add = T)
```

---

[2] Due to the different parameterization of the Gamma distribution in R – see ?dgamma – we specify the scale through the rate input argument.

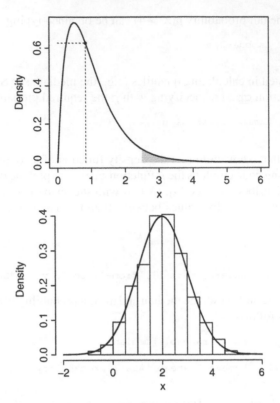

Figure 4.1   Density function of the Gamma($a = 2, b = 2$) distribution (top). The black dot denotes the median of the distribution while the gray area corresponds to the tail area $p(X > 2.5)$. Histogram of the m simulated values drawn from the Normal($\mu = 2, \sigma^2 = 1$) distribution (bottom); the solid black line refers to the true density function.

4.4   Examples of Monte Carlo simulation

In this section, we present three examples with simulated data in order to illustrate how the MC method can be employed for Bayesian inference. In the first example, we consider an Exponential likelihood[3] combined with a Gamma prior – which together give rise to a conjugate Gamma posterior distribution – and compare the MC approximations with the exact values obtained analytically. In the second example, we are interested in the approximation to the log-odds function of

---

[3] The Exponential distribution is a Gamma distribution with the shape parameter $a = 1$ and the scale parameter $b = \lambda$. Its probability density function is given by $p(y|\lambda) = \lambda \exp(-\lambda y)$ for $\lambda, y > 0$.

the probability of a Binomial distribution. Finally, the last example regards joint inference for the mean and the variance in a Gaussian setting.

Exponential–Gamma conjugate model

As illustrated in Table 3.2, when the observations $y = (y_1, \ldots, y_n)$ come from an Exponential distribution with parameter λ and the prior distribution for λ is Gamma(a, b), the posterior distribution is conjugate and is a Gamma with parameters $a_1 = a + n$ and $b_1 = b + n\bar{y}$. Thus, following Eq. (3.15) the *exact* posterior mean $E(\lambda|y)$ is computed as $a_1/b_1 = (a + n)/(b + n\bar{y})$.

We show here how to approximate the posterior mean of λ using a MC sample, given m independent values drawn directly from the Gamma(a_1, b_1) posterior distribution. Moreover, the accuracy of the MC approximation is evaluated with respect to the exact posterior mean. First of all, we simulate our data vector y of size $n = 50$ from an Exponential distribution with parameter $\lambda = 2$ (through the `rexp` function). We consider a Gamma distribution with the shape parameter $a = 8$ and the scale parameter $b = 4$ as the prior for λ.

```
> set.seed(6789)
> n <- 50
> lambda <- 2
> y <- rexp(n=n, rate=lambda)
> a <- 8
> b <- 4
> a1 <- a + n
> b1 <- b + n*mean(y)
> a1
[1] 58
> b1
[1] 28.58578
> a1/b1
[1] 2.028981
```

As reported above, this setting leads to an exact posterior mean for λ equal to 2.029.

To generate the independent values $\{\lambda^{(1)}, \ldots, \lambda^{(m)}\}$ of the MC sample from the known posterior distribution, we run the `rgamma` function with sample size m equal to 10, 100 and 1000. We save the random values in three vectors:

```
> sim10 <- rgamma(n=10, shape=a1, rate=b1)
> sim100 <- rgamma(n=100, shape=a1, rate=b1)
> sim1000 <- rgamma(n=1000, shape=a1, rate=b1)
```

The empirical distributions of the simulated values are represented by the histograms in Figure 4.2 together with the exact posterior Gamma density function with the shape parameter $a_1 = 58$ and the scale parameter $b_1 = 28.586$. The code used for obtaining the first plot in Figure 4.2, which refers to $m = 10$, is the following:

```
> hist(sim10, freq=F, main="", xlim=c(0,4), ylim=c(0,3),
        xlab=expression(lambda))
> curve(dgamma(x, shape=a1, rate=b1), from=0, to=4, add=T)
```

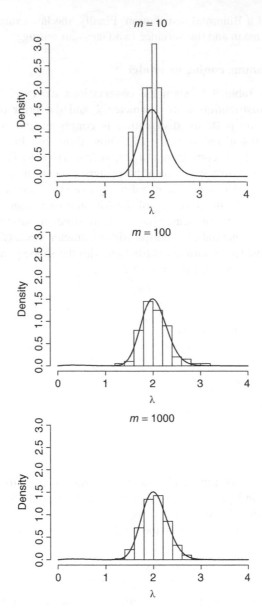

Figure 4.2   Histograms of the empirical distribution of the MC samples of λ for different sample size m. The solid line refers to the exact posterior distribution $\lambda | y \sim Gamma(a_1 = 58, b_1 = 28.586)$.

When the MC sample size m increases the empirical distribution is closer to the exact posterior distribution $\lambda|y \sim \text{Gamma}(a_1 = 58, b_1 = 28.586)$.

We now consider the MC sample with size $m = 1000$ in order to compute the approximated posterior mean and median of λ together with the approximated tail posterior probability $p(\lambda > 2.5|y)$, and to compare them with the corresponding exact values:

```
> mean(sim1000) #approx. mean
[1] 2.032811
> a1/b1 #exact mean
[1] 2.028981
> quantile(sim1000, p=0.5) #approx. median
     50%
2.022984
> qgamma(p=0.5, shape=a1, rate=b1) #exact median
[1] 2.017332
> mean(sim1000>2.5) #approx. tail prob.
[1] 0.043
> 1-pgamma(q=2.5, shape=a1, rate=b1) #exact tail prob.
[1] 0.04550062
```

As expected, the MC approximations to the posterior summaries for λ (mean, median, and tail probability) are close to the corresponding exact values. The MC standard error (see Eq. (4.3)) can be obtained with the following command:

```
> sqrt(sum((sim1000-mean(sim1000))^2)/(1000^2)) #standard error
[1] 0.008386994
```

To monitor the convergence of the MC approximation to the posterior mean $E(\lambda|y)$, in Figure 4.3 we depict the running posterior mean of λ (for different values of m from 1 to 1000) together with the 95% asymptotic (frequentist) confidence interval given in Eq. (4.1). This plot can help assess the sample size m which provides an accurate approximation to the posterior mean.

Monte Carlo approximation to the log-odds

In this example, we consider the case discussed in Section 3.6.1 focusing on a Binomial likelihood

$$y|\pi \sim \text{Binomial}(\pi, n)$$

combined with a Beta(a, b) distribution as prior for the probability of success π. We know that in this case the posterior distribution of π (see Table 3.2) is given by

$$\pi|y \sim \text{Beta}(a_1 = y + a, b_1 = n - y + b).$$

Here we are interested in the log-odds function of π defined as $\log\left(\frac{\pi}{1-\pi}\right)$ (Van Belle et al., 2004). The log-odds is commonly used in epidemiological and biostatistical applications to measure the ratio of the probability of experiencing and nonexperiencing health outcome, typically when exposed (or not) to some

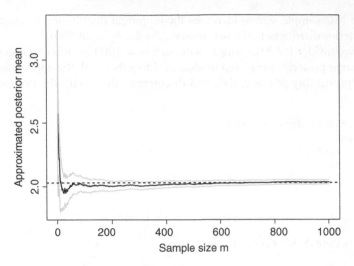

Figure 4.3   Convergence of the MC approximation to the posterior mean. The black solid line is the running approximated mean of λ, the dashed black line is the exact posterior mean $a_1/b_1 = 2.029$ and the gray lines define the 95% confidence interval based on the Normal asymptotic approximation as in Eq. (4.1).

particular risk factors (e.g., asthma attack in the case of air pollution exposure, side effects in the case of drug treatment, etc.). In this framework, y is the number of exposed individuals who experience the health outcome with probability π. The posterior mean of the log-odds is

$$\int_0^1 \log\left(\frac{\pi}{1-\pi}\right) p(\pi|y)\mathrm{d}\pi. \tag{4.6}$$

This integral cannot be computed analytically and thus we resort to MC approximation as in Eq. (4.5), with $h(\theta) = \log\left(\frac{\pi}{1-\pi}\right)$. Practically, we simulate m independent values $\{\pi^{(1)}, \dots, \pi^{(m)}\}$ from the Beta(a_1, b_1) posterior distribution. Then, we apply the log-odds transformation to each of these obtaining the set of values $\left\{\log\left(\frac{\pi^{(1)}}{1-\pi^{(1)}}\right), \dots, \log\left(\frac{\pi^{(m)}}{1-\pi^{(m)}}\right)\right\}$. Finally, we compute the sample mean

$$\frac{\sum_{i=1}^m \log\left(\frac{\pi^{(i)}}{1-\pi^{(i)}}\right)}{m},$$

which is the MC approximation to $\log\left(\frac{\pi}{1-\pi}\right)$.

To implement the example, we simulate data from a Binomial distribution with size $n = 1000$ and probability $\pi = 0.8$ using the function rbinom. The parameters for the Beta prior distribution are $a = b = 1$.

```
> set.seed(65423)
> pi <- 0.8
> n <- 1000
> y <- rbinom(n=1, size=n, p=pi)
> y
[1] 778
> a <- 1
> b <- 1
> a1 <- a + y
> b1 <- b + n - y
> a1
[1] 779
> b1
[1] 223
```

With this setting, the exact posterior distribution of π is Beta($a_1 = 779, b_1 = 223$). To approximate the log-odds, we simulate $m = 50\,000$ values from this Beta posterior distribution using the rbeta function. The empirical distribution of the MC sample is plotted in Figure 4.4 (top) together with the exact posterior distribution of π.

```
> sim <- rbeta(n=50000, shape1=a1, shape2=b1)
> hist(sim, freq=F, main="", xlab=expression(pi))
> curve(dbeta(x, shape1=a1, shape2=b1), from=0, to=1, add=T, n=1000)
```

The MC approximation to the posterior distribution of the log-odds is obtained simply by typing

```
> log.odds <- log(sim/(1-sim))
```

and the corresponding histogram is plotted in Figure 4.4 (bottom). The approximated posterior mean of the log-odds is

```
> mean(log.odds)
[1] 1.252131
```

To assess the quality of this approximation, we use the R function integrate, which computes integrals by means of numerical integration routines (see ?integrate for details). To run integrate, we need to write the mathematical function we want to integrate as an R function (see Section 2.5). The following R function, named logodds_integral

```
> logodds_integral <- function(pi,a,b){
    log(pi/(1-pi)) * pi^(a-1) * (1-pi)^(b-1)/beta(a,b)
  }
```

is the equivalent of the function in Eq. (4.6), with $p(\pi|y)$ replaced by the corresponding Beta distribution defined in Eq. (3.8), and has to be integrated in [0, 1]. Then, we compute the integral numerically

```
> integrate(logodds_integral, lower=0, upper=1, a=a1, b=b1)
1.252441 with absolute error < 1.1e-07
```

obtaining the value 1.252441 which is very close to the corresponding MC approximation to the log-odds posterior mean.

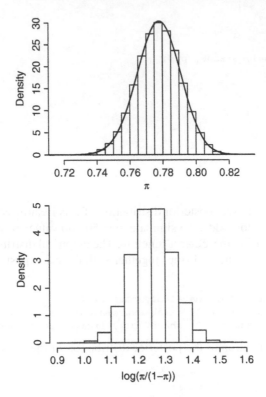

Figure 4.4   Histogram of the empirical distribution of the MC sample of π with $m = 50\,000$ (top). The solid line refers to exact posterior distribution which is a Beta density function with parameters $a_1 = 779$ and $b_1 = 223$. Histogram of the empirical distribution of the MC sample of $\log\left(\frac{\theta}{1-\theta}\right)$ with $m = 50\,000$ (bottom).

Monte Carlo approximation to a joint distribution using a noninformative prior

Up to now we have considered the case of likelihood functions depending only on a generic parameter θ (e.g., the probability π for the Binonial distribution or the mean μ for the Gaussian case with known variance). We now deal with a multidimensional parameter set θ for the case of n iid observations from a Normal(μ, σ^2) distribution with unknown mean and variance (in this case $\theta = \{\mu, \sigma^2\}$). In particular, we illustrate how to use the MC principle to simulate values from the joint posterior distribution $\mu, \sigma^2 | y$, defined as the product of a conditional and a marginal distribution.

We first specify the likelihood function as

$$p(y|\mu, \sigma^2) = \left(\frac{1}{\sqrt{2\pi\sigma^2}}\right)^n \exp\left(-\frac{1}{2\sigma^2}\sum_{i=1}^{n}(y_i - \mu)^2\right)$$

and then we choose a noninformative (and improper) prior for μ and σ^2 given by $p(\mu, \sigma^2) \propto \frac{1}{\sigma^2}$, as proposed in Gelman *et al.* (2003, Chapter 3). Hence, we obtain the following joint posterior distribution:

$$p(\mu, \sigma^2 | y) = p(y | \mu, \sigma^2) p(\mu, \sigma^2) \tag{4.7}$$

$$\propto (\sigma)^{-n-2} \exp\left(-\frac{1}{2\sigma^2} \left(\sum_{i=1}^{n} (y_i - \bar{y})^2 + n(\bar{y} - \mu)^2\right)\right)$$

$$\propto (\sigma)^{-n-2} \exp\left(-\frac{1}{2\sigma^2} \left((n-1)s^2 + n(\bar{y} - \mu)^2\right)\right),$$

where $\bar{y} = \sum_{i=1}^{n} y_i / n$ and $s^2 = \sum_{i=1}^{n} (y_i - \bar{y})^2 / (n-1)$ are the sample mean and variance, respectively.

Using the basic probability rules given in Section 3.2.3, it is possible to express the joint posterior distribution as the product of a conditional and a marginal distribution:

$$p(\mu, \sigma^2 | y) = p(\mu | \sigma^2, y) \times p(\sigma^2 | y).$$

The conditional posterior distribution of μ (given σ^2 and y) corresponds to the Normal–Normal conjugate case included in Table 3.2 with a flat prior on μ (i.e., $\sigma_0^2 \to +\infty$). Thus, the conditional distribution is given by

$$\mu | \sigma^2, y \sim \text{Normal}\left(\bar{y}, \frac{\sigma^2}{n}\right).$$

The marginal posterior distribution of σ^2 is obtained by integrating out μ from the joint posterior density as follows:

$$p(\sigma^2 | y) = \int_{-\infty}^{+\infty} p(\mu, \sigma^2 | y) d\mu$$

$$\propto \int_{-\infty}^{+\infty} (\sigma)^{-n-2} \exp\left(-\frac{1}{2\sigma^2} \left((n-1)s^2 + n(\bar{y} - \mu)^2\right)\right) d\mu$$

$$\propto (\sigma)^{-n-2} \exp\left(-\frac{(n-1)s^2}{2\sigma^2}\right)$$

$$\times \underbrace{\int_{-\infty}^{+\infty} \exp\left(-\frac{n}{2\sigma^2}(\bar{y} - \mu)^2\right) d\mu}$$

Divide and multiply by $\sqrt{2\pi\sigma^2/n}$ to get the density of $N(\mu, \sigma^2/n)$

$$= (\sigma)^{-n-2} \exp\left(-\frac{(n-1)s^2}{2\sigma^2}\right) \sqrt{2\pi \frac{\sigma^2}{n}}$$

$$\propto (\sigma^2)^{-\frac{n+1}{2}} \exp\left(-\frac{(n-1)s^2}{2\sigma^2}\right).$$

This is the functional form of a scaled inverse Chi-square distribution[4] with $(n-1)$ degrees of freedom and scale parameter s, denoted as $\text{invChi}(n-1, s^2)$.

In this framework, the MC approximation to the joint posterior distribution $p(\mu, \sigma^2 | y)$ is performed iteratively, by alternating a simulation from the marginal posterior distribution $p(\sigma^2 | y)$ with a simulation from the conditional posterior distribution $p(\mu | \sigma^2, y)$ (this is also known as *method of composition*, Tanner, 1993). In particular, the ith iteration of the MC algorithm (for $i = 1, \dots, m$) is structured as follows:

1. sample the value $\sigma^{2(i)}$ from the marginal posterior distribution $\sigma^2 | y \sim \text{invChi}(n-1, s^2)$;

2. sample the value $\mu^{(i)}$ from the conditional posterior distribution $\mu | \sigma^2, y \sim \text{Normal}\left(\bar{y}, \frac{\sigma^{2(i)}}{n}\right)$.

   This creates the set $\left\{\left(\mu^{(1)}, \sigma^{2(1)}\right), \dots, \left(\mu^{(i)}, \sigma^{2(i)}\right), \dots, \left(\mu^{(m)}, \sigma^{2(m)}\right)\right\}$ which is a MC sample from the joint posterior distribution $\mu, \sigma^2 | y$. Additionally, the sequence $\{\mu^{(1)}, \dots, \mu^{(i)}, \dots, \mu^{(m)}\}$ constitutes a MC sample from the marginal posterior distribution $\mu | y$.

As an example, consider a vector of data y of size $n = 100$ simulated from a Normal distribution with mean $\mu = 10$ and variance $\sigma^2 = 1.5$.

```
> set.seed(44566)
> mu <- 10
> sigma2 <- 1.5
> n <- 100
> y <- rnorm(n=n, mean=mu, sd=sqrt(sigma2))
```

To approximate the joint posterior distribution $\mu, \sigma^2 | y$, we generate a MC sample of size $m = 1000$ following the steps described previously. In particular, we collect the values drawn from the marginal scaled inverse Chi-square distribution, simulated using the `rchisq` function[4], in a R vector named `sigma2.sim`. These values

---

[4] A Chi-square distribution with v degrees of freedom, denoted by $\chi^2(v)$, is a particolar case of the Gamma distribution with shape $a = v/2$ and scale $b = 1/2$. If $y \sim \chi^2(v)$ its density function is given by

$$p(y|v) = \frac{2^{-v/2}}{\Gamma(v/2)} \exp(-y/2) y^{v/2-1}$$

for $y > 0$ and $v > 0$. As described in Gelman *et al.* (2003), the transformed variable $\omega = vs^2/y$ is distributed as a scaled inverse Chi-square distribution with v degrees of freedom and scale parameter s. This distribution is denoted by $\text{invChi}(v, s^2)$ as is characterized by the following density function:

$$p(\omega|v) = \frac{(v/2)^{v/2}}{\Gamma(v/2)} s^v \omega^{-(v/2+1)} \exp(-vs^2/(2\omega))$$

with $\omega > 0$, $v > 0$ and $s > 0$.

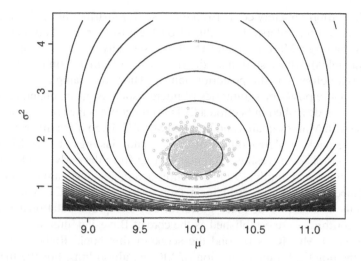

Figure 4.5   Contour plot of the bivariate joint posterior distribution $\mu, \sigma^2 | y$ and MC sample given by the pairs $(\mu^{(i)}, \sigma^{2(i)})$ for $i = 1, \ldots, m = 1000$ (gray dots).

represent the variances $\{\sigma^{2(1)}, \ldots, \sigma^{2(m)}\}$ required for generating random numbers from the Normal conditional distribution, saved in the mu.sim vector.

```
> m <- 1000
> sigma2.sim <- (n-1)*var(y)/rchisq(n=m,df=n-1)
> mu.sim <- rnorm(n=m, mean=mean(y), sd=sqrt(sigma2.sim/n))
```

The pairs $(\mu^{(i)}, \sigma^{2(i)})$ for $i = 1, \ldots, 1000$ are displayed as gray points in Figure 4.5. The black contour lines refer to the bivariate joint posterior density $\mu, \sigma^2 | y$ obtained by evaluating Eq. (4.7) for each pairs of values on the regular grid given by $\mu \in [8.8, 11.2] \times \sigma^2 \in [0.5, 4.5]$. The posterior means for μ and σ^2 are computed typing

```
> mean(mu.sim)
[1] 9.984053
> mean(sigma2.sim)
[1] 1.679223
```

which are very close to the true values $\mu = 10$ and $\sigma^2 = 1.5$.

4.5   Markov chain Monte Carlo methods

For all but trivial examples, it will be difficult to draw an iid MC sample directly from the posterior distribution. This happens, for example, when the dimension of the parameter vector θ is high or the posterior distribution is a nonstandard density function difficult to sample from. More importantly, MC methods presuppose that the posterior distribution is in a known form, which is not always the case. In these situations, an alternative solution consists in generating a sample of *correlated* values which approximately come from the posterior distribution. This means that, instead of simulating independent values from the posterior distribution, we draw a sample by running a Markov chain (which is essentially a collection of dependent random variables), whose stationary distribution – a formal definition for stationarity is given below – is the posterior density. Then, this sample can be used as usual to compute posterior summaries of interest such as mean, quantiles, and tail probabilities, as described in Section 4.2. This procedure is the combination of MC integration with Markov chains and is called MCMC. Even if the first MCMC publications date back to Metropolis *et al.* (1953) and Hastings (1970), MCMC has emerged as a tool for Bayesian inference starting from the early 1990s, when the paper by Gelfand and Smith (1990) was published in a mainstream statistical journal (see Robert and Casella, 2011 for a short history of MCMC). After that, also thanks to the availability of more powerful and cheap computational resources, MCMC algorithms were established as the core of Bayesian inference.

The theory of MCMC is beyond the scope of this book. Rather, we want to focus on the practical implementation of MCMC algorithms. For the theoretical basics of MCMC refer to Robert and Casella (2004, Chapter 6) or Brooks *et al.* (2011), a handbook including also many applications and case studies involving MCMC. Here, we just recall that a collection of dependent random variables $\{X^{(0)}, X^{(1)}, \ldots, X^{(t)}, \ldots\}$, each defined on the state-space χ, is a Markov chain if the conditional distribution of $X^{(t)}$ given $X^{(0)}, X^{(1)}, \ldots, X^{(t-1)}$ depends on the previous value $X^{(t-1)}$ only and is conditionally independent of all the previous components. Thanks to this property, we can write

$$p(X^{(t)}|X^{(0)}, X^{(1)}, \ldots, X^{(t-1)}) = p(X^{(t)}|X^{(t-1)}),$$

where $p(X^{(t)}|X^{(t-1)})$ is usually denoted as transition probability. The general idea behind MCMC is that in order to simulate realizations from a given target distribution π, it is sufficient to draw values from a Markov chain whose *stationary* (or *equilibrium* or *invariant*) distribution is exactly π. Given that π is the stationary distribution, it holds that if $X^{(t)} \sim \pi$ then $X^{(t+1)} \sim \pi$; in other words, this means that, once the chain has reached its stationary distribution π, the marginal distribution of $X^{(t)}$ does not change with t.

The existence of a unique stationary distribution requires that the Markov chain satisfies the following properties: *irreducibility* (regardless of the initial value $X^{(0)}$ the chain has a positive probability of reaching any region of the state-space χ), *recurrency* (the expected number of return of the chain to a set $A \subset \chi$ is infinite or, in a stricter sense, the limit of the probability of visiting A infinitely often is 1) and *aperiodicity* (the chain follows no cycles in exploring the state-space). Under these regularity conditions, the stationary distribution π is also a limiting distribution in the sense that $X^{(t)}$ converges in distribution to π:

$$X^{(t)} \xrightarrow{d} \pi$$

for $t \to +\infty$, no matter what the starting value is. Thus, the probability $\pi(A) = \int_A \pi(x)dx$ can be approximated by $p(X^{(t)} \in A)$ for all $A \subset \chi$. A consequence of this convergence property is the *ergodicity theorem*, which states that the empirical average converges almost surely to the expected value $E(h(X)) = \int_\chi h(x)\pi(x)dx$ for $m \to +\infty$:

$$\frac{1}{m} \sum_{t=1}^{m} h(X^{(t)}) \xrightarrow{as} E(h(X)).$$

Note that this theorem is the equivalent to the law of large numbers used for iid MC samples in Section 4.1.

In the Bayesian inferential framework, our target distribution π is usually the posterior density $p(\theta|y)$. Thus, a sequence of values $\{\theta^{(1)}, \theta^{(2)}, \ldots\}$ generated from a Markov chain that has reached its invariant distribution (i.e., has converged) can be considered as an approximation to the posterior distribution $p(\theta|y)$ and can be used to compute all the posterior summaries of interest.

The following sections provide a brief description and an example of the standard MCMC algorithms, the Gibbs sampler, and the Metropolis–Hastings (MH) algorithm, which define Markov chains whose stationary distribution is by construction the chosen posterior distribution.

4.5.1   Gibbs sampler

The Gibbs sampler was first introduced by Geman and Geman (1984) in the context of image processing models and then proposed by Gelfand and Smith (1990) as a sampling-based approach for calculating marginal densities within a Bayesian inference framework. A clear and simple explanation of the algorithm is given by Casella and George (1992).

We are interested in the posterior distribution $p(\theta|y)$ of a generic P-dimensional parameter set $\theta = \{\theta_1, \ldots, \theta_P\}$. To implement the Gibbs sampler, we need for each parameter θ_i the *full conditional* distribution, i.e., the posterior conditional distribution of θ_i given all the other parameters, denoted by $p(\theta_i|\theta_{j\neq i}, y)$ for $i, j = 1, \ldots, P$. To simulate values from the joint posterior $p(\theta|y)$, the Gibbs sampler draws values iteratively from all the conditional distributions. In practice, it means that we start with a set of initial values for all the parameters $\theta^{(0)} = \{\theta_1^{(0)}, \ldots, \theta_P^{(0)}\}$. Then, at the tth iteration, given the parameter vector $\theta^{(t-1)}$ obtained at the previous step, we proceed as follows:

1. sample $\theta_1^{(t)}$ from the full conditional distribution $p(\theta_1|\theta_2^{(t-1)}, \ldots, \theta_P^{(t-1)}, y)$;

2. sample $\theta_2^{(t)}$ from the full conditional distribution $p(\theta_2|\theta_1^{(t)}, \ldots, \theta_P^{(t-1)}, y)$, with $\theta_1^{(t-1)}$ replaced by $\theta_1^{(t)}$;

3. …;

4. sample $\theta_P^{(t)}$ from the full conditional distribution $p(\theta_P|\theta_1^{(t)}, \ldots, \theta_{P-1}^{(t)}, y)$, with $\theta_1^{(t-1)}, \ldots, \theta_{P-1}^{(t-1)}$ replaced by $\theta_1^{(t)}, \ldots, \theta_{P-1}^{(t)}$;

5. let $\theta^{(t+1)} = \{\theta_1^{(t+1)}, \ldots, \theta_P^{(t+1)}\}$.

Under regularity conditions, it is possible to prove that the tth realization $\theta^{(t)} = \{\theta_1^{(t)}, \ldots, \theta_P^{(t)}\}$ converges in distribution to the target distribution $\pi = p(\theta|y)$ (Robert and Casella, 2004, Chapter 10). This happens after a sufficiently large number of iterations, say for $t > t_0$. Thus, the sets $\{\theta^{(t)}, t = t_0 + 1, \ldots, m\}$ and $\{\theta_i^{(t)}, t = t_0 + 1, \ldots, m; i = 1, \ldots, P\}$ can be considered as samples from the joint posterior distribution $p(\theta|y)$ and from the marginal distributions $p(\theta_i|y)$, respectively. The discarded t_0 iterations are known as the *burn-in* period.

As an illustration of the Gibbs algorithm, we consider the case introduced in Section 4.4 concerning a Normal distribution with unknown mean μ and variance σ^2. Here, instead of a noninformative prior, we specify informative independent priors such that $p(\mu, \sigma^2) = p(\mu)p(\sigma^2)$. In particular, we choose a Normal prior for the mean

$$\mu \sim \text{Normal}(\mu_0, \sigma_0^2)$$

and an inverse Gamma prior distribution[5] for the variance

$$\sigma^2 \sim \text{invGamma}(a, b).$$

It follows that the joint posterior distribution is given by

$$p(\mu, \sigma^2|y) \propto (\sigma^2)^{-n/2} \exp\left(-\frac{1}{2\sigma^2} \sum_{i=1}^{n} (y_i - \mu)^2\right)$$

$$\times (\sigma_0^2)^{-1/2} \exp\left(-\frac{1}{2\sigma_0^2}(\mu - \mu_0)^2\right)$$

$$\times (\sigma^2)^{-(a+1)} \exp\left(-\frac{b}{\sigma^2}\right),$$

with σ_0^2, a, b positive and $-\infty < \mu_0 < +\infty$. Note that in this case it is not possible to adopt the composition method introduced in Section 4.4 as the marginal posterior density of the variance is not a standard distribution from which it is simple to sample; thus, we resort to the Gibbs sampler. The full conditional distribution of the mean μ is

$$p(\mu|\sigma^2, y) \propto \exp\left(-\frac{1}{2\sigma^2} \sum_{i=1}^{n} (y_i - \mu)^2\right) \times \exp\left(-\frac{1}{2\sigma_0^2}(\mu - \mu_0)^2\right)$$

---

[5] An inverse Gamma distribution $y \sim \text{invGamma}(a, b)$ with shape $a > 0$ an scale $b > 0$ has density function given by

$$p(y) = \frac{b^a}{\Gamma(a)} y^{-(a+1)} \exp(-b/y)$$

for $y > 0$. Note that if $y \sim \text{invGamma}(a, b)$, then $1/y \sim \text{Gamma}(a, b)$. Moreover, there is a relationship with the scaled inverse Chi-square distribution since $\text{invChi}(\nu, s^2)$ is equivalent to $\text{invGamma}(\nu/2, \nu/2s^2)$.

$$= \exp\left(-\frac{1}{2}\left(\frac{\sum_{i=1}^{n} y_i^2 + n\mu^2 - 2\mu \sum_{i=1}^{n} y_i}{\sigma^2} + \frac{\mu^2 + \mu_0^2 - 2\mu_0\mu}{\sigma_0^2}\right)\right)$$

$$\propto \exp\left(-\frac{1}{2}\left[\mu^2\left(\frac{n}{\sigma^2} + \frac{1}{\sigma_0^2}\right) - 2\mu\left(\frac{\sum_{i=1}^{n} y_i}{\sigma^2} + \frac{\mu_0}{\sigma_0^2}\right)\right]\right).$$

With some simple calculations[6], it can be derived that the full conditional distribution has a Gaussian form

$$\mu|\sigma^2, y \sim \text{Normal}\left(\frac{\frac{\sum_{i=1}^{n} y_i}{\sigma^2} + \frac{\mu_0}{\sigma_0^2}}{\frac{n}{\sigma^2} + \frac{1}{\sigma_0^2}}, \frac{1}{\frac{n}{\sigma^2} + \frac{1}{\sigma_0^2}}\right). \tag{4.8}$$

With regard to the full conditional distribution of the variance σ^2, it holds that

$$p(\sigma^2|\mu, y) \propto (\sigma^2)^{-n/2} \exp\left(-\frac{1}{2\sigma^2}\sum_{i=1}^{n}(y_i - \mu)^2\right) \times (\sigma^2)^{-(a+1)} \exp\left(-\frac{b}{\sigma^2}\right)$$

$$\propto (\sigma^2)^{-n/2-(a+1)} \exp\left(-\frac{1}{\sigma^2}\left(b + \frac{\sum_{i=1}^{n}(y_i - \mu)^2}{2}\right)\right),$$

which is the functional form of the following inverse Gamma distribution:

$$\sigma^2|\mu, y \sim \text{invGamma}\left(\frac{n}{2} + a, b + \frac{\sum_{i=1}^{n}(y_i - \mu)^2}{2}\right). \tag{4.9}$$

In order to perform Gibbs sampling in R, we need to implement a `for` loop (see Section 2.5) as at each iteration the algorithm requires to sample from the full conditionals where the values for the conditioning parameters are taken from the previous iteration. To run the example, we consider the same data and setting used in Section 4.4:

```
> set.seed(44566)
> mu <- 10
> sigma2 <- 1.5
> n <- 100
> y <- rnorm(n=n, mean=mu, sd=sqrt(sigma2))
```

Moreover, we choose over dispersed initial values which are quite far from the true ones such as $\mu^{(0)} = 1$ and $\sigma^{2(0)} = 5$. This is a particular situation as we do know the true values. In general, we select initial values that are sensible and over dispersed, with respect to some knowledge of the prior distribution. Finally, we set $\mu_0 = 3$, $\sigma_0^2 = 10$, $a = 2.5$, $b = 0.5$, which correspond to noninformative prior distributions.

---

[6] Generally speaking, if $p(\theta) \propto \exp\left(-\frac{1}{2}(a\theta^2 - 2b\theta)\right)$, then $\theta \sim \text{Normal}\left(\frac{b}{a}, \frac{1}{a}\right)$.

```
> mu.init <- 1
> sigma2.init <- 5
> mu.0 <- 3
> sigma2.0 <- 10
> a <- 2.5
> b <- 0.5
```

At each iteration, we sample from the full conditional distributions in Eqs. (4.8) and (4.9) (using the rnorm and rgamma function) and we save iteratively the generated values in two vectors named mu.sim and sigma2.sim. We set $m = 5000$ and consider a burn-in period of $t_0 = 1000$ iterations.

```
> m <- 5000
> mu.sim <- c()
> sigma2.sim <- c()
> #Set the initial values
> mu.sim[1] <- mu.init
> sigma2.sim[1] <- sigma2.init
> #Run the for loop
> for(i in 2:m){
    mu.sim[i] <- rnorm(1,
                  mean = (sum(y)/sigma2.sim[i-1] + mu.0/sigma2.0) /
                          (n/sigma2.sim[i-1] + 1/sigma2.0),
                  sd = sqrt(1/(n/sigma2.sim[i-1] + 1/sigma2.0)))

    sigma2.sim[i] <- 1/rgamma(1, shape = n/2 + a,
                       scale = 1 / (sum((y-mu.sim[i-1])^2)/2 + b))
}
```

We discard the first t_0 burn-in iterations

```
> t0 <- 1000
> mu.sim <- mu.sim[-c(1:t0)]
> sigma2.sim <- sigma2.sim[-c(1:t0)]
```

and plot the simulated values for both parameters

```
> plot(mu.sim,t="l",xlab="Iteration",ylab=expression(mu))
> plot(sigma2.sim,t="l",xlab="Iteration", ylab=expression(sigma^2))
```

The trace plots represented in Figures 4.6 and 4.7 (top) display the iteration number versus the chain value and are a useful graphical diagnostic tool for assessing the convergence of the chain. As the simulated values do not show upward or downward trends but look like a random scatter around a stable mean value, the chain appears to have converged. Hence, we can compute the empirical means

```
> mean(mu.sim)
[1] 9.968405
> mean(sigma2.sim)
[1] 1.602073
```

and plot the empirical distribution of the simulated values (obtained using the hist function), which are reported in Figures 4.6 and 4.7 (bottom).

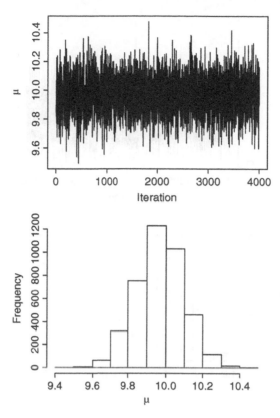

Figure 4.6   Trace plot (top) and histogram (bottom) of the simulated values of μ through the Gibbs sampler.

As suggested by Gilks *et al.* (1996, Chapter 8), when only one chain is run it may happen that the lack of convergence is not apparent (in the case, for example, of a slow moving chain). To avoid this, the suggestion is to run multiple independent chains, starting from different initial values, and check if the resulting trace plots overlap. In our example, we run again the Gibbs sampler starting from $\mu^{(0)} = 5$ and $\sigma^{2(0)} = 0.1$. In Figure 4.8, the resulting chains for μ and σ^2 – with the first t_0 iterations discarded – are superimposed with gray lines to the previous trace plots (with $\mu^{(0)} = 1$ and $\sigma^{2(0)} = 5$ as starting values). It can be noted that, in this example characterized by well mixing chains, the trace plots overlap indicating that the choice of the starting values does not affect the chain convergence to the posterior distribution.

For the MCMC method, the correlation between iterations needs to be checked as it could signal lack of convergence to the target distribution. Generally speaking, for the *i*th parameter θ_i ($i = 1, \ldots, P$) the empirical autocorrelation at lag l (distance

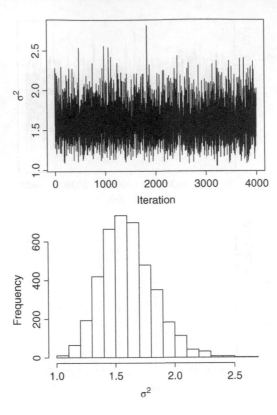

Figure 4.7   Trace plot (top) and histogram (bottom) of simulated values of σ^2 through the Gibbs sampler.

between values) is defined as

$$\mathrm{acf}_l = \frac{\sum_{t=l+1}^{m}(\theta_i^{(t)} - \bar{\theta}_i)(\theta_i^{(t-l)} - \bar{\theta}_i)}{\sum_{t=1}^{m}(\theta_i^{(t)} - \bar{\theta}_i)^2}$$

for $l = 1, 2, \ldots$, with $\bar{\theta}_i$ given by the sample mean of the considered parameter. The `acf` function in R computes the autocorrelation for several lags:

```
> acf(mu.sim,ylab=expression(mu),main="")
> acf(sigma2.sim,ylab=expression(sigma^2),main="").
```

The resulting autocorrelation plots are reported in Figure 4.9 and show that for any lag the autocorrelation is close to zero, suggesting that the simulated values can be considered almost independent.

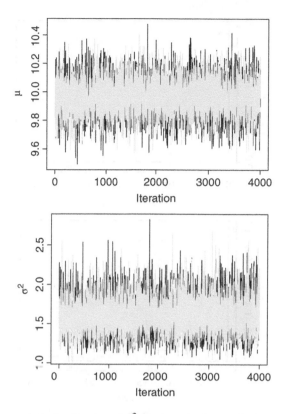

Figure 4.8   Trace plot of μ (top) and σ² (bottom) of two chains run with different starting values. The black line refers to the chain with $\mu^{(0)} = 1$ and $\sigma^{2(0)} = 5$, while the light gray line is for the chain starting from $\mu^{(0)} = 5$ and $\sigma^{2(0)} = 0.1$.

4.5.2   Metropolis–Hastings algorithm

The MH algorithm was first proposed by Metropolis *et al.* (1953) and then generalized by Hastings (1970). A description of the algorithm is provided by Chib and Greenberg (1995).

We consider here the case of a single generic parameter θ. Starting from an initial value $\theta^{(0)}$, the tth iteration of the algorithm is structured as follows:

1. Sample a candidate value $\theta^\star$ from a proposal distribution $q(\theta^\star | \theta^{(t-1)})$. Some examples of density functions for generating candidate values will be given below.

2. Compute the acceptance ratio

$$r = \frac{p(\theta^\star | y)}{p(\theta^{(t-1)} | y)} = \frac{p(y | \theta^\star)p(\theta^\star)}{p(y | \theta^{(t-1)})p(\theta^{(t-1)})}.$$

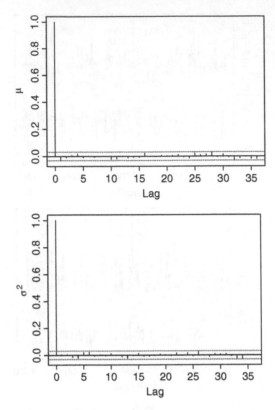

Figure 4.9   Autocorrelation plot of simulated values of μ (top) and σ^2 (bottom).

3. Let

$$\theta^{(t)} = \begin{cases} \theta^\star & \text{with probability} \quad \min(r, 1) \\ \theta^{(t-1)} & \text{with probability} \quad 1 - \min(r, 1) \end{cases}.$$

In practice, we draw a random number u from a Uniform(0,1) distribution and set $\theta^{(t)} = \theta^\star$ if $u < r$ (accept the candidate value $\theta^\star$) or $\theta^{(t)} = \theta^{(t-1)}$ if $u \geq r$ (refuse $\theta^\star$ and keep the previous value $\theta^{(t-1)}$).

As demonstrated by Robert and Casella (2004, Chapter 7), a Markov chain simulated following the above defined scheme converges, by construction, to the stationary distribution $p(\theta|y)$. To implement the MH algorithm, a proposal distribution is required for simulating candidate values. Usually, a symmetric density is preferred, such that $q(\theta^\star|\theta^{(t-1)}) = q(\theta^{(t-1)}|\theta^\star)$. In this case, a possible choice is the Uniform or the Gaussian distribution centered around the previous value:

$$q(\theta^\star|\theta^{(t-1)}) \sim \text{Uniform}(\theta^{(t-1)} - \gamma; \theta^{(t-1)} + \gamma) \qquad \text{or}$$

$$q(\theta^\star|\theta^{(t-1)}) \sim \text{Normal}(\theta^{(t-1)}, \gamma^2),$$

Table 4.2   Observed frequencies y_i and probabilities $p(y_i|\pi)$ for $i = 1, \ldots, 4$ categories of 197 animals of the genetic linkage model illustrated by Tanner (1993, Page 40).

Category	1	2	3	4
Frequency y_i	125	18	20	34
Probability $p(y_i|\pi)$	$\frac{1}{2} + \frac{\pi}{4}$	$\frac{1}{4}(1 - \pi)$	$\frac{1}{4}(1 - \pi)$	$\frac{\pi}{4}$

where γ is a tuning parameter chosen appropriately with respect to the algorithm efficiency (we will discuss this later). Note, that the Gibbs sampler defined in the previous section is a particular case of the MH algorithm, when the full conditional distribution is chosen as proposal density.

For illustrating the MH algorithm, we consider the example given by Tanner (1993, Page 40) concerning a genetic linkage model. The data consider 197 animals that are distributed into four categories with frequencies y_i and probabilities $p(y_i|\pi)$ for $i = 1, \ldots, 4$, as reported in Table 4.2.

The goal is the estimation of the posterior distribution $p(\pi|y)$, where π is the parameter defining the category probabilities reported in Table 4.2. By setting Uniform(0, 1) as a prior distribution[7] for π, the posterior distribution can be derived easily:

$$p(\pi|y) = p(y|\pi)p(\pi)$$

$$= \left(\frac{1}{2} + \frac{\pi}{4}\right)^{125} \left(\frac{1}{4}(1 - \pi)\right)^{18+20} \left(\frac{\pi}{4}\right)^{34} \times 1$$

$$= \left(\frac{1}{4}\right)^{197} (2 + \pi)^{125}(1 - \pi)^{38}\pi^{34}.$$

As proposal density, we adopt a Normal distribution with mean given by the previous value $\pi^{(t-1)}$ and standard deviation equal to $\sigma = 0.1$ (which corresponds to the tuning parameter γ introduced before):

$$q(\pi^\star|\pi^{(t-1)}) \sim \text{Normal}(\pi^{(t-1)}, \gamma^2 = \sigma^2 = 0.01).$$

We store the values of the Markov chain in the vector named pi.sim whose first element is equal to the starting value $\pi^{(0)} = 0.5$. Moreover, we create an auxiliary variable named acceptance as a counter for the number of times the proposal value $\pi^\star$ is accepted (it is initialized to 0). Finally, the number of iterations m is fixed to 10 000.

```
> y <- c(125,18,20,34)
> pi.sim <- c()
```

---

[7] The density function of the Uniform(a, b) distribution is equal to $f(\pi) = 1/(b - a)$ for $a < \pi < b$ and 0 elsewhere.

```
> pi.sim[1] <- 0.5
> acceptance <- 0
> sigma <- 0.1
> m <-10000
```

To implement the MH algorithm, we need a `for` loop to iterate and a conditional `if` statement for updating the chain (see Section 2.5). The R code for running the MH example is the following:

```
> for (i in 2:m){

    #Draw a value from the proposal distribution
    pi.star <- rnorm(n=1, mean=pi.sim[i-1], sd=sigma)

    #Compute the acceptance ratio
    r.numerator <-
        (2+pi.star)^y[1] * (1-pi.star)^(y[2]+y[3]) * pi.star^y[4]
    r.denominator <-
        (2+pi.sim[i-1])^y[1] * (1-pi.sim[i-1])^(y[2]+y[3]) *
        pi.sim[i-1]^y[4]
    r <- r.numerator/r.denominator

    #Draw a value from the Uniform distribution
    u <- runif(n=1, min=0, max=1)

    #Compare u and r and accept/refuse the candidate value
    if(u < r){
        pi.sim[i]   <- pi.star #Accept
        #Update the counter
        acceptance <- acceptance+1
    } else {
        pi.sim[i] <- pi.sim[i-1] #Refuse
    }
}
```

We discard $t_0 = 2000$ simulated values as burn-in period:

```
> t0 <- 2000
> pi.sim <- pi.sim[-c(1:t0)]
```

The resulting chain for π plotted in Figure 4.10 (top) is obtained using the following code:

```
> plot(pi.sim, t="l", xlab="Iteration", ylab=expression(pi))
```

The chain mixes well and no anomalies or trends are detected in the trace plot; thus, the chain appears to have reached convergence giving rise to a posterior mean equal to

```
> mean(pi.sim)
[1] 0.624185
```

As a diagnostic tool for convergence, another Markov chain with different initial values should be run, as shown previously for the Gibbs sampler. In this example,

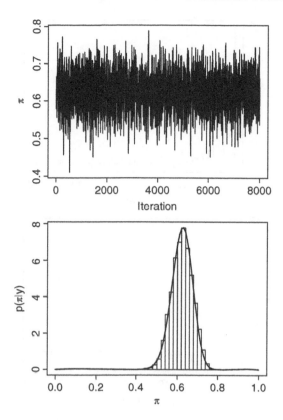

Figure 4.10   Trace plot of the simulated values of π (top) through the MH algorithm. Empirical distribution of the simulated values of π with the exact posterior distribution superimposed (bottom).

however, since the exact posterior distribution can be derived analytically, we compare the histogram of the simulated values with the curve of $p(\pi|y)$ (see Figure 4.10, bottom). Note that the histogram and the curve basically coincide.

It is interesting to compute the *acceptance rate* given by the value of the `acceptance` variable over the total number m of iterations.

```
> acceptance/m
[1] 0.5126
```

As illustrated by Hoff (2009), commonly an acceptance rate between 0.20 and 0.50 is considered a good choice. Note that the acceptance rate can be calibrated by adjusting the standard deviation σ of the proposal distribution (i.e., the tuning parameter γ). On one hand, if we increase σ then the proposed values will be sparser and the algorithm will tend to refuse too often; on the other hand, for small values of σ the Markov chain will accept too often giving rise to a stronger autocorrelation of the Markov chain and to a lower convergence speed. In the considered example,

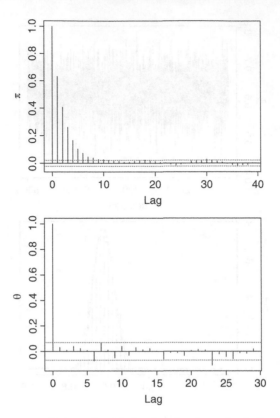

Figure 4.11   Autocorrelation plot of simulated value of π before (top) and after (bottom) thinning (one value every 10).

by rerunning the algorithm with $\sigma = 4$ and $\sigma = 0.01$, we get an acceptance rate equal to 0.1755 and 0.9404, respectively.

The autocorrelation function of the original setting with $\sigma = 0.1$ is plotted in the top panel of Figure 4.11 using the following code:

```
> acf(pi.sim,  ylab=expression(pi), main="")
```

The plot highlights a certain degree of correlation between consecutive values of the Markov chain (the autocorrelation seems to be significantly different from 0 for the first 10 lags); this is consistent with the obtained acceptance rate of 0.506 which is slightly high.

In order to reduce the correlation, it is possible to *thin* the Markov chain by taking one value of π every δ (e.g., $\delta = 10$). To do this, firstly we create a vector containing the index of the values to be chosen, and then we proceed with the selection:

```
> thinning.position <- seq(from=1, to=length(pi.sim), by=10)
> pi.sim <- pi.sim[thinning.position]
```

The autocorrelation function of the thinned Markov chain is plotted in Figure 4.11 (bottom); here no correlation can be detected. The new posterior mean of π is

```
> mean(pi.sim)
[1] 0.6233673
```

The disadvantage of thinning is that it increases the variance of the chain (in this case the posterior variance of π increases from 0.00267 to 0.00268).

4.5.3   MCMC implementation: software and output analysis

MCMC methods are powerful computational tools for Bayesian inference. In particular, the Gibbs sampler and the MH algorithm are extremely flexible and can be easily adapted for the estimation of complex models that involve a large number of parameters or are characterized by nonstandard posterior distributions. This ease of implementation is enhanced when, instead of developing new ad-hoc R code, black-box software or R packages are used. The most used software, especially among applied statisticians, is WinBUGS (Lunn *et al.*, 2000, Ntzoufras, 2009), which is part of the BUGS (Bayesian inference using Gibbs sampling) project for the Bayesian analysis of complex statistical models using MCMC methods. When using WinBUGS the user needs only to specify the model (using a *proto-type*), provide the data and the initial values; then the software will automatically select the sampling methods to generate values from the posterior distributions of the specified model. A very similar software package for performing Bayesian inference using MCMC is JAGS (just another Gibbs sampler, proposed by Plummer, 2003). JAGS is developed as a cross-platform engine for the BUGS language and has the advantage of allowing the users to define their own functions, distributions and samplers. Another ready-to-use software tool is BayesX (Belitz *et al.*, 2012), which is designed for MCMC-based Bayesian inference for a class of regression models. WinBUGS, JAGS and BayesX can be linked to R by means of the packages named R2WinBUGS, R2jags, and R2BayesX, respectively. Through these interfaces, it is possible to access the functions and facilities of the three software using R language. Finally, many R packages are available in the CRAN archive for Bayesian estimation functions and Bayesian model fitting (such as, for example, MCMCpack). All the packages are listed and described in the CRAN task view about Bayesian inference (http://cran.r-project.org/web/views/Bayesian.html), see Park *et al.* (2012).

Independently of the programming strategy or software used to implement MCMC methods, particular attention should be paid to the analysis of MCMC output. In fact, even though the MCMC theory, briefly sketched out in Section 4.5, states that the distribution of the simulated values converges to the target density (i.e., the posterior distribution) when the iteration number goes to infinity, it is not feasible to run a Markov chain infinitely. Thus, we run it long enough in order to achieve convergence, even if no stopping rule exists suggesting how many MCMC iterations are required for convergence or how long the burn-in period should be for eliminating the influence of starting values. The usual practice consists in employing convergence diagnostic tools (Cowles and Carlin, 1996), on a single or multiple chains, in order to explore the MCMC output and detect a failure in convergence (unfortunately, even when no problems are observed, we are not guaranteed that convergence has successfully occured). The convergence diagnostics comprise graphs, such as the trace and the autocorrelation plot, and indexes such as the acceptance rate and some test statistics (the most used are the Geweke, the Gelman–Rubin and the Raftery–Lewis methods which are also available in a R package named coda by Plummer *et al.*, 2006). As shown in the previous sections, the trace plot is a straightforward graphical tool that can be used to diagnose poor mixing occuring when the chain explores the posterior distribution very slowly. The consequence is that the simulated values are highly correlated and it takes a long time to achieve convergence. Moreover, correlation affects the accuracy of the posterior approximations because, as demonstrated by Geyer (1992), the variance of the MCMC approximation is given by the sum of the MC variance (see Section 4.1) and a positive term that depends on the correlation of the Markov chain. So, the higher the correlation, the lower the accuracy of the MCMC posterior estimates. Autocorrelation can be reduced by thinning the set of simulated valued or by improving the algorithm efficiency (e.g., through reparameterization for the Gibbs sampler or by tuning the MH proposal distribution).

The key point is that, when making inference with MCMC, great care (and a lot of time) is devoted to the tuning and monitoring convergence phases in order to find the best setting (in terms of parameterization, prior distributions, initial values, and MH proposal distributions) that produces the most reliable and accurate MCMC output (see Brooks *et al.*, 2011, Chapter 6 and references therein for recommendations about MCMC implementation). Another crucial aspect that cannot be ignored concerns the computational costs of MCMC methods. When models are complex (especially when designed in a hierarchical fashion as described in Chapter 5) or we deal with massive datasets, MCMC algorithms may be extremely slow and even become computationally unfeasible. This computational burden occurs particulary in the case of spatial and spatio-temporal models (discussed later in Chapters 6 and 7) and is usually known as "big n problem" (Banerjee *et al.*, 2004, Page 387; Jona Lasinio *et al.*, 2012). A viable alternative to MCMC methods able to reduce the computional costs of Bayesian inference is the INLA algorithm described in the following section.

4.6   The integrated nested Laplace approximations algorithm

The INLA algorithm, proposed by Rue *et al.* (2009), is a deterministic algorithm for Bayesian inference (rather than simulation based, such as MC and MCMC). INLA is especially designed for latent Gaussian models and, compared to MCMC, it provides accurate results in shorter computing time.

In this section, we introduce first the Laplace approximation which is the core of the INLA approach; then we formalize the INLA setting and describe the details of the INLA algorithm. In order to be consistent with the rest of the book, we adopt here a notation which is slightly different from the one used by Rue and Martino (2007) and Rue *et al.* (2009).

4.7   Laplace approximation

An alternative approach to the simulation-based MC integration is analytic approximation with the Laplace method. Suppose we are interested in computing the following integral:

$$\int f(x)dx = \int \exp(\log f(x))dx,$$

where $f(x)$ is the density function of a random variable X. We represent $\log f(x)$ by means of a Taylor series expansion evaluated in $x = x_0$:

$$\log f(x) \approx \log f(x_0) + (x - x_0)\left.\frac{\partial \log f(x)}{\partial x}\right|_{x=x_0} + \frac{(x - x_0)^2}{2}\left.\frac{\partial^2 \log f(x)}{\partial x^2}\right|_{x=x_0}.$$

If x_0 is set equal to the mode $x^* = \text{argmax}_x \log f(x)$, then $\left.\frac{\partial \log f(x)}{\partial x}\right|_{x=x^*} = 0$ and the approximation becomes

$$\log f(x) \approx \log f(x^*) + \frac{(x - x^*)^2}{2}\left.\frac{\partial^2 \log f(x)}{\partial x^2}\right|_{x=x^*}.$$

The integral of interest is then approximated as follows:

$$\int f(x)dx \approx \int \exp\left(\log f(x^*) + \frac{(x - x^*)^2}{2}\left.\frac{\partial^2 \log f(x)}{\partial x^2}\right|_{x=x^*}\right)dx$$

$$= \exp(\log f(x^*))\int \exp\left(\frac{(x - x^*)^2}{2}\left.\frac{\partial^2 \log f(x)}{\partial x^2}\right|_{x=x^*}\right)dx,$$

where the integrand can be associated with the density of a Normal distribution. In fact, by setting $\sigma^{2*} = -1/\left.\frac{\partial^2 \log f(x)}{\partial x^2}\right|_{x=x^*}$ we obtain

$$\int f(x)dx \approx \exp(\log f(x^*))\int \exp\left(-\frac{(x - x^*)^2}{2\sigma^{2*}}\right)dx,$$

where the integrand is the kernel of a Normal distribution with mean equal to x^* and variance σ^{2*}. More precisely, the integral evaluated in the interval (α, β) is approximated by

$$\int_\alpha^\beta f(x)dx \approx f(x^*)\sqrt{2\pi\sigma^{2*}}(\Phi(\beta) - \Phi(\alpha)), \qquad (4.10)$$

Table 4.3   Exact and approximated values of the integral $\int_\alpha^\beta f(x)dx$ where $f(x)$ is the density function of the Gamma(a, b) distribution.

(a, b)	(α, β)	Exact value	Approximated value
$(5, 1)$	$(2, 6)$	0.6622905	0.6686424
$(5, 1)$	$(1, 10)$	0.9670875	0.9126693
$(10, 0.5)$	$(18, 22)$	0.2468976	0.2452272
$(10, 0.5)$	$(10, 40)$	0.9631765	0.9002946

where $\Phi(\cdot)$ denotes the cumulative density function of the Normal(x^*, σ^{2*}) distribution.

As an example, we consider the case of the Gamma distribution with the density function

$$f(x) = \frac{b^a}{\Gamma(a)} \exp(-bx)x^{a-1} \qquad x, a, b > 0. \tag{4.11}$$

For computing the Laplace approximation, we need the following quantities:

$$\log f(x) = (a - 1)\log x - bx + \text{constant},$$

$$\frac{\partial \log f(x)}{\partial x} = \frac{a - 1}{x} - b,$$

$$\frac{\partial^2 \log f(x)}{\partial x^2} = -\frac{a - 1}{x^2}.$$

By solving $\frac{\partial \log f(x)}{\partial x} = 0$, we obtain the mode $x^* = \frac{a-1}{b}$ (for $a > 1$). Moreover, the variance σ^{2*}, which is obtained by evaluating $-1/\frac{\partial^2 \log f(x)}{\partial x^2}$ at the mode x^*, is equal to $\sigma^{2*} = \frac{a-1}{b^2}$. Thus, the Laplace approximation of the Gamma distribution is

$$\text{Gamma}(a, b) \approx \text{Normal}\left(x^* = \frac{a - 1}{b}, \sigma^{2*} = \frac{a - 1}{b^2}\right).$$

For evaluating the approximation, we consider different values for the Gamma parameters a and b and for the interval of integration (α, β); see Table 4.3. We report in the following the R commands for computing the Laplace approximation for the case with $a = 5, b = 1, \alpha = 2, \beta = 6$.

```
> #Gammma parameters:
> a=5
> b=1
> #Approximation parameters:
> star.x = (a-1)/b #mode
> star.x
[1] 4
> star.sigma2 = (a-1)/b^2 #variance
> star.sigma2
[1] 4
```

```
> #Integral extremes:
> alpha = 2
> beta = 6
```

The *exact* value of the integral $\int_2^6 f(x)\mathrm{d}x$, where $f(x)$ is the Gamma density function of Eq. (4.11) and is computed as difference of the cumulative density function values evaluated in β and in α:

```
> pgamma(beta,shape=a,rate=b) - pgamma(alpha,shape=a,rate=b)
[1] 0.6622905
```

while the approximated value of the integral is obtained as in Eq. (4.10):

```
> dgamma(star.x, shape=a,rate=b)*
    sqrt(2*pi*star.sigma2)*
      (pnorm(beta,mean=star.x,sd=sqrt(star.sigma2)) -
       pnorm(alpha,mean=star.x,sd=sqrt(star.sigma2)))
[1] 0.6686424
```

See Figure 4.12 (top) for a comparison of the true Gamma$(5, 1)$ density and the approximating Normal$(4, 4)$, obtained with the following code:

```
> xx=seq(0,20,l=100)
> plot(xx,dgamma(xx, shape=a,rate=b),t="l",ylab="Density",xlab="x")
> lines(xx,dnorm(xx,mean=star.x,sd=sqrt(star.sigma2)),lty=2)
```

Note that with $\alpha = 1$ and $\beta = 10$ the integral interval is wider and includes the tails of the Gamma distribution; in this case the Laplace approximation does not perform as well (the approximated value is equal to 0.9126693 while the exact one is 0.9670875). The same happens with the Gamma$(10, 0.5)$ (see the bottom panel of Figure 4.12): the Laplace approximation is close to the exact value when the integral is computed in the central part of the distribution (with $\alpha = 18$ and $\beta = 22$) and is poorer when the interval increases (with $\alpha = 10$ and $\beta = 40$).

4.7.1   INLA setting: the class of latent Gaussian models

The first step in defining a latent Gaussian model within the Bayesian framework is to identify a distribution for the observed data $y = (y_1, \dots, y_n)$. A very general approach consists in specifying a distribution for y_i characterized by a parameter ϕ_i (usually the mean $E(y_i)$) defined as a function of a structured additive predictor η_i through a link function $g(\cdot)$, such that $g(\phi_i) = \eta_i$. The additive linear predictor η_i is defined as follows:

$$\eta_i = \beta_0 + \sum_{m=1}^{M} \beta_m x_{mi} + \sum_{l=1}^{L} f_l(z_{li}). \tag{4.12}$$

Here β_0 is a scalar representing the intercept; the coefficients $\boldsymbol{\beta} = \{\beta_1, \dots, \beta_M\}$ quantify the (linear) effect of some covariates $\boldsymbol{x} = (x_1, \dots, x_M)$ on the response; and $\boldsymbol{f} = \{f_1(\cdot), \dots, f_L(\cdot)\}$ is a collection of functions defined in terms of a set of covariates $\boldsymbol{z} = (z_1, \dots, z_L)$. The terms $f_l(\cdot)$ can assume different forms such as smooth and

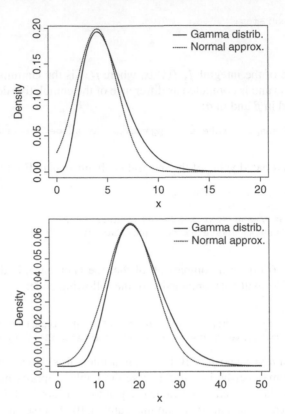

Figure 4.12   Gamma density function with parameter a = 5, b = 1 (top) and a = 10, b = 0.5 (bottom). The dashed line refers to the corresponding Normal approximation obtained using the Laplace method.

nonlinear effects of covariates, time trends and seasonal effects, random intercept and slopes as well as temporal or spatial random effects. For this reason, the class of latent Gaussian models is very flexible and can accomodate a wide range of models ranging from generalized and dynamic linear models to spatial and spatio-temporal models (see Martins *et al.*, 2013 for a review).

We collect all the latent (nonobservable) components of interest for the inference in a set of parameters named θ defined as $\theta = \{\beta_0, \beta, f\}$. Moreover, we denote with $\psi = \{\psi_1, \ldots, \psi_K\}$ the vector of the K hyperparameters. By assuming conditional independence, the distribution of the n observations (all coming from the same distribution family) is given by the likelihood

$$p(y|\theta, \psi) = \prod_{i=1}^{n} p(y_i|\theta_i, \psi), \tag{4.13}$$

where each data point y_i is connected to only one element θ_i in the latent field θ. Martins *et al.* (2013) discuss the possibility of relaxing this assumption assuming that each observation may be connected with a linear combination of elements in $\boldsymbol{\theta}$; moreover, they take into account the case when the data belong to several distributions, i.e., the multiple likelihoods case.

We assume a multivariate Normal prior on $\boldsymbol{\theta}$ with mean $\mathbf{0}$ and precision matrix $\boldsymbol{Q}(\boldsymbol{\psi})$, i.e., $\boldsymbol{\theta} \sim \text{Normal}(\mathbf{0}, \boldsymbol{Q}^{-1}(\boldsymbol{\psi}))$ with density function given by

$$p(\boldsymbol{\theta}|\boldsymbol{\psi}) = (2\pi)^{-n/2}|\boldsymbol{Q}(\boldsymbol{\psi})|^{1/2} \exp\left(-\frac{1}{2}\boldsymbol{\theta}'\boldsymbol{Q}(\boldsymbol{\psi})\boldsymbol{\theta}\right), \qquad (4.14)$$

where $|\cdot|$ denotes the matrix determinant and $'$ is used for the transpose operation. The components of the latent Gaussian field $\boldsymbol{\theta}$ are supposed to be conditionally independent with the consequence that $\boldsymbol{Q}(\boldsymbol{\psi})$ is a sparse precision matrix.[8] This specification is known as *Gaussian Markov random field* (GMRF, Rue and Held, 2005). Note that the sparsity of the precision matrix gives rise to computational benefits when making inference with GMRFs. In fact, linear algebra operations can be performed using numerical methods for sparse matrices, resulting in a considerable computational gain (see Rue and Held, 2005 for algorithms).

The joint posterior distribution of $\boldsymbol{\theta}$ and $\boldsymbol{\psi}$ is given by the product of the likelihood (4.13), of the GMRF density (4.14) and of the hyperparameter prior distribution $p(\boldsymbol{\psi})$:

$$p(\boldsymbol{\theta}, \boldsymbol{\psi}|\boldsymbol{y}) \propto p(\boldsymbol{\psi}) \times p(\boldsymbol{\theta}|\boldsymbol{\psi}) \times p(\boldsymbol{y}|\boldsymbol{\theta}, \boldsymbol{\psi}) \qquad (4.15)$$

$$\propto p(\boldsymbol{\psi}) \times p(\boldsymbol{\theta}|\boldsymbol{\psi}) \times \prod_{i=1}^{n} p(y_i|\theta_i, \boldsymbol{\psi})$$

$$\propto p(\boldsymbol{\psi}) \times |\boldsymbol{Q}(\boldsymbol{\psi})|^{1/2} \exp\left(-\frac{1}{2}\boldsymbol{\theta}'\boldsymbol{Q}(\boldsymbol{\psi})\boldsymbol{\theta}\right) \times \prod_{i=1}^{n} \exp(\log(p(y_i|\theta_i, \boldsymbol{\psi})))$$

$$\propto p(\boldsymbol{\psi}) \times |\boldsymbol{Q}(\boldsymbol{\psi})|^{1/2} \exp\left(-\frac{1}{2}\boldsymbol{\theta}'\boldsymbol{Q}(\boldsymbol{\psi})\boldsymbol{\theta} + \sum_{i=1}^{n} \log\left(p(y_i|\theta_i, \boldsymbol{\psi})\right)\right).$$

4.7.2   Approximate Bayesian inference with INLA

The objectives of Bayesian inference are the marginal posterior distributions for each element of the parameter vector

---

[8] If the components θ_i are θ_j are conditionally independent given all the other components $\boldsymbol{\theta}_{-i,j}$, the joint conditional distribution can be factorized as follows:

$$p(\theta_i, \theta_j|\boldsymbol{\theta}_{-i,j}) = p(\theta_i|\boldsymbol{\theta}_{-i,j})p(\theta_j|\boldsymbol{\theta}_{-i,j}).$$

We write this as $\theta_i \perp\!\!\!\perp \theta_j|\boldsymbol{\theta}_{-i,j}$. This conditional independence property defines the zero pattern of the precision matrix $\boldsymbol{Q}(\boldsymbol{\psi})$ because, for a general pair i and j with $j \neq i$, it holds that the corresponding element of the precision matrix is null:

$$\theta_i \perp\!\!\!\perp \theta_j|\boldsymbol{\theta}_{-i,j} \iff Q_{ij}(\boldsymbol{\psi}) = 0.$$

$$p(\theta_i|y) = \int p(\theta_i, \psi|y)\mathrm{d}\psi = \int p(\theta_i|\psi,y)p(\psi|y)\mathrm{d}\psi, \qquad (4.16)$$

and for each element of the hyperparameter vector

$$p(\psi_k|y) = \int p(\psi|y)\mathrm{d}\psi_{-k}.$$

Thus, we need to perform the following tasks:

(i) compute $p(\psi|y)$, from which also all the relevant marginals $p(\psi_k|y)$ can be obtained;

(ii) compute $p(\theta_i|\psi,y)$, which is needed to compute the parameter marginal posteriors $p(\theta_i|y)$.

The INLA approach exploits the assumptions of the model to produce a numerical approximation to the posteriors of interest based on the Laplace approximation method introduced in Section 4.7 (Tierney and Kadane, 1986).

The first task (i) consists of the computation of an approximation to the joint posterior of the hyperparameters as

$$
\begin{aligned}
p(\psi|y) &= \frac{p(\theta, \psi|y)}{p(\theta|\psi,y)} \qquad (4.17)\\[2mm]
&= \frac{p(y|\theta, \psi)p(\theta, \psi)}{p(y)} \frac{1}{p(\theta|\psi,y)}\\[2mm]
&= \frac{p(y|\theta, \psi)p(\theta|\psi)p(\psi)}{p(y)} \frac{1}{p(\theta|\psi,y)}\\[2mm]
&\propto \frac{p(y|\theta, \psi)p(\theta|\psi)p(\psi)}{p(\theta|\psi,y)}\\[2mm]
&\approx \frac{p(y|\theta, \psi)p(\theta|\psi)p(\psi)}{\tilde{p}(\theta|\psi,y)}\bigg|_{\theta=\theta^*(\psi)} =: \tilde{p}(\psi|y), \qquad (4.18)
\end{aligned}
$$

where $\tilde{p}(\theta|\psi,y)$ is the Gaussian approximation – given by the Laplace method – of $p(\theta|\psi,y)$ and $\theta^*(\psi)$ is the mode for a given ψ. The Gaussian approximation turns out to be accurate since $p(\theta|\psi,y)$ appears to be almost Gaussian as it is a priori distributed like a GMRF, y is generally not informative and the observation distribution is usually well-behaved.

The second task (ii) is slightly more complex, because in general there will be more elements in θ than in ψ, and thus this computation is more expensive. A first easy possibility is to approximate the posterior conditional distributions $p(\theta_i|\psi,y)$ directly as the marginals from $\tilde{p}(\theta|\psi,y)$, i.e. using a Normal distribution, where the Cholesky decomposition is used for the precision matrix (Rue and Martino, 2007). While this is very fast, the approximation is generally not very good. The second possibility is to rewrite the vector of parameters as

$\theta = (\theta_i, \theta_{-i})$ and use again Laplace approximation to obtain

$$p(\theta_i|\psi,y) = \frac{p((\theta_i,\theta_{-i})|\psi,y)}{p(\theta_{-i}|\theta_i,\psi,y)} \tag{4.19}$$

$$= \frac{p(\theta,\psi|y)}{p(\psi|y)}\frac{1}{p(\theta_{-i}|\theta_i,\psi,y)}$$

$$\propto \frac{p(\theta,\psi|y)}{p(\theta_{-i}|\theta_i,\psi,y)}$$

$$\approx \frac{p(\theta,\psi|y)}{\tilde{p}(\theta_{-i}|\theta_i,\psi,y)}\bigg|_{\theta_{-i}=\theta^*_{-i}(\theta_i,\psi)} =: \tilde{p}(\theta_i|\psi,y), \tag{4.20}$$

where $\tilde{p}(\theta_{-i}|\theta_i,\psi,y)$ is the Laplace Gaussian approximation to $p(\theta_{-i}|\theta_i,\psi,y)$ and $\theta^*_{-i}(\theta_i,\psi)$ is its mode. Because the random variables $\theta_{-i}|\theta_i,\psi,y$ are in general reasonably Normal, the approximation provided by (4.20) typically works very well. This strategy, however, can be very expensive in computational terms as $\tilde{p}(\theta_{-i}|\theta_i,\psi,y)$ must be recomputed for each value of θ and ψ (some modifications to the Laplace approximation in order to reduce the computational costs are described in Rue et al., 2009).

A third option is the *simplified Laplace approximation*, which is based on a Taylor's series expansion of the Laplace approximation $\tilde{p}(\theta_i|\psi,y)$ in Eq. (4.20). This is usually "corrected" by including a mixing term (e.g. spline), to increase the fit to the required distribution. The accuracy of this approximation is sufficient in many applied cases and given that the time needed for the computation is considerably shorter, this is the standard option.

Once we get $\tilde{p}(\theta_i|\psi,y)$ and $\tilde{p}(\psi|y)$, the marginal posterior distributions $p(\theta_i|y)$ – introduced in Eq. (4.16) – are then approximated by

$$\tilde{p}(\theta_i|y) \approx \int \tilde{p}(\theta_i|\psi,y)\tilde{p}(\psi|y)d\psi, \tag{4.21}$$

where the integral can be solved numerically through a finite weighted sum:

$$\tilde{p}(\theta_i|y) \approx \sum_j \tilde{p}(\theta_i|\psi^{(j)},y)\tilde{p}(\psi^{(j)}|y)\Delta_j \tag{4.22}$$

for some relevant integration points $\{\psi^{(j)}\}$ with a corresponding set of weights $\{\Delta_j\}$. Operationally, INLA proceeds as follows:

(i) first it explores the hyperparameter joint posterior distribution $\tilde{p}(\psi|y)$ of Eq. (4.18) in a nonparametric way, in order to detect good points $\{\psi^{(j)}\}$ for the numerical integration required in Eq. (4.22). Rue et al. (2009) propose two different exploration schemes, both requiring a reparameterization of the ψ-space – in order to deal with more regular densities – through the following steps:

a) Locate the mode ψ^* of $\tilde{p}(\psi|y)$ by optimizing $\log \tilde{p}(\psi|y)$ with respect to ψ (e.g., through the Newton–Raphson method).

b) Compute the negative Hessian H at the modal configuration.

c) Compute the eigen-decomposition $\Sigma = V\Lambda^{1/2}V'$, with $\Sigma = H^{-1}$.

d) Define the new variable z, with standardized and mutually orthogonal components, such that

$$\psi(z) = \psi^* + V\Lambda^{1/2}z.$$

The first exploration scheme (named *grid strategy*) builds, using the z-parameterization, a grid of points associated with the bulk of the mass of $\tilde{p}(\psi|y)$. This approach has a computational cost which grows exponentially with the number of hyperparameters; therefore the advice is to adopt it when K, the dimension of ψ, is lower than 4. Otherwise, the second exploration scheme, named *central composite design* (CCD) strategy, should be used as it reduces the computational costs. With the CCD approach, the integration problem is seen as a design problem; using the mode ψ^* and the Hessian H, some relevant points in the ψ-space are selected for performing a second-order approximation to a response variable (see Section 6.5 of Rue *et al.*, 2009 for details). In general, the CCD strategy uses much less points, but still is able to capture the variability of the hyperparameter distribution. For this reason it is the default option in R-INLA.

Figure 4.13 illustrates an example of bivariate joint distribution for the case of $\psi = \{\psi_1, \psi_2\}$, together with the integration points detected with the grid and CCD strategy.

After the grid exploration, each marginal posterior $\tilde{p}(\psi_k|y)$ can be obtained using an interpolation algorithm based on the values of the density $\tilde{p}(\psi|y)$ evaluated in the set of integration points $\{\psi_k^{(j)}\}$. See Martins *et al.* (2013) for the details about the interpolation strategy which can be used (the default one is the so-called numerical integration free algorithm).

(ii) For each value in $\{\psi_k^{(j)}\}$, the conditional posteriors $\tilde{p}(\theta_i|\psi^{(j)},y)$ are then evaluated on a grid of selected values for θ_i and the marginal posteriors $\tilde{p}(\theta_i|y)$ are obtained by numerical integration as in Eq. (4.22).

4.8   The R-INLA package

R-INLA is the R package to implement approximate Bayesian inference using the INLA approach (Martino and Rue, 2010a). The package, which substitutes the standalone INLA program build upon the GMRFLib library (Martino and Rue, 2010b), is available for Linux, Mac, and Windows operating systems and can be

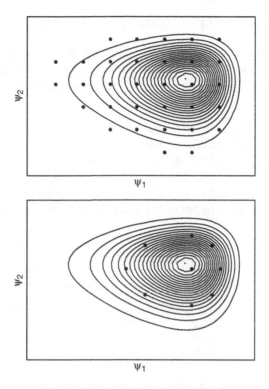

Figure 4.13   Joint posterior distribution of ψ_1 and ψ_2. The black dots denote the location of the integration points identified with the grid (top) and CCD (bottom) strategy.

downloaded and installed typing in the R console

```
> source("http://www.math.ntnu.no/inla/givemeINLA.R")
```

Then, as described in Chapter 2, the package can be loaded with the command

```
> library(INLA)
```

The INLA function

```
> inla.upgrade(testing=TRUE)
```

is used to upgrade the package to the latest test version (type `inla.version()` to find out the installed version[9]). Note that there are frequent upgrades and our suggestion is to download the more stable version of the package with the command `inla.upgrade(testing=FALSE)`. The website `http://www.r-inla.org/` provides documentation for the package as well as many worked examples and a discussion forum. Additionally, the

---

[9] The R-INLA version for running all the code of this book is 0.0-1402298691 released on Mon 9 Jun 09:24:51 CEST 2014.

^{TM}Google Code project `http://code.google.com/p/inla/` hosts all the source code.

For introducing the R-INLA syntax, we consider the case of two covariates $x = (x_1, x_2)$ and a function $f(\cdot)$ indexed by a third covariate z_1; the linear predictor as presented in Eq. (4.12) is reproduced in R-INLA through the command

```
> formula <- y ~ 1 + x1 + x2 + f(z1, model="...")
```

where y, x1, x2, and z1 are the column names of the dataframe containing the data (for simplicity the dataframe name is data). The term 1 is not mandatory as an intercept would be included by default. In the R function f() the string model="..." specifies the type of $f(\cdot)$ function. The default choice is model="iid" which refers to independent and Gaussian distributed random variables indexed by z1. The list of the other alternatives is available typing

```
> names(inla.models()$latent)
 [1] "linear"       "iid"           "mec"            "meb"
 [5] "rgeneric"     "rw1"           "rw2"            "crw2"
 [9] "seasonal"     "besag"         "besag2"         "bym"
[13] "bym2"         "besagproper"   "besagproper2"   "ar1"
[17] "ar"           "ou"            "generic"        "generic0"
[21] "generic1"     "generic2"      "spde"           "spde2"
[25] "spde3"        "iid1d"         "iid2d"          "iid3d"
[29] "iid4d"        "iid5d"         "2diid"          "z"
[33] "rw2d"         "rw2diid"       "slm"            "matern2d"
[37] "copy"         "clinear"       "sigm"           "revsigm"
```

and a description of each of them is given at `http://www.r-inla.org/models/latent-models`. Of course, it is possible to include in the formula several f() terms specifying them separately, as for example in

```
> formula <- y ~ x1 + x2 + f1(z1) + f2(z2) + f3(z3)
```

provided that the dataset has three columns named z1, z2 and z3 containing the covariate values.

There are some other options that can be specified in the f() term, such as, for example, hyper, replicate, constr (see the help page ?f); some of the options will be discussed in the following chapters when real data applications are presented.

Finally, we run the INLA algorithm using the inla function as follows:

```
> inla(formula, family = "...", data),
```

where the formula has been defined previously, data is the dataframe containing all the variables included in the formula and family is a string that specifies the distribution of the data (i.e., the likelihood). Some of the available distributions are

```
> names(inla.models()$likelihood) #output partially omitted

[1] "poisson"            "gpoisson"
[3] "binomial"           "testbinomial1"
[5] "gamma"              "beta"
```

```
[7]  "betabinomial"              "cbinomial"
[9]  "nbinomial"                 "simplex"
[11] "gaussian"                  "normal"
[13] "circularnormal"            "wrappedcauchy"
[15] "iidgamma"                  "iidlogitbeta"
[17] "sas"                       "loggammafrailty"
[19] "logistic"                  "skewnormal"
[21] "sn"                        "gev"
[23] "laplace"                   "lognormal"
[25] "exponential"               "coxph"
[27] "weibull"                   "loglogistic"
[29] "zeroinflatednbinomial0"
```

and complete descriptions with examples are provided at http://www.r-inla
.org/models/likelihoods. The inla function includes many other
options; see ?inla for a complete list.

To provide a first application with R-INLA, we consider the linear regression
example introduced in Section 2.6 for the iris dataset and the model

```
> lm1 <- lm(Petal.Length ~ Petal.Width, data=iris)
```

that considers Petal.Length as a function of Petal.Width. This model,[10]
which comprises only the linear effects β_0 and β_1, can be implemented in R-INLA
simply typing the following commands:

```
> formula <- Petal.Length ~ 1 + Petal.Width
> output <- inla(formula, family="gaussian", data=iris)
```

The inla function returns an object, here named output, of class inla. This
is a list containing many objects which can be explored with names(output).
For a general summary of the results use

```
> summary(output)
Call:
"inla(formula = formula, family = \"gaussian\", data = iris)"

Time used:
  Preprocessing    Running inla Post-processing          Total
          0.112           0.104           0.090          0.306

Fixed effects:
               mean      sd 0.025quant 0.5quant 0.975quant    mode kld
(Intercept) 1.0836  0.0727     0.9407   1.0836     1.2263  1.0836   0
Petal.Width 2.2299  0.0512     2.1293   2.2299     2.3305  2.2299   0

The model has no random effects
```

---

[10] Using the notation introduced in Section 4.7.1, in this example we have $y_i \sim \text{Normal}(\eta_i = \beta_0 + \beta_1 x_i, \sigma^2)$, $g(\cdot)$ is the identity function, $\theta = \{\beta_0, \beta_1\}$ and $\psi = \{1/\sigma^2\}$.

```
Model hyperparameters:
                    mean      sd  0.025quant  0.5quant  0.975quant   mode
Precision for the   4.43  0.5117       3.495     4.408       5.501  4.368
Gaussian observations

Expected number of effective parameters(std dev): 2.011(0.001)
Number of equivalent replicates : 74.59

Marginal likelihood:  -119.59
```

This summary includes some statistics about the computing times as well as the posterior mean, the standard deviation, the quartiles of the fixed effects (β_0 and β_1) and of the hyperparameter (denoted by Precision for the Gaussian observations). The same output can be obtained by means of these single commands (as we are dealing with a list we make use of the $ sign to access the output):

```
> output$summary.fixed
> output$summary.hyperpar
```

The posterior marginal distributions of parameters and hyperparameters can be extracted through

```
> output$marginals.fixed
> output$marginals.hyperpar
```

As an example, suppose we want to plot the posterior marginal distribution of β_1 (the Petal.width coefficient). First of all, we note that the object output$marginals.fixed is a list formed by two objects whose names are recovered with

```
> names(output$marginals.fixed)
[1] "(Intercept)" "Petal.Width"
```

Each element of the list is a matrix with column names given by x and y. Thus, the following commands

```
> beta1_post <- output$marginals.fixed$Petal.Width
> plot(beta1_post, type="l",xlab=expression(beta[1]),
      ylab=expression(tilde(p) (paste(beta[1],"|",y))))
```

produce the desidered plot which is reported in Figure 4.14 (top).

The R-INLA library includes also a set of functions for manipulating marginal distributions (see ?marginal). For example inla.dmarginal, inla.pmarginal and inla.qmarginal compute the density, the distribution and the quantile function, respectively. Going back to β_1, the following syntax provides its 95% credibility interval (as defined in Section 3.5):

```
> inla.qmarginal(0.025,beta1_post)
[1] 2.129255
```

```
> inla.qmarginal(0.975,beta1_post)
[1] 2.330128
```

which could have been deduced using the results in the general summary, as well. It is also possible to get the values q_1 and q_2 that define the *highest posterior density* confidence interval such that $\int_{q_1}^{q_2} \tilde{p}(\beta_1|y)d\beta_1 = 0.95$, with

```
> inla.hpdmarginal(0.95,beta1_post)
                low       high
level:0.95 2.129256 2.330129
```

Another interesting case regards the calculation of the expected value of a function of the original parameters. For example, we may be interested in the posterior mean of the variance of the observations σ^2, instead of the precision which is given by default in the summary of the hyperparameters. In this case, we employ the R-INLA function `inla.emarginal` which computes the expected value of a function `fun` applied to the marginal distribution `marg` (in this case the inverse of the precision):

```
> names(output$marginals.hyperpar)
[1] "Precision for the Gaussian observations"
> prec_post <- output$marginals.hyperpar$"Precision for the
Gaussian observations"
> # an equivalent command is
> # prec_post <- output$marginals.hyperpar[[1]]
> inla.emarginal(fun=function(x) 1/x, marg=prec_post)
[1] 0.2287445
```

Additionaly, the approximated posterior standard deviation of the variance σ^2, given by the square root of $E((\sigma^2)^2) - (E(\sigma^2))^2$ (Tierney and Kadane, 1986), can be computed using twice the `inla.emarginal` function as follows:

```
> m1 <- inla.emarginal(function(x) 1/x, prec_post)
> m2 <- inla.emarginal(function(x) (1/x)^2, prec_post)
> sd <- sqrt(m2 - m1^2)
> sd
[1] 0.02660479
```

Thus, 0.2287 and 0.0266 are the approximated posterior mean and standard deviation of the variance. To plot the approximate posterior distribution of the variance, we run the following command[11]

```
> plot.default(inla.tmarginal(function(x) 1/x,prec_post),
      type="l",xlab=expression(sigma^2),
      ylab=expression(tilde(p) (paste(sigma^2,"|",y))))
```

where the inner function `inla.tmarginal` transforms a given marginal distribution (see the bottom panel in Figure 4.14).

---

[11] We use `plot.default` instead of `plot` in order to reset the plot options set by R-INLA and to be able to customize axes labels.

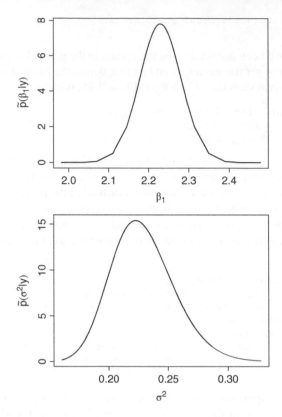

Figure 4.14   Approximate marginal posterior distribution of the fixed effect β_1 (top) and of the observation variance σ^2 (bottom).

4.9   How INLA works: step-by-step example

In this section, we consider the example introduced in Section 4.5.1 regarding normally distributed data with independent prior distributions and we illustrate how the INLA approach works step by step.

The observations $\mathbf{y} = (y_1, \dots, y_n)$ are assumed independent and normally distributed with $y_i|\mu, \sigma^2 \sim \text{Normal}(\mu, \sigma^2)$. Moreover, we choose independent prior distributions for μ and $\psi = 1/\sigma^2$ with

$$\mu \sim \text{Normal}(\mu_0, \sigma_0^2),$$

$$\psi \sim \text{Gamma}(a, b).$$

Using the INLA notation, this setting corresponds to the observation distribution

$$y_i|\theta, \psi \sim \text{Normal}(\eta_i, \sigma^2)$$

where $\eta_i = \theta = \mu$ and $\psi = 1/\sigma^2$. In the following, we use a Gamma(a, b) as a prior distribution for ψ.

The first task concerns the posterior distribution of the hyperparameter ψ which can be computed integrating out θ from the joint posterior distribution:

$$p(\psi|y) \propto \int p(\theta, \psi|y)d\theta,$$

where $p(\theta, \psi|y) \propto p(y|\theta, \psi)p(\theta)p(\psi)$. To avoid the integration, the same approach adopted by INLA in Eq. (4.17) can be used and the posterior distribution can be defined as follows:

$$p(\psi|y) = \frac{p(\theta, \psi|y)}{p(\theta|\psi, y)}$$

$$\propto \frac{p(y|\theta, \psi)p(\theta)p(\psi)}{p(\theta|\psi, y)}, \tag{4.23}$$

where the involved distributions are

$$y|\theta, \psi \sim \prod_{i=1}^{n} \text{Normal}(\theta, 1/\psi)$$

$$\theta \sim \text{Normal}(\mu_0, \sigma_0^2)$$

$$\psi \sim \text{Gamma}(a, b)$$

$$\theta|\psi, y \sim \text{Normal}\left(\theta_n = \frac{\psi \sum_{i=1}^{n} y_i + \frac{\mu_0}{\sigma_0^2}}{n\psi + \frac{1}{\sigma_0^2}}, \sigma_n^2 = \frac{1}{n\psi + \frac{1}{\sigma_0^2}}\right) \quad \text{(see Eq. (4.8))}.$$

The point here is that, in this particular case with normally distributed observations, the Laplace approximation is not required for the denominator in Eq. (4.23). Moreover, even if the posterior distribution in (4.23) does not have any known form (i.e., it is not conjugate), it is valid for any value of θ. This means that the terms depending on θ in the numerator and denominator have to cancel out. The consequence is that we can fix and choose any arbitrary value for θ in Eq. (4.23) and a convenient choice is $\theta = \theta_n$ (i.e., the conditional posterior mode of θ). Given this, it follows that $p(\theta = \theta_n|\psi, y) = 1/\sqrt{2\pi\sigma_n^2}$ and

$$p(\psi|y) \propto \left. \frac{p(y|\theta, \psi)p(\theta)p(\psi)}{p(\theta|\psi, y)} \right|_{\theta=\theta_n} = \frac{1}{1/\sqrt{2\pi\sigma_n^2}} p(y|\theta, \psi)p(\theta)p(\psi)|_{\theta=\theta_n}. \tag{4.24}$$

In order to evaluate the (unnormalized) posterior distribution (4.24), some values for ψ are chosen,[12] included in the set $\{\psi^{(j)}\}$, and for each of them the value of the

---

[12] In this example with simulated data we choose for simplicity the most probable values for ψ whereas INLA adopts the grid strategy or CCD strategy described in Section 4.7.1.

density function is computed:

$$p(\psi^{(j)} \mid y) \propto \underbrace{\frac{1}{1/\sqrt{2\pi\sigma_n^2}}}_{} \underbrace{p(y \mid \theta = \theta_n, \sigma^2 = 1/\psi^{(j)})}_{\prod_{i=1}^{n} \text{Normal}(\theta_n, 1/\psi^{(j)})} \underbrace{p(\theta = \theta_n)}_{\text{Normal}(\mu_0, \sigma_0^2)} \underbrace{p(\psi^{(j)})}_{\text{Gamma}(a,b)} \quad (4.25)$$

where

$$\theta_n = \frac{\psi^{(j)} \sum_{i=1}^{n} y_i + \frac{\mu_0}{\sigma_0^2}}{n\psi^{(j)} + \frac{1}{\sigma_0^2}}$$

and

$$\sigma_n^2 = \frac{1}{n\psi^{(j)} + \frac{1}{\sigma_0^2}}.$$

We report here below the R code for computing the marginal posterior for ψ as in Eq. (4.25) with reference to some simulated data contained in the data vector y.

```
> # Load the data
> y <- c(1.2697,7.7637,2.2532,3.4557,4.1776,6.4320,-3.6623,7.7567,
  5.9032,7.2671,-2.3447,8.0160,3.5013,2.8495,0.6467,3.2371,
  5.8573,-3.3749,4.1507,4.3092,11.7327,2.6174,9.4942,-2.7639,
  -1.5859,3.6986,2.4544,-0.3294,0.2329,5.2846)
> n <- length(y)
> ybar <- mean(y)


> # Define the parameters of the prior distributions
> mu0 <- -3
> sigma2_0 <- 4
> a <- 1.6
> b <- 0.4


> # Select H grid points for the hyperparameter psi
> H <- 25
> psi.min <- 0.001
> psi.max <- 0.3
> psi.grid <- seq(psi.min,psi.max,length.out=H)
> hprior <- dgamma(psi.grid,shape=a,rate=b)


> # Compute quantities in Eq. (4.24)
> theta.n <- sigma2.n <- lik <- num <- den <- prior <- c()
> for (h in 1:H) {
    theta.n[h]    <- (psi.grid[h]*n*ybar + mu0/sigma2_0) /
                     (psi.grid[h]*n + 1/sigma2_0)
    sigma2.n[h]   <- 1 / (n*psi.grid[h] + 1/sigma2_0)
    prior[h]   <- dnorm(theta.n[h], mu0, sd=sqrt(sigma2_0))
    lik[h]     <- prod(dnorm(y, theta.n[h], sd=1/sqrt(psi.grid[h])))
    num[h]     <- hprior[h] * prior[h] * lik[h]
    den[h]     <- dnorm(theta.n[h], theta.n[h], sd=sqrt(sigma2.n[h]))
  }
```

```
> # Unnormalized marginal posterior for psi
> post.psi <- num/den
```

```
> # Normalise the density
> f.psi <- approxfun(psi.grid, post.psi,
                     yleft=min(psi.grid), yright=max(psi.grid))
> const <- integrate(f.psi, min(psi.grid), max(psi.grid))
> post.psi <- post.psi/const$value
```

The normalized posterior distribution for ψ (post.psi) is depicted in the top panel of Figure 4.15. It can be seen that the distribution is quite skewed: this is an effect of not transforming ψ into some more normal-shaped distribution, using, for example, the logarithm transformation. Note that INLA adopts suitable transformation in order to make everything smoother and the choice of integration points easier (avoiding in this way numerical problems).

The second task concerns the evaluation of the full conditional distribution $p(\theta|\psi,y)$ for each value of ψ in $\{\psi^{(j)}\}$ and of θ in the set $\{\theta^{(l)}\}$. This consists in evaluating $p(\theta = \theta^{(l)}|\psi = \psi^{(j)},y)$ using the Normal(θ_n, σ_n^2) distribution. Then the marginal posterior distribution $p(\theta|y)$ can be obtained by integrating out ψ from the joint posterior $p(\theta, \psi|y)$ through a finite weighted mean as in Eq. (4.22):

$$p(\theta = \theta^{(l)}|y) \propto \sum_j p(\theta^{(l)} \mid \psi^{(j)},y)p(\psi^{(j)} \mid y)\Delta_j, \qquad (4.26)$$

where in this case $\Delta_j = \Delta = \frac{1}{\sum_j p(\psi^{(j)}|y)}$. The code for the second task is as follows:

```
> # Select J grid points for the parameter theta
> J <- 50
> min.theta <- -8
> max.theta <- 5
> theta.grid <- seq(min.theta,max.theta,length.out=J)
```

```
> # Full conditional distributions theta | psi,y
> full.cond.theta <- matrix(NA,J,H)
> for (j in 1:J) {
    for (h in 1:H) {
      full.cond.theta[j,h] <- dnorm(theta.grid[j], theta.n[h],
                               sd=sqrt(sigma2.n[h]))
    }
  }
```

```
> # Weighted joint posterior for theta and psi
> Delta <- 1/sum(post.psi)
> joint.post.theta.psi <- matrix(NA,J,H)
> for (h in 1:H) {
    joint.post.theta.psi[,h] <- full.cond.theta[,h] * post.psi[h]*
                                Delta
  }
```

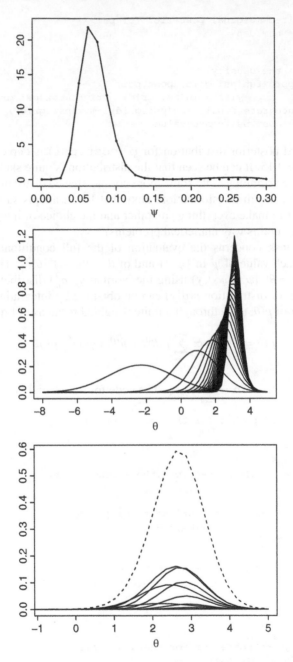

Figure 4.15   Top panel: posterior distribution of ψ with black dots denoting the set of values {ψ^(j)}. Middle panel: full conditional distributions of θ|ψ^(j), y for each values of ψ in {ψ^(j)}. Bottom panel: the dashed curve denotes the posterior distribution of θ given by Eq. (4.26), computed as finite sum of the weighted joint posterior distributions – given by p(θ^(l)|ψ^(j),y)p(ψ^(j))Δ_j – which are depicted with solid lines.

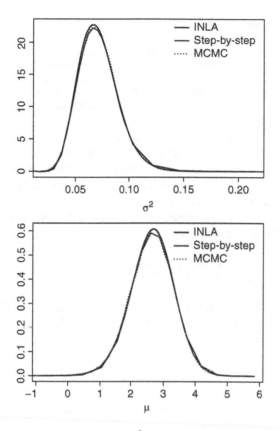

Figure 4.16   Posterior distribution of σ^2 (top) and μ (bottom) obtained with the step-by-step approach, an MCMC algorithm, and R-INLA.

```
> # Integrate out psi to obtain the marginal posterior of theta
> marg.post.theta <- rowSums(joint.post.theta.psi)


> # Now normalise the density
> f.theta <- approxfun(theta.grid,marg.post.theta,
                     yleft=min(theta.grid), yright=max(theta.grid))
> const <- integrate(f.theta,min(theta.grid),max(theta.grid))
> marg.post.theta <- marg.post.theta/const$value
```

The full conditional distributions (full.cond.theta) and the weighted joint posterior distributions (joint.post.theta.psi) as well as the normalized posterior distribution of θ (marg.post.theta) are represented in the central and bottom panels of Figure 4.15.

We compare the results obtained here with the step-by-step approach with the output of R-INLA and of a MCMC-based approach via Gibbs sampling (as described in Section 4.5.1). We first define the INLA formula just including the intercept

```
> formula <- y ~ 1
```

and finally we run the `inla` function

```
> inla.output <- inla(formula, data = data.frame(y = y),
                       control.family = list(hyper = list(prec =
                       list(prior = "loggamma", param = c(a, b)))),
                       control.fixed = list(mean.intercept = mu0,
                                         prec.intercept = 1/sigma2_0))
```

where we use the `control.family` and `control.fixed` options in order to specify the prior distributions for ψ and θ, respectively.

Note that R-INLA specifies a logGamma(a, b) distribution on the logarithm of the precision $\log(\psi)$, which is equivalent to fix a Gamma(a, b) on the precision ψ (with the same a and b parameters).

The marginal posterior distributions are retrieved from the `inla.output` object with the following commands:

```
> inla.output$marginals.hyperpar[[1]]
> inla.output$marginals.fixed$"(Intercept)"
```

and are represented in Figure 4.16 together with the corresponding distributions obtained with the step-by-step approach and with MCMC; as expected the curves are almost identical.

References

Banerjee, S., Carlin, B., and Gelfand, A. (2004). *Hierarchical Modeling and Analysis for Spatial Data*. Chapman & Hall.

Belitz, C., Brezger, A., Kneib, T., Lang, S., and Umlauf, N. (2012). BayesX – Software for Bayesian inference in structured additive regression model. Version 2.1. Available from `http://www.stat.uni-muenchen.de/~bayesx`.

Brooks, S., Gelman, A., Jones, G., and Meng, X., editors (2011). *Handbook of Markov Chain Monte Carlo*. CRC Press, Taylor & Francis Group.

Casella, G. and Berger, R. (2002). *Statistical Inference*. Duxbury, Thomson Learning.

Casella, G. and George, E. (1992). Explaining the Gibbs Sampler. *The American Statistician*, **46**, 167–174.

Chib, S. and Greenberg, E. (1995). Understanding the Metropolis–Hastings algorithm. *The American Statistician*, **49**, 327–335.

Cowles, M. and Carlin, B. (1996). Markov chain Monte Carlo convergence diagnostics: A comparative review. *Journal of the American Statistical Association*, **91**, 883–904.

Gelfand, A. and Smith, A. (1990). Sampling-based approaches to calculating marginal densities. *Journal of the American Statistical Association*, **85**, 398–409.

Gelman, A., Carlin, J., Stern, H., and Rubin, D. (2003). *Bayesian Data Analysis, Second Edition*. Chapman & Hall/CRC.

Geman, S. and Geman, D. (1984). Stochastic relaxation, Gibbs distributions and the Bayesian restoration of images. *IEEE Transactions on Pattern Analysis and Machine Intelligence*, **6**, 721–741.

Gentle, J. (2009). *Computational Statistics*. Springer.

Geyer, C. J. (1992). Practical Markov chain Monte Carlo. *Statistical Science*, **7**(4), pp. 473–483.

Gilks, W., Richardson, S., and Spiegelhalter, D. (1996). *Markov Chain Monte Carlo in Practice*. Chapman & Hall/CRC.

Hastings, W. (1970). Monte Carlo sampling methods using Markov chains and their application. *Biometrika*, **57**, 97–109.

Hoff, P. (2009). *A First Course in Bayesian Statistical Methods*. Springer.

Jona Lasinio, G., Mastrantonio, G., and Pollice, A. (2012). Discussing the "big n problem." *Statistical Methods & Applications*, pp. 1–16.

Lange, K. (2010). *Numerical Analysis for Statisticians*. Springer.

Lunn, D., Thomas, A., Best, N., and Spiegelhalter, D. (2000). WinBUGS – a Bayesian modelling framework: Concepts, structure, and extensibility. *Statistics and Computing*, **10**, 325–337.

Martino, S. and Rue, H. (2010a). Case studies in Bayesian computation using INLA. In P. Mantovan and P. Secchi, editors, *Complex Data Modeling and Computationally Intensive Statistical Methods*, Contributions to Statistics.

Martino, S. and Rue, H. (2010b). *Implementing Approximate Bayesian Inference using Integrated Nested Laplace Approximation: A manual for the INLA program*.

Martins, T. G., Simpson, D., Lindgren, F., and Rue, H. (2013). Bayesian computing with INLA: New features. *Computational Statistics & Data Analysis*, **67**, 68–83.

Metropolis, N., Rosenbluth, A., Teller, A., and Teller, E. (1953). Equation of state calculations by fast computing machines. *Journal of Chemical Physics*, **21**(6), 1087–1092.

Ntzoufras, I. (2009). *Bayesian Modeling Using WinBUGS*. John Wiley and Sons.

Park, J., Martn, A., and Quinn, K. (2012). CRAN task view: Bayesian inference. http://cran.r-project.org/web/views/Bayesian.html.

Plummer, M. (2003). JAGS: A program for analysis of Bayesian graphical models using Gibbs sampling. In *Proceedings of the 3rd International Workshop on Distributed Statistical Computing*.

Plummer, M., Best, N., Cowles, K., and Vines, K. (2006). Coda: Convergence diagnosis and output analysis for MCMC. *R News*, **6**, 7–11.

Press, W., Teukolsky, S., Vetterling, W., and Flannery, B. (2007). *Numerical Recipes. The Art of Scientific Computing*. Cambridge University Press.

Ripley, B., editor (1987). *Stochastic Simulation*. John Wiley and Sons.

Robert, C. and Casella, G. (2004). *Monte Carlo Statistical Methods*. Springer.

Robert, C. and Casella, G. (2011). A short history of Markov chain Monte Carlo: Subjective recollections from incomplete data. *Statistical Science*, **26**, 102–115.

Rue, H. and Held, L. (2005). *Gaussian Markov Random Fields. Theory and Applications*. Chapman & Hall.

Rue, H. and Martino, S. (2007). Approximate Bayesian inference for hierarchical Gaussian Markov random fields models. *Journal of Statistical Planning and Inference*, **137**, 3177–3192.

Rue, H., Martino, S., and Chopin, N. (2009). Approximate Bayesian inference for latent Gaussian model by using integrated nested Laplace approximations (with discussion). *Journal of Royal Statistical Society, Series B*, **71**, 319–392.

Tanner, M. (1993). *Tools for Statistical Inference.Methods for the Exploration of Posterior Distribution and Likelihood Functions*. Springer.

Tierney, L. and Kadane, J. (1986). Accurate approximations for posterior moments and marginal densities. *Journal of the American Statistical Association*, **81**, 82–86.

Van Belle, G., Fisher, L., Heagerty, P., and Lumley, T. (2004). *Biostatistics: A Methodology for the Health Sciences*. John Wiley and Sons.

5

Bayesian regression and hierarchical models

Regression models are nowadays probably the statistical methods most commonly used to assess the presence of a relationship between a dependent variable and one or more independent variables (also called predictors). They were originally proposed by Galton (1886), who developed the first linear regression to explain how stature was hereditary between generations. In the Bayesian framework, one of the first applications of regression models can be found in econometrics (Zellner, 1971) to work with lognormal distributions. In the last three decades, other important contributions have appeared on generalized linear models (see for instance Ibrahim and Purushottam, 1991; Dellaportas and Smith, 1993), or on complex nonlinear structures like in pharmacokinetics models (Gelman *et al.*, 1996). Nowadays, the Bayesian approach to regression models is universally accepted and widely used as seen in many publications such as Gelman *et al.* (2004) and Congdon (2007), who extensively present Bayesian regression models with applications to different fields, from sociology to epidemiology.

Given a vector of n observations $\boldsymbol{y} = (y_1, y_2, \ldots, y_n)$ (also called outcome or response), in a typical regression model there are two steps which need to be followed: first we have to specify a suitable probability distribution for the observations and second we need to identify the type of relationship between the predictor(s) and $\boldsymbol{y}$, or, in other words, how the distribution of the outcome depends on the predictor(s). In the Bayesian approach, additionally to these two steps, we need to specify the prior distribution for the regression coefficients, as well as for any other unknown nuisance parameters (e.g., the variance of the outcome if appropriate).

Spatial and Spatio-temporal Bayesian Models with R-INLA, First Edition.
Marta Blangiardo and Michela Cameletti.
© 2015 John Wiley & Sons, Ltd. Published 2015 by John Wiley & Sons, Ltd.

5.1 Linear regression

The simplest regression model assumes a linear relationship between the predictors and the outcome; each outcome y_i is normally distributed as follows:

$$y_i \sim \text{Normal}(\mu_i, \sigma^2). \tag{5.1}$$

Using the INLA notation, as presented in Section 4.7.1, we can specify the linear predictor η_i as a function of μ_i through the identity link $\eta_i = g(\mu_i) = \mu_i$ so that

$$\eta_i = \beta_0 + \sum_{m=1}^{M} \beta_m x_{im},$$

where x_{im} is the value of the mth predictor (or covariate) for the ith unit. This is equivalent to the more commonly presented form:

$$E(y_i \mid \beta_0, \dots, \beta_M, x_{i1}, \dots, x_{iM}) = \beta_0 + \sum_{m=1}^{M} \beta_m x_{im}.$$

A prior distribution needs to be specified on the regression parameters $\beta = \{\beta_0, \dots, \beta_M\}$ and on the variance σ^2 of the outcome. In the absence of information, the typical choice of prior is a vague one (recall Section 3.6.3 for a discussion on the common choices of prior distribution) such as

$$\beta_m \sim \text{Normal}(0, 10^6), \qquad m = 1, \dots, M \tag{5.2}$$

$$\log(\tau) = \log(1/\sigma^2) \sim \text{logGamma}(1, 10^{-5}). \tag{5.3}$$

The aim is to perform the inferential process and to obtain the posterior distribution for β and σ^2.

5.1.1 Comparing the Bayesian to the classical regression model

Let y be the $n \times 1$ vector of outcomes and X the $n \times (1 + M)$ matrix of covariates, with generic element x_{im} and with the first column given by a vector of 1's for the intercept β_0; in the classical frequentist approach the maximum likelihood estimate of β is

$$\hat{\beta} = (X'X)^{-1}X'y$$

with standard error

$$\text{se}(\hat{\beta}) = \sqrt{s^2(X'X)^{-1}},$$

where $s^2 = (y - X\hat{\beta})'(y - X\hat{\beta})/(n - M)$ is the estimate of σ^2. For more details on the maximum likelihood estimates, refer to Casella and Berger (2002). To obtain the $(100 - \alpha)\%$ confidence interval for the mth regression coefficient the following formula is used:

$$\hat{\beta}_m \pm t_{n-M, \alpha/2} \, \text{se}(\hat{\beta}_m),$$

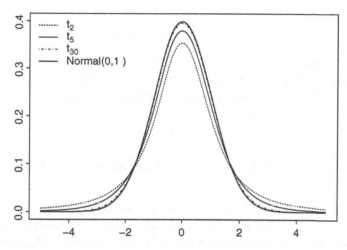

Figure 5.1   Density function for a zero mean Student t with different degrees of freedom (df). As the number of degrees of freedom increases, the Student t tends to a standard Normal distribution and approaches it for df≥ 30.

where $\hat{\beta}_m$ is the mth element of $\hat{\beta}$, $t_{n-M,\alpha/2}$ is the $\alpha/2$ quantile of a Student t distribution with mean equal to 0, variance equal to 1 and $n - M$ degrees of freedom (df), while se($\hat{\beta}_m$) is the mth element on the diagonal of se($\hat{\beta}$).

The Student t distribution, denoted by $t_{\text{df}}(\mu, \sigma^2)$, is symmetric and bell shaped as the Gaussian distribution, but it is characterized by three parameters: the mean, the variance, and the degrees of freedom, which govern how heavy the tails are, or in other words, how likely values far from the mean will occur. Smaller degrees of freedom correspond to a distribution with heavier tails, while when df ≥ 30 the Student t approaches the standard Normal distribution. See Figure 5.1 for the density function of a Student t with different degrees of freedom.

In the Bayesian approach, assuming noninformative priors on β and σ^2, so that $p(\beta_m) \propto 1$ for each m and $p(\log(\sigma^2)) \propto 1$,[1] the conditional posterior for β has a multivariate Normal distribution:

$$\beta \mid \sigma^2, y, X \sim \text{MVNormal}((X'X)^{-1}X'y, \sigma^2(X'X)^{-1}),$$

whose parameters are equivalent to those of the classical regression formulation (Casella and Berger, 2002). In addition, to obtain the marginal posterior for β_m, we need to integrate out σ^2:

$$p(\beta_m \mid y, X) = \int_0^{+\infty} p(\beta_m \mid \sigma^2, y, X) d\sigma^2, \tag{5.4}$$

---

[1] In general, the notation $p(\theta) \propto 1$ is equivalent to specify a Uniform prior on the appropriate scale (e.g., $(0, +\infty)$ for a precision).

which leads to

$$\beta_m \mid y, X \sim t_{n-M}(\hat{\beta}_m, \text{se}(\hat{\beta}_m)^2)$$

showing the same results as the classical regression. However, recall that the interpretation is diametrically different, as in the Bayesian framework β_m is characterized by a proability distribution, while in the frequentist framework it is a fixed unknown quantity and only its estimator, which is a function of the data used to infer values about β_m, is a random variable.

5.1.2 Example: studying the relationship between temperature and PM_{10}

In this section, we use the National Morbidity and Mortality Air Pollution Study described in Section 1.4.1 to assess the presence of a linear relationship between temperature and air pollution concentration. We consider daily PM_{10} concentration ($\mu g/m^3$) and temperature (°F) in Salt Lake City between 1987 and 2000 (the name of the dataframe is dataNMMAPS). The distribution of the data was presented in Figure 1.1. The model considered is

$$PM_{10i} \sim \text{Normal}(\mu_i, \sigma^2); \qquad \eta_i = \mu_i = \beta_0 + \beta_1 \text{Temp}_i; \qquad i = 1, \ldots, n \text{ days}$$

with a vague prior on β_0, β_1, and σ^2. This model can be run in R-INLA using the following commands:

```
> formula <-  pm10 ~ 1 + temperature
```

where 1 means that the model includes the intercept and

```
> model.linear <- inla(formula,family="gaussian",data=dataNMMAPS)
> round(model.linear$summary.fixed[,1:5],3)
              Mean     SD 0.025quant 0.5quant 0.975quant
(Intercept) 38.725 0.984     36.793   38.725     40.655
temperature -0.094 0.017     -0.128   -0.094     -0.060
```

which returns estimates of the marginal posterior mean, standard deviation (mean and SD) and 95% credibility intervals. The command model.linear $marginals.fixed returns a list with the posterior densities of the regression coefficients, which are shown in Figure 5.2.

If we compare this model with the following standard regression model obtained running the R function lm (see Section 2.6):

```
> summary(lm(formula,data=dataNMMAPS))
Call:
lm(formula = formula, data = dataNMMAPS)

Residuals:
    Min      1Q  Median      3Q     Max
-50.584 -14.941  -4.029   9.222 273.208
```

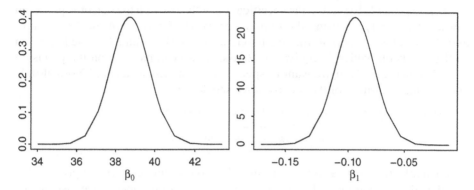

Figure 5.2   Posterior density plot for the intercept β_0 and slope β_1 of the linear regression model for the NMMAPS data.

```
Coefficients:
              Estimate Std. Error t value Pr(>|t|)
(Intercept) 38.72517    0.98373  39.366  < 2e-16 ***
temperature -0.09400    0.01746  -5.384 7.62e-08 ***
- - -
Signif. codes:  0 '***' 0.001 '**' 0.01 '*' 0.05 '.' 0.1 ' ' 1

Residual standard error: 22.84 on 5060 degrees of freedom
  (52 observations deleted due to missingness)
Multiple R-squared:  0.005696, Adjusted R-squared:  0.005499
F-statistic: 28.98 on 1 and 5060 DF,  p-value: 7.625e-08
```

we essentially obtain the same results as we are assuming noninformative prior distributions on all the parameters and we are not specifying any hierarchical structure, which will be seen in Section 5.4.3.

If we are interested in changing the prior for the regression parameters, for instance, reducing the variability on the prior for β_0 and β_1, specifying $\beta_0 \sim \text{Normal}(0, 10000)$ and $\beta_1 \sim \text{Normal}(0, 1)$, we can achieve it in R-INLA using the option control.fixed:

```
> model.linear <- inla(formula,family="gaussian", data=dataNMMAPS,
                  control.fixed=list(mean=0, prec=1,
                  mean.intercept=0, prec.intercept=0.0001))
```

where mean and prec represent the mean and precision of the regression parameters, respectively (excluding the intercept, whose parameters can be accessed through mean.intercept and prec.intercept).[2]

---

[2] Note that when the model includes more than one fixed effect, a list has to be specified. For example, control.fixed=list(mean=list(a=1, b=2, default=0)) assigns prior mean equal to 1 for fixed effect a and equal to 2 for b; all the other fixed effects have a zero prior mean. The same holds for the precision prec.

It is also possible to modify the specification of the prior on the outcome precision (remember $\tau = 1/\sigma^2$) using the option `control.family` of the `inla` command. By default, a noninformative logGamma prior is assumed on the logarithm of the precision, which is equivalent to assume a Gamma prior on the precision $\tau \sim \text{Gamma}(1, 10^{-5})$; if we want to specify, for instance, a standard Normal$(0, 1)$ prior on the logarithm of the precision we should write:

```
> model.linear <- inla(formula,family="gaussian",
                        data=dataNMMAPS,
                        control.family=list(hyper=list(
                        prec=list(prior="gaussian",param=c(0,1))))))
```

When information is available, it might be more intuitive to set the prior on the standard deviation σ instead of on the log precision. For instance, if we assume that the standard deviation of the observations is uniformly distributed between 2 and 14, we could use this simple R code to obtain the equivalent values of the parameters on the log precision scale to be included in the `inla` function[3]:

```
> #Parameters for sigma
> a1 <- 2
> b1 <- 14
> #Simulate sigma from a Uniform distribution
> sigma <- runif(n=10000,min=a1,max=b1)
> #Check the mean and variance of sigma
> mean(sigma); var(sigma)
[1] 8.005617
[1] 12.13075
> #Obtain the precision
> tau <- 1/sigma^2
> #Calculate the values of a and b for the distribution of the
  #precision
> a2 <- mean(tau)^2/var(tau)
> b2 <- a2/mean(tau)
> #Plot the values of the precision
> plot(density(tau))
> #Plot the distribution of a Gamma with a and b parameters
> curve(dgamma(x,a2,rate=b2), from=0, to=max(tau), add=T, lty=2)
```

So simply setting in R-INLA

```
> inla(...,control.family=list(hyper=list(
      prec=list(prior="loggamma",param=c(a2,b2))))))
```

will specify the prior obtained above on the log precision.

5.2 Nonlinear regression: random walk

The results from the linear regression seen in the previous section seem counter-intuitive as they show a small average decrease in PM_{10} (-0.09 µg/m^3) when the

---

[3] Note that for a generic Gamma distribution X with given mean $E(X)$ and variance $Var(X)$ the shape and scale parameters can be computed as $a = E(X)^2/Var(X)$ and $b = a/E(X)$, see Eq. (3.15).

temperature increases by 1°F. The standardized residuals, calculated as $\frac{y_i - \hat{\mu}_i}{\hat{\sigma}_i}$ with $\hat{\mu}_i = \hat{\beta}_0 + \hat{\beta}_1 \text{Temp}_i$, can also be used to evaluate the departure of the model from the observations. The code to obtain these quantities is the following:

```
> model.linear <- inla(formula,family="gaussian",
                       data=dataNMMAPS,
                       control.predictor=list(compute=TRUE))
> res.lin <- (dataNMMAPS$pm10 -
              model.linear$summary.fitted.values$mean) /
              model.linear$summary.fitted.values$sd
```

where `summary.fitted.values` is an object of the `inla` outcome when the option `control.predictor` is set to `TRUE` and reports the summary of the predicted values $\hat{\mu}_i$ as follows:

```
> #output partially omitted (only first 5 rows are shown)
> round(model.linear$summary.fitted.values[1:5,1:5],3)
                       Mean    SD 0.025quant 0.5quant 0.975quant
fitted.predictor.0001 35.952 0.525    34.924   35.952     36.981
fitted.predictor.0002 35.529 0.465    34.618   35.529     36.441
fitted.predictor.0003 35.247 0.429    34.407   35.247     36.088
fitted.predictor.0004 34.730 0.372    34.001   34.730     35.460
fitted.predictor.0005 35.435 0.453    34.548   35.435     36.323
```

Looking at the residuals on a plot (Figure 5.3, top), it is clear how they are characterized by a cyclic pattern, which could be explained by the seasonality of temperature that has not been taken into account in the model and can confound the true relationship with PM_{10}. A relatively crude and easy way to allow for this is to include a month effect as a categorical variable in the regression (recall that a categorical variable is specified as a `factor` in R; see Section 2.2):

```
> month <- substring(as.character(dataNMMAPS$date), first=4, last=6)
> dataNMMAPS$month <- factor(month,
                levels=c("Jan","Feb","Mar","Apr","May","Jun",
                         "Jul","Aug","Sep","Oct","Nov","Dec"))
> formula.inla2 <- pm10 ~ 1 + temperature + month
> model.linear2 <- inla(formula.inla2,family="gaussian",
                        data=dataNMMAPS,
                        control.predictor = list(compute = TRUE))
> round(model.linear2$summary.fixed[,1:5],3)
                Mean     SD 0.025quant 0.5quant 0.975quant
(Intercept)   39.661  1.613     36.495   39.661     42.825
temperature    0.129  0.040      0.052    0.129      0.207
monthFeb      -3.592  1.535     -6.607   -3.592     -0.580
monthMar     -18.879  1.584    -21.989  -18.879    -15.772
monthApr     -22.199  1.712    -25.560  -22.199    -18.841
monthMay     -23.632  1.892    -27.348  -23.632    -19.920
monthJun     -18.159  2.149    -22.378  -18.159    -13.942
monthJul     -14.214  2.389    -18.904  -14.214     -9.527
monthAug     -14.381  2.366    -19.027  -14.381     -9.739
```

```
monthSep      -12.754 2.064     -16.806  -12.755      -8.706
monthOct      -12.900 1.747     -16.329  -12.900      -9.474
monthNov      -12.302 1.545     -15.335  -12.302      -9.272
monthDec       -0.741 1.491      -3.669   -0.741       2.185
```

Taking into account the month leads to a substantial change in the temperature coefficient: now an average increment in PM_{10} (0.13 µg/m^3) occurs when the temperature increases by 1°F. The residuals are smaller and the cyclic pattern is reduced (Figure 5.3, centre).

A more realistic and complex model assumes that the levels of PM_{10} are likely to change slowly and to show a degree of temporal correlation (e.g., to be similar in consecutive days); this is a structure which will be seen extensively in Chapter 7 in relation to space–time models. There are different ways of specifying the temporal correlation and we consider here the commonly used *random walk* (RW).

Given a time ordered vector $z_1, \ldots, z_T$, a random walk is a model defined by an order r so that z_t only depends on the previous $t - r$ elements (Feller, 1968). The simplest RW model is defined when $r = 1$, so that the conditional distribution of z_t given all the other elements of the vector is

$$z_t \mid z_{t-1} \sim \text{Normal}(z_{t-1}, \sigma^2). \tag{5.5}$$

We include a RW of order 1 in the model to explain the residual temporal effect of PM_{10}, so that the formula changes as follows:

```
> formula.inla3 <- pm10 ~ 1 + temperature + month +
                 f(id, model="rw1",
                   hyper = list(prec = list(
                   prior="loggamma",param=c(1,0.01)))))
```

where f(id, model="rw1") specifies the nonlinear function (random walk structure) on the days in the period under study, identified by id. See Section 4.8 for the list of the available nonlinear functions in R-INLA. Note that, as shown in Eq. (5.5), the random walk structure is characterized by a variance parameter, on which we need to specify a prior distribution. R-INLA models the precision using the option hyper of f(), as shown in the code above.

```
> model.linear3 <- inla(formula.inla3,family="gaussian",
                  data=dataNMMAPS,
                  control.predictor = list(compute = TRUE))
> round(model.linear3$summary.fixed[,1:5],3)
               Mean     SD 0.025quant 0.5quant 0.975quant
(Intercept)  12.282 4.433      3.578   12.282     20.976
temperature   0.511 0.047      0.419    0.511      0.603
monthFeb     -3.925 3.935    -11.651   -3.925      3.794
monthMar     -6.648 5.175    -16.809   -6.649      3.505
monthApr     -9.971 5.920    -21.593   -9.971      1.644
monthMay     -6.053 6.351    -18.520   -6.053      6.407
monthJun     -3.617 6.589    -16.552   -3.617      9.309
monthJul     -8.195 6.663    -21.278   -8.195      4.877
monthAug     -5.852 6.589    -18.789   -5.852      7.075
```

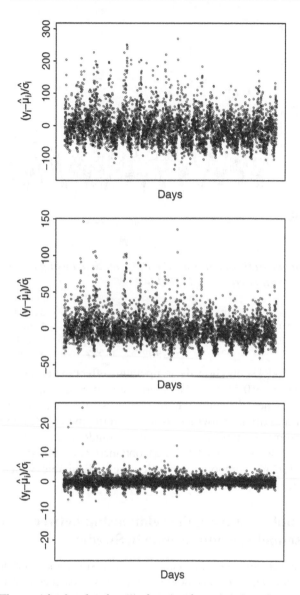

Figure 5.3   The residuals plot for (i) the simple univariate linear regression to explain PM$_{10}$ as a function of temperature (top), (ii) the linear regression adding the month as predictor (centre) and (iii) the linear regression including also a nonlinear effect of time (bottom). Note that a different scale is maintained in the three plots to make them readable.

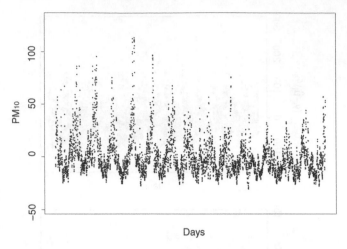

Figure 5.4   The posterior means for the PM$_{10}$ modeled using a random walk spec-ification. A temporal correlation is visible.

```
monthSep      -8.890 6.361    -21.379    -8.891    3.588
monthOct     -10.145 5.943    -21.812   -10.145    1.514
monthNov      -8.603 5.247    -18.904    -8.603    1.692
monthDec       1.522 4.070     -6.469     1.522    9.506
```

Running this model shows how the temperature effect increases further: the poste-rior mean reaches now 0.51 µg/m^3 indicating an increase of around half microgram per cubic meter when the temperature increases of 1°F; in addition the residu-als are smaller and do not show a seasonal pattern anymore (Figure 5.3, bottom). Figure 5.4 presents the posterior mean of the random walk of order 1 specified through f(id, model="rw1", ...) obtained using the summary.random function of R-INLA: a temporal correlation is clearly visible, which is expected as a result of the random walk structure.

5.2.1   Example: studying the relationship between average household age and income in Sweden

We use the dataset described in Section 1.4.2 to study the relationship between average age of the head of household (x) and the standardized average household income for 284 municipalities in Sweden (y). A standard linear regression model is specified as follows for $i = 1, \ldots, n$:

$$y_i \sim \text{Normal}(\mu_i, \sigma^2) \tag{5.6}$$

$$\eta_i = \mu_i = \beta_0 + \beta_1(\text{Age}_i - \overline{\text{Age}}),$$

where y is standardized removing the sample mean and dividing by the sample stan-dard deviation through the R command scale, while the age is centered around its mean. To implement this model in R-INLA the following code is used:

```
> data.income$age.centered <- scale(data.income$age, scale=FALSE)
> data.income$income.scaled <- scale(data.income$income, scale=TRUE)
> formula.inla <- income.scaled ~ 1 + age.centered
> model.linear <- inla(formula.inla,family="gaussian",
                    data=data.income,
                    control.predictor=list(compute=TRUE))
```

The regression coefficients are presented in Table 5.1 (left) showing how the average income tends to be higher for older head of households, with a posterior mean for β_1 equal to 0.136. Figure 5.5 (top) shows the scatterplot of the average household income versus average age of the head of household. The fitted regression line is also plotted. An extreme point is visible on the right bottom end of the plot, corresponding to the municipality with the highest average head age but the lowest average income. To avoid that this data point influences the regression estimates too strongly, it is possible to *robustify* the model, specifying Student t errors (or equivalently a Student t distribution) instead of Normal ones (or equivalently a Gaussian distribution), changing the first line of Eq. (5.6) into $y_i \sim t_{df}(\mu_i, \sigma^2)$ (and in R-INLA using family="T").

Note that to run this model in R-INLA, a function of the degrees of freedom, $\log(df - 2)$ is included as an additional parameter, called dof and by default is characterized by a Gamma(1, 0.5) distribution. If instead we want to fix the degrees of freedom, the option control.family needs to be called as follows:

```
> model.linearT <- inla(formula.inla, family="T",
                    data=data.income,
                    control.family=list(hyper=list(dof=
                                list(initial=0.693,fixed=TRUE))),
                    control.predictor=list(compute=TRUE))
```

Fixing dof to 0.693 is equivalent to assume that the degrees of freedom are 4, as $df = \exp(dof) + 2$. Looking at the results, presented in Table 5.1 (right), it can be appreciated that the association between age and income increases and the posterior mean of β_1 reaches now 0.183. This happens because the Student t has heavier tails, thus the presence of extreme observations has a smaller influence on its parameters, as can be seen in Figure 5.5 (bottom), where the regression line shows a steeper slope than observed using a Gaussian likelihood.

Table 5.1   Parameters of the regression model to explain the average household income as a function of age of the household head. The model with the Gaussian likelihood is on the left and the one with the Student t likelihood is on the right.

	Normal distribution Post. Mean (95% CI)	Robustified distribution Post. Mean (95% CI)
β_0 (Intercept)	0.000 (−0.108;0.107)	−0.003 (−0.099;0.092)
β_1 (Age-centered)	0.136 (−0.098;0.174)	0.183 (0.148;0.219)

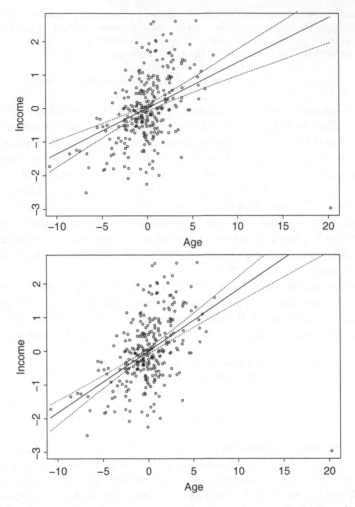

Figure 5.5   Scatter plot of average age and average income in the Swedish munic-ipalities when the likelihood is assumed Gaussian (top) or Student t (bottom). The solid line represents the posterior mean of the fitted values μ_i, while the dashed lines corresponds to the 95% credibility intervals for μ_i. Note how the regression line has a steeper slope when the Student t is specified.

5.3   Generalized linear models

Generalized linear models (GLM) is a class of models introduced by Nelder and Wedderburn (1972) and by McCullagh and Nelder (1989) with the aim of extending the linear regression to the case when the dependent variable is not necessarily normally distributed, but its distribution still belongs to the exponential family.[4] As all the commonly used random variables belong to this family, this assures that GLM can be widely used in (almost) any statistical analysis.

In Section 2.6, we have introduced how to run GLM models in R. In the next paragraphs, we present the two GLM mostly used in epidemiology and social science: logistic regression and Poisson regression and we show their use in R-INLA.

Logistic regression

Logistic regression is the standard model for binary outcomes (e.g., death); if $(y_1, \ldots, y_n)$ represent data for individual units (e.g., a person experiences or not death), then y_i will be distributed as a Bernoulli, which can only assume values 0 or 1. Alternatively, if $(y_1, \ldots, y_n)$ represent the counts of the event under study over a specified number of trials for n groups, then y_i will be distributed as a Binomial, which can assume values $0, 1, 2, \ldots, n_i$, where n_i represents the number of individual units for the ith group.

The parameter of interest is $\pi_i = p(y_i = 1 \mid x_i)$, where $x_i = (x_{i1}, \ldots, x_{iM})$ is the vector of M predictors for the ith individual or group. The link function is the $logit$, defined as

$$\text{logit}(\pi_i) = \log\left(\frac{\pi_i}{1 - \pi_i}\right) = x_i\beta$$

so that

$$\pi_i = \text{logit}^{-1}(x_i\beta) = \frac{\exp(x_i\beta)}{(1 + \exp(x_i\beta))}.$$

In other words, the antilogit function (i.e., logit^{-1}) transforms the continuous values obtained from $x_i\beta$ back into probabilities, the scale for the π_i parameter. The logistic regression model, also including an intercept β_0, can be written as follows:

$$y_i \sim \text{Binomial}(\pi_i, n_i) \tag{5.8}$$

$$\eta_i = \text{logit}(\pi_i) = \beta_0 + \sum_{m=1}^{M} \beta_m x_{im}.$$

To complete it, priors on $\{\beta_0, \beta_1, \ldots, \beta_M\}$ are specified typically as Normal distributions characterized by a large variability if no information is available from previous studies or expert opinion, similarly to Eq. (5.2).

---

[4] The Exponential family (Casella and Berger, 2002) is a class of random variables whose probability (if discrete) or density (if continuous) is given by

$$p(y) = \exp(s(y)\theta + \kappa(\theta) + c(y)). \tag{5.7}$$

The logarithm of $p(y)$ can be written as the sum of three components: a function of y, a function of the parameter θ and a function of both. Note that all the commonly used random variables belong to the Exponential family.

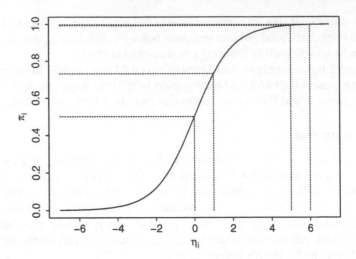

Figure 5.6   Inverse logit function $logit^{-1}(\eta_i)$. *The plot shows how the linear pre-dictor* η_i *is transformed to the probability scale with* $\pi_i = logit^{-1}(\eta_i)$.

It is important to note that the increase (or decrease) in π_i is not constant for all the differences in the values of the predictors. Figure 5.6 shows the $logit^{-1}$ as a function of the linear predictor η_i: in the middle of the curve the change in π_i is steeper, so for instance if η_i increases from 0 and 1, then π_i will change of 0.23 as

$$logit^{-1}(x_i\beta = 0) = 0.5 \text{ and } logit^{-1}(x_i\beta = 1) = 0.73.$$

On the other hand, an increase of one unit in η_i in the extreme part of the plot, e.g., between 5 and 6, corresponds to a 0.005 change in π_i as

$$logit^{-1}(x_i\beta = 5) = 0.993 \text{ and } logit^{-1}(x_i\beta = 6) = 0.998.$$

Using the $logit^{-1}(\beta_0)$ function only for the regression coefficient β_0, the output can be interpreted as the average probability of $y_i = 1$ when all the predictors are at their reference category (if categorical) or 0 (if numerical). The interpretation of the remaining parameters $\{\beta_1, \dots, \beta_M\}$ can also be obtained using the $logit^{-1}$ function. Assuming the simple case of only one predictor, $logit(\pi_i) = \beta_0 + \beta_1 x_i$, so when the predictor changes from x_i to $x_i + 1$ we have

$$p(y_i = 1 \mid x_i + 1) = logit^{-1}(\beta_0 + \beta_1(x_i + 1))$$
$$p(y_i = 1 \mid x_i) = logit^{-1}(\beta_0 + \beta_1(x_i)),$$

then calculating $p(y_i = 1 \mid x_i + 1) - p(y_i = 1 \mid x_i)$ gives the difference in the probability that we are interested in.

Alternatively, the odds ratio can be used to interpret β. Using the definition of logit, and considering again the simple case of one predictor, we can define the following log odds:

$$\text{log odds}(x+1) : \log\left(\frac{p(y_i = 1 \mid x_i + 1)}{p(y_i = 0 \mid x_i + 1)}\right) = \beta_0 + \beta_1(x_i + 1),$$

$$\text{log odds}(x) : \log\left(\frac{p(y_i = 1 \mid x_i)}{p(y_i = 0 \mid x_i)}\right) = \beta_0 + \beta_1(x_i).$$

Then the difference between the two log odds is β_1 and, exponentiating it we get the so-called odds-ratio (OR):

$$\exp\left(\frac{\text{log odds}(x+1)}{\text{log odds}(x)}\right) = \exp(\beta_1),$$

so the exponential of β_1 represents the change in the odds ratio when x_i increases by one unit. This second type of interpretation is the most used in epidemiological studies and we will see it extensively in Chapters 6 and 7.

Example: studying stroke mortality in Sheffield (UK)

Using the data presented in Chapter 1.4.3, we want to assess the presence of an association between levels of NOx and stroke mortality in Sheffield, UK. We consider annual NOx concentration measured in $\mu g/m^3$ in quintiles (denoted by Qu_k), averaged over the period 1994–1999, and number of deaths for stroke in each enumeration district in Sheffield. Recall from the previous section that as y is a count of events it follows a Binomial distribution, so that we can specify the following logistic regression:

$$y_i \sim \text{Binomial}(\pi_i, n_i) \tag{5.9}$$

$$\eta_i = \text{logit}(\pi_i) = \beta_0 + \sum_{k=2}^{5} \beta_{1k} I(\text{NOx}_i \in Qu_k) + \sum_{h=2}^{5} \beta_{2h} I(Z_i \in Qu_h) + \text{logit}(\tilde{p}_i),$$

where n_i is the population for the ith enumeration district and Z is the Townsend index of disadvantage and deprivation (in quintiles denoted by Qu_h) proposed by Townsend (1987) to measure social deprivation of the area (the higher the category, the more severe the deprivation) and that we include as a potential confounder. The term $\tilde{p}_i$ represents age-sex adjusted risk of stroke mortality calculated using indirect standardization with internal reference rates based on 18 strata (9 for age classes and 2 for genders) and which is used as baseline risk in the model (Maheswaran et al., 2006):

```
> Stroke$Adjusted.prob <- Stroke$stroke_exp/Stroke$pop
Stroke$logit.adjusted.prob <- log(Stroke$Adjusted.prob/
                                  (1-Stroke$Adjusted.prob))
```

This is a very simplistic model as it does not include area-specific coefficients; we will use a more complex model to analyze these data in the hierarchical models Section 5.4.6. This model can be run in R-INLA using the following command:

```
> formula.inla <- y ~ 1 + factor(NOx) + factor(Townsend) +
                      offset(logit.adjusted.prob)
> model.logistic <- inla(formula.inla,
                         family="binomial", Ntrials=pop, data=Stroke)
```

where `Ntrials` specifies the population at risk for each area (n_i in Eq. (5.9)). As we want to make the areas comparable in terms of demographic structure, we include the standardized risks of stroke mortality as offset with `offset(logit.adjusted.prob)`, so that $\tilde{p}_i$ is treated as a known component in the regression, characterized by a fixed coefficient equal to 1. The results are the following:

```
> round(model.logistic$summary.fixed[,1:5],3)
                    mean     SD 0.025quant 0.5quant 0.975quant
(Intercept)       -0.181  0.057     -0.293   -0.180     -0.071
factor(NOx)2       0.132  0.059      0.016    0.132      0.248
factor(NOx)3       0.105  0.061     -0.014    0.105      0.225
factor(NOx)4       0.261  0.059      0.144    0.261      0.377
factor(NOx)5       0.425  0.062      0.302    0.425      0.547
factor(Townsend)2  0.077  0.061     -0.043    0.077      0.198
factor(Townsend)3  0.137  0.060      0.020    0.137      0.255
factor(Townsend)4 -0.132  0.063     -0.255   -0.132     -0.009
factor(Townsend)5 -0.118  0.067     -0.250   -0.118      0.014
```

Note that as NOx and Townsend index are treated as categorical variables (using `factor`), their first categories are used as reference and no coefficients are estimated for these. To obtain the average probability of stroke mortality we need to apply the logit^{-1} function on the entire posterior marginal of the intercept. This could be done using the command `inla.tmarginal`, which calculates the posterior marginal for any transformation of the original parameter:

```
> prob.stroke <- inla.tmarginal(function(x) exp(x)/(1+exp(x)),
                       model.logistic$marginals.fixed[[1]])
```

Moreover, the function `inla.zmarginal` provides a table with summary statistics of the transformed posterior marginal:

```
> inla.zmarginal(prob.stroke)
Mean              0.455023
Stdev             0.0138584
Quantile  0.025  0.427566
Quantile  0.25   0.445596
Quantile  0.5    0.455045
Quantile  0.75   0.464434
Quantile  0.975  0.482031
```

If we simply apply the antilogit transformation to the posterior mean of the intercept obtained above ($\exp(-0.181)/(1 + \exp(-0.181))$ =0.455), we would get very similar results. This happens when the posterior distribution for the parameter is Gaussian, and such distribution is invariant to transformations. Notwithstanding this, as a general rule it is recommended to apply the required transformation on the entire posterior distribution (using `inla.tmarginal`), to avoid biases in the results.

In addition to the probability of stroke mortality, it is interesting to transform the coefficients of the models on the natural scale (e.g., exponentiate them), to provide an easier interpretation of the association between predictors and outcome. For instance, to assess the effect of NOx exposure on the probability of stroke mortality, we can simply exponentiate the corresponding β distribution, using again `inla.tmarginal` and then `inla.zmarginal`. Alternatively, if we are solely interested in the posterior mean we could simply apply the `inla.emarginal` function:

```
> inla.emarginal(exp, model.logistic$marginals.fixed$"factor(NOx)2")
[1] 1.142787
```

which reports an increment of 14.3 % in the probability of stroke mortality when the NOx exposure goes from the first to the second category. Similarly for the other categories we obtain a 11.3%, 30%, and 53.2% increase in the probability of stroke mortality going from the first to the third class, to the fourth and to the fifth class of exposure, respectively.

Poisson regression

In the previous section, we have described how the logistic regression can be used with count of successes over number of trials. Similarly, the Poisson regression is used when the outcome variable represents count data, so that it can assume discrete value between 0 and $+\infty$ (0, 1, 2, 3, ...), but there is no running limit equivalent to the number of trials. A typical epidemiological example considers the number of hospitalizations or deaths in different areas or hospitals during a specific period of time.

The parameter of interest is the average number of events, $\lambda_i = E(y_i)$, and the link function is the *logarithm*, so that, considering only one predictor:

$$\eta_i = \log(\lambda_i) = x_i\beta \qquad \text{and} \qquad \lambda_i = \exp(x_i\beta).$$

In other words, the exponential (or antilog) function transforms the continuous values obtained applying $x_i\beta$ into the range of values of λ_i (see Figure 5.7).

A Poisson regression model can be specified as follows:

$$y_i \sim \text{Poisson}(\lambda_i) \tag{5.10}$$

$$\eta_i = \log(\lambda_i) = \beta_0 + \sum_{m=1}^{M} \beta_m x_{im}. \tag{5.11}$$

As seen before, to complete the model, priors on β are specified, typically as Normal distribution, characterized by a large variability if no information is available from previous studies or expert opinion.

The interpretation of the coefficients is done through the exponential function: exponentiating the intercept β_0, using `inla.tmarginal` or `inla.emarginal`, shows the average count of events in the area or period under

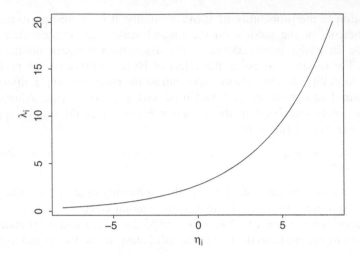

Figure 5.7   Inverse logarithmic function $\lambda_i = \log^{-1}(\eta_i)$. The plot shows how the linear regression function $x_i\beta$ is transformed to the original scale of λ_i.

study when the predictors are at their reference category (if categorical) or at 0 (if numerical). Similarly, exponentiating the generic β_m returns the change in the average of y when x_m changes by one unit.

Most of the times, when using Poisson regression, the interest lays on rates or relative risks more than on the average number of cases (indicated as λ_i in Eq. (5.10)). To change the scale, an offset can be used as a correction factor in the model specification. It represents the denominator of the rate, enters the regression on the logarithmic scale and is assumed to have a regression coefficient fixed to 1, so that from

$$\eta_i = \log(\lambda_i) = \beta_0 + \sum_{m=1}^{M} \beta_m x_{im} + \log(\text{Offset}_i)$$

the log relative risk can be obtained as

$$\log\left(\frac{\lambda_i}{\text{Offset}_i}\right) = \beta_0 + \sum_{m=1}^{M} \beta_m x_{im}$$

and the coefficients β can be interpreted on the risk scale rather than on the absolute scale. In this case, exponentiating the intercept returns the baseline rate while the exponential of β_m represents the change in the rate (or relative risk), for one unit change in the corresponding predictor.

Example: incidents in ships

We use the data introduced in Section 1.4.4 to evaluate the monthly rate of incidents in ships ($i = 1, \ldots, 34$). The potential risk factors are the construction period (built), the operation period (oper) and the type of ship (type). The outcome that we are going to use is the number of incidents for each ship. The model can be written in R-INLA as follows:

```
> formula.inla <- y ~ 1 + built + oper + type
> model.poisson <- inla(formula.inla,family="poisson",
                     data=ShipsIncidents, offset=log(months))
```

In this formulation, we include months as an offset in the linear predictor η_i, thus on the logarithmic scale. An alternative way is to use in the inla function E=months (instead of offset=log(months)) which represents the offset on the natural scale, so that the Poisson distribution in Eq. (5.10) becomes

$$y_i \sim \text{Poisson}(E_i \rho_i),$$

where $\eta_i = \log(\rho_i)$ is the linear predictor, and the average number of incidents λ_i is $E_i \rho_i$. Note that in this case the offset is not included in the linear predictor η_i. The results of the model are the following:

```
> round(model.poisson$summary.fixed[,1:5],3)
```

	mean	SD	0.025quant	0.5quant	0.975quant
(Intercept)	-6.416	0.217	-6.852	-6.413	-5.997
built65-69	0.696	0.150	0.406	0.695	0.993
built70-74	0.819	0.170	0.487	0.818	1.153
built75-79	0.452	0.233	-0.012	0.455	0.904
oper75-79	0.384	0.118	0.153	0.384	0.617
typeB	-0.543	0.178	-0.882	-0.546	-0.185
typeC	-0.688	0.329	-1.366	-0.677	-0.072
typeD	-0.075	0.291	-0.664	-0.068	0.478
typeE	0.326	0.236	-0.141	0.327	0.785

For interpreting the coefficients we exponentiate them: for the intercept $\exp(-6.416) = 0.002$ represents the average monthly incident rate among the ships when built=60-64, oper=60-74 and type=A (the reference categories). The exponential function applied to the coefficients of the risk factors provides the relative risk of incident for different types of ships; for example $\exp(0.326) = 1.385$, thus there is a 38.5% increase in the monthly rate of incidents for ships of type E compared to type A. The same interpretation can be extended to the other factors.

5.4   Hierarchical models

In many statistical applications, the model is characterized by several parameters. For instance, when in a study the interest lies on a treatment effect, we might want to specify parameters for different age group, sex, state of diseases, etc.; in a meta-analysis there could be a parameter for a study specific effect; carrying out a small area study for the risk of a particular disease, we might want to allow for area or time-specific parameters; in a cohort study with repeated measures, we might be interested in including a baseline for each individual.

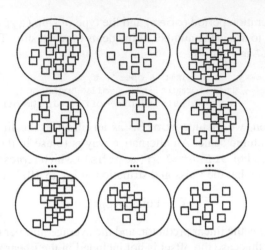

*Figure 5.8   Graphical representation of hierarchical structured data: the squares identify the observations, which could be at the individual level (e.g., disease status) or at the area level (e.g., number of hospitalizations in a particular period) and are called the **first level** unit. These units are nested within the **second level** unit, represented by the circles, which identify clusters (e.g., individuals attending the same hospital, areas within the same region, etc.).*

In this situation, there are two levels as shown in Figure 5.8 the first level is identified by the observations (the squares in the figure), which follow a probability distribution (the *sampling model*). Each unit belongs to one of the groups which could be age classes, hospitals, schools, cities, etc. These are also called *second level units* and are represented by circles in the figure. The observations $y = (y_1, \dots, y_j, \dots, y_J)$ can be written as follows:

$$y_1 = (y_{11}, \dots, y_{n_1 1})$$
$$y_2 = (y_{12}, \dots, y_{n_2 2})$$
$$\dots$$
$$y_j = (y_{1j}, \dots, y_{n_j j})$$
$$\dots$$
$$y_J = (y_{1J}, \dots, y_{n_J J}),$$

where $i = 1, \dots, n_j$ identifies the first level and $j = 1, \dots, J$ the second level units. For this setting, the parameters of interest are $\theta = \{\theta_1, \dots, \theta_J\}$, where the index identifies the group so that all the units in the same group share the same parameter. This type of structure is hierarchical: the idea is that y_{1j} and y_{2j} are more similar than y_{1j} and $y_{2(j+1)}$ as they both belong to the same second level unit j.

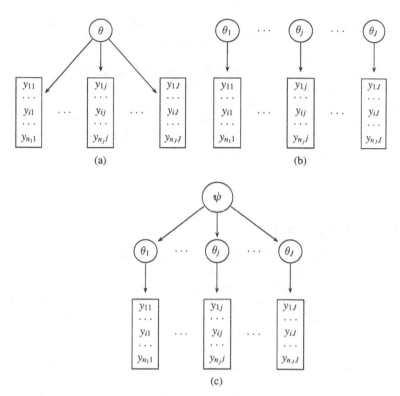

Figure 5.9   The figure shows the directed acyclic graphs (DAG) when (a) θ_j are assumed to be the same for all the statistical units $\theta_j = \theta$ for each j (pooled model), (b) the θ_j are independent from each other (independent model) and (c) the θ_j are modeled through a hierarchical structure (hierarchical model).

An easy representation of a hierarchical structure can be obtained through a particular type of graph, called directed acyclic graph (DAG); see Whittaker (1990), Gilks and Spiegelhalter (1996) and Edwards (2000) for a less technical introduction. In a DAG, the nodes can be represented as circles, if they are unobservable quantities characterized by a probability distribution, or squares if they are observable quantities (i.e., data). The arrows connecting the nodes represent stochastic (solid) or logical (dashed) dependences. As there are several ways of dealing with hierarchical data, we introduce them below and report the corresponding DAGs in Figure 5.9 to help the reader with their comparison. Inference on θ can be trivially performed assuming that all the parameters are equal, so $\theta_j = \theta$ for each j and then specifying a distribution, typically Normal, on θ; in other words this means ignoring the second level units and assuming that all the first level units are a sample from the same population. This simplifies the model as only one parameter θ characterizes the distribution of the observations, which is estimated using all the available data y (Figure 5.9(a)). This is also called *pooled* model. However, such model can be unrealistic as it dismisses an important data feature, which is the information on the second level units.

At the other extreme, it is also possible to perform a stratified analysis by second level units; in this case θ_j is independent from θ_r ($r \neq j$) and the data nested in each second level unit can be analyzed independently, for instance, through a fully specified probability distribution, like $\theta_j \sim$ Normal(0, 1000) in case of no prior information available (Figure 5.9(b)). The main drawback of such an approach is that, unless the sample size for each group is large enough, the estimates for θ can be highly variable. In addition, if the θ_j's are considered independent there is no exchange of information between them.

5.4.1   Exchangeability

To fully take into account the hierarchical structure of the data, $\{\theta_1, \ldots, \theta_J\}$ can be assumed to be similar in the sense that they come from a distribution $p(\theta_j \mid \psi)$ characterized by the same hyperparameters $\psi = \{\psi_1, \ldots, \psi_K\}$. This model framework is depicted in Figure 5.9(c): it is clear that there are now two different levels of analysis, one directly of interest regarding the θ_j's and the upper one identified by ψ. As the θ_j's are generated by a common distribution, this model also allows for an exchange of information between θ_j and θ_r ($r \neq j$), differently from the models presented before, which either assumed them to be identical or to be totally independent.

To better understand how these model structures differ from each other, we will focus on the definition of an *iid* sample (as for the Monte Carlo method of Section 4.1) commonly used in the frequentist approach for specifying the distribution of the data. We can write the joint prior distribution for $\theta = \{\theta_1, \ldots, \theta_J\}$ as the product of the marginal distributions:

$$p(\theta_1, \ldots, \theta_J) = \prod_{j=1}^{J} p(\theta_j) = p(\theta)^J, \qquad (5.12)$$

since the θ_j's are characterized by the same distribution $p(\theta)$.

In alternative, when a hierarchical structure is specified on $\{\theta_1, \ldots, \theta_J\}$, Eq. (5.12) is transformed to

$$p(\theta_1, \ldots, \theta_J \mid \psi) = \int \prod_{j=1}^{J} p(\theta_j \mid \psi) p(\psi) d\psi \qquad (5.13)$$

and the parameters θ are said to be *similar* with respect to the common random generating process. In other words all the θ_j's share the same distribution characterized by hyperparameters ψ, which are in turn characterized by a prior distribution. This means that the elements of θ are conditionally independent given ψ: if the components of ψ were fixed quantities and we knew their actual values, then θ would

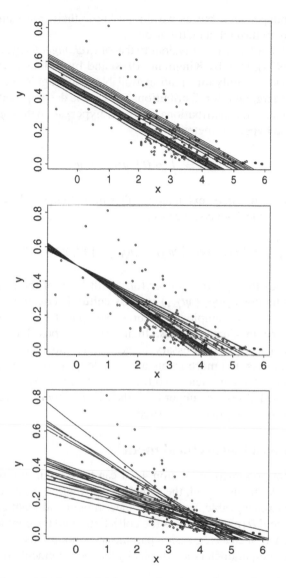

*Figure 5.10   Hierarchical models: the top plot shows the **random intercept** model, which assumes exchangeable β_{0j}; the plot in the centre represents the **random slope** model, which specifies exchangeable β_{1j}; the bottom plot shows the **random intercept and slope** model, which assumes exchangeable β_{0j} and β_{1j}.*

be marginally independent, but as we do not know their true values we include uncertainty on them through a distribution.

The concept of similarity is equivalent to that of *exchangeability*, first introduced by De Finetti (1974), then by Kingman (1978) and by Aldous (1981). Assuming that the data provide the only information available to distinguish between θ_j and θ_r ($r \neq j$), then the marginal prior distributions of θ can be decomposed in the product of their conditional prior distributions given the hyperparameters ψ and the prior distribution of the hyperparameters $p(\psi)$:

$$p(\theta) = \int p(\theta \mid \psi)p(\psi)\mathrm{d}\psi. \tag{5.14}$$

Note that this structure can be extended to allow more than two levels of hierarchy. For instance, assuming L levels, we have

$$p(\theta) = \int p(\theta \mid \psi_1)p(\psi_1 \mid \psi_2)\dots p(\psi_{L-1} \mid \psi_L)p(\psi_L)\mathrm{d}\psi_1\dots\mathrm{d}\psi_L,$$

where ψ_l identifies the hyperparameter for the lth level of the hierarchy and the conditional distributions $p(\psi_l \mid \psi_{l+1})$ express cultural judgements, for instance, exchangeability or more complex structures like spatial or temporal correlation which we will see in Chapters 6–8. In theory, it is possible to allow for as many hierarchical levels as necessary to accurately model the structure of the problem. Nevertheless, the more levels are included, the more complex becomes the interpretation of the parameters, so that in practice a maximum of three levels are usually included. As on the upper level there is no structure on the parameters, usually a noninformative prior is specified.

5.4.2   INLA as a hierarchical model

The INLA model presented in Section 4.7.1 can be written in terms of a hierarchical structure. At the first level, the sampling distribution for y can be factorized as $y_1, \dots, y_n$ are exchangeable, so they are independent and identically distributed given the latent field θ (recall that it is the collection of all the components of interest for the inference, such as regression parameters, smooth functions of covariates, etc.) and some hyperparameters ψ_1 (typically the measurement error precision):

$$y \mid \theta, \psi_1 \sim p(y \mid \theta, \psi_1) = \prod_{i=1}^{n} p(y_i \mid \theta_i, \psi_1).$$

Then at the second level the latent field θ is characterized by a multivariate Normal distribution given the remaining hyperparameters ψ_2 (again recall Section 4.7.1):

$$\theta \mid \psi_2 \sim \text{MVNormal}(0, Q^{-1}(\psi_2)).$$

Finally, the hyperparameters $\psi = \{\psi_1, \psi_2\}$ have some prior distribution given by $\psi \sim p(\psi)$.

5.4.3   Hierarchical regression

It is easy to apply exchangeability on the parameters of linear or generalized linear models, such as the ones presented in Sections 5.1 and 5.3. Given a vector of data $y = (y_1, \ldots, y_n)$, where each element has a probability distribution specified by $p(y_i \mid \theta_i)$, recalling the definition of GLM as described in Section 5.3 and the notation presented in Section 4.7.1, we can write the linear predictor using the link function

$$\eta_i = g(\theta_i) = \beta_0 + \sum_{m=1}^{M} \beta_m x_{im},$$

where we assume a pooled model with the same regression coefficients shared amongst all the observations. If we now assume that the n observations come from J groups (e.g., individuals within administrative areas, pupils within schools, etc.), we can rewrite y in the vectorial form presented in Section 5.4; the regression model would include a group-specific intercept and/or slopes, specifying an exchangeable structure on these, which would take advantage of the hierarchical structure present in the data.

For instance, considering the following linear regression:

$$y_{ij} \sim \text{Normal}(\mu_{ij}, \sigma^2)$$

$$\eta_{ij} = \mu_{ij}$$

and assuming only one predictor, the three following hierarchical structures can be specified:

$$\mu_{ij} = \beta_{0j} + \beta_1 x_{ij}; \qquad \beta_{0j} = b_0 + \upsilon_{0j} \tag{5.15}$$

$$\mu_{ij} = \beta_0 + \beta_{1i} x_{ij}; \qquad \beta_{1j} = b_1 + \upsilon_{1j} \tag{5.16}$$

$$\mu_{ij} = \beta_{0j} + \beta_{1i} x_{ij}; \qquad \beta_{0j} = b_0 + \upsilon_{0j}; \qquad \beta_{1j} = b_1 + \upsilon_{1j}, \tag{5.17}$$

where b_0 and b_1 are called *fixed effects* and are typically normally distributed, centered on 0 and with a large variance, while υ_{0j} and υ_{1j} are called *random effects* and are typically normally distributed with an exchangeable structure, i.e., $\upsilon_{0j} \sim \text{Normal}(0, \sigma_{\upsilon_0}^2)$ and $\upsilon_{1j} \sim \text{Normal}(0, \sigma_{\upsilon_1}^2)$. In these three models θ contains, respectively, $\{b_0, \{\upsilon_{0j}\}, \beta_1\}$, $\{\beta_0, b_1, \{\upsilon_{1j}\}\}$, and $\{b_0, b_1, \{\upsilon_{0j}\}, \{\upsilon_{1j}\}\}$.

Equation (5.15) assumes that the J groups are characterized by a different intercept, but by the same slope (this is also called a random intercept model); thus belonging to different groups only impacts the average (or baseline) outcome, but has no effect on the coefficient of the predictor. This specification is equivalent to assume that the regression lines are parallel (see Figure 5.10, top).

Equation (5.16) assumes that the J groups are characterized by the same intercept but a different slope (this is also called a random slope model); in this case belonging to different groups only leads to a different effect of the predictor on the outcome. This is represented in Figure 5.10 (centre) and shows regression lines with the same starting point, but with slopes diverging from each other.

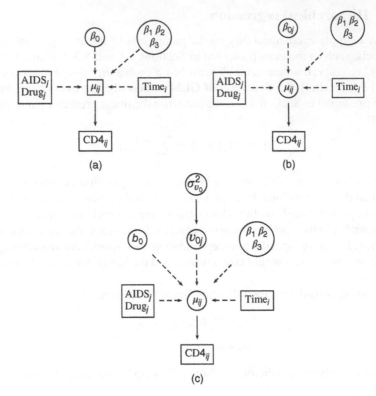

Figure 5.11   CD4 example: graphical structure (DAG) of the pooled model (a), independent model (b) and hierarchical model (c).

Finally, Eq. (5.17) refers to the J groups having different intercept and slope (also called a random intercept and slope model), thus assuming that belonging to different groups has an impact on both the average outcome and on the effect of the predictor on the outcome. This case is depicted in Figure 5.10 (bottom), which shows diverging regression lines with different starting points.

We illustrate how to include a hierarchical structure in R-INLA through a simple example. We assume $J = 100$ groups, simulate $n = 10000$ values for an exposure variable $x_{ij} \sim$ Normal$(0, 1)$ and assume that each individual belongs to one of the 100 groups ($j = 1, \ldots, 100$).

```
> m <- 10000
> set.seed(123)
> x <- rnorm(m)
> group <- sample(seq(1,100), size=m, replace=T)
```

Then we simulate n values for y from a Normal distribution specifying a linear relationship with the exposure x and allowing for a random group intercept

$v_{0j} \sim \text{Normal}(0, \sigma_{v_0}^2 = 1/0.25)$:

$$y_{ij} \sim \text{Normal}(5 + v_{0j} + 2x_{ij}, \sigma^2 = 1/3).$$

```
> #Simulate Random effect (recall that beta_0 = b_0 + v_j)
> tau.v0 <- 0.25
> set.seed(4455)
> v <- rnorm(length(unique(group)), 0, sqrt(1/tau.v0))
> #Assign the group random effect to each individual
> vj <- v[group]
> #Simulate y
> tau <- 3
> set.seed(334455)
> b0 <- 5
> beta1 <- 2
> y <- rnorm(m, b0 + vj + beta1*x, 1/sqrt(tau))
```

After having simulated the data we can now run R-INLA. Note that the latent field θ comprises the regression coefficients b_0 and β_1 and the random effects $v_0 = \{v_{0j}\}$. The hyperparameters are the random effect precision $1/\sigma_{v_0}^2$ and the inverse of the measurement error $1/\sigma^2$:

```
> formula <- y ~ 1 + x + f(group, model="iid")
> output <- inla(formula, family="gaussian",
              data=data.frame(y,x,group))
```

The `f(group, model="iid")` specifies that an exchangeable structure (`iid`) is included on the variable group. Note that the default prior on $1/\sigma_{v_0}^2$ is logGamma(1, 0.00005) but if different parameters are more suitable for the particular case study considered, a similar reasoning as introduced at the end of Section 5.1.2 can be applied. For instance, recalling that the true value for the random effect standard deviation is `sigma.v <- 1/sqrt(tau.v)` which is equal to 2, we can use this information to set a Uniform prior between 1.5 and 2.5 on `sigma.v` as follows:

```
> a1 <- 1.5
> b1 <- 2.5
> #Standard deviation
> sigma.v0 <- runif(n=10000,min=a1,max=b1)
> #Precision
> tau.v <- 1/sigma.v0^2
> mean(tau.v)
[1] 0.2678099
```

and then obtain the corresponding parameters for the log precision `log(tau.v)` as

```
> a2 <- mean(tau.v)^2/var(tau.v)
> b2 <- a2/mean(tau.v)
> a2
[1] 11.27762
```

```
> b2
[1] 42.11054
```

to be used in the f() within the formula environment

```
> f(group,model="iid",hyper=list(prec=list(prior="loggamma",
                                    param=c(a2,b2))))
```

The output shows that the estimates of the regression coefficients are very close to the true values, as well as the values of the hyperparameters:

```
> round(output$summary.fixed[,1:5],2)
            Mean   SD 0.025quant 0.5quant 0.975quant
(Intercept) 4.98 0.18       4.62     4.98       5.34
x           2.00 0.01       1.99     2.00       2.01
> round(output$summary.hyperpar[,1:5],2)
                                     Mean   SD 0.025quant 0.5quant
Precision for the Gaussian observations 3.02 0.04       2.94     3.02
Precision for group                     0.30 0.04       0.22     0.30
                                     0.975quant
Precision for the Gaussian observations     3.11
Precision for group                         0.39
```

5.4.4   Example: a hierarchical model for studying CD4 counts in AIDS patients

We use the dataset presented in Section 1.4.5 to evaluate the association of drug use and AIDS diagnosis on the CD4 counts for 80 HIV-positive patients. Counts of CD4 (specialized cells which are part of the immune system) collected at four different times ($i = 1, 2, 3, 4$) are available for each patient.

We first specify two nonhierarchical models: the first does not take into account the fact that for each patient ($j = 1, \ldots, J$) repeated measures of CD4 counts are available, but pools all the data and assumes a global intercept and slope. The pooled model is the following:

$$CD4_{ij} \sim \text{Normal}(\mu_{ij}, \sigma^2) \tag{5.18}$$

$$\eta_{ij} = \mu_{ij} = \beta_0 + \beta_1 \text{Time}_i + \beta_2 \text{Drug}_j + \beta_3 \text{AIDS}_j \tag{5.19}$$

with $\log(\tau) = \log(1/\sigma^2) \sim \text{logGamma}(0, 0.0001)$ and with noninformative Normal distributions on β_0, β_1, β_2, and β_3.

The second model considers each unit as an independent sample and does not assume any similarity between them:

$$CD4_{ij} \sim \text{Normal}(\mu_{ij}, \sigma^2) \tag{5.20}$$

$$\eta_{ij} = \mu_{ij} = \beta_{0j} + \beta_1 \text{Time}_i + \beta_2 \text{Drug}_j + \beta_3 \text{AIDS}_j. \tag{5.21}$$

It specifies an intercept for each individual characterized by an independent prior $\beta_{0j} \sim \text{Normal}(0, 0.0001)$.

Then we also specify a hierarchical structure, which assumes an intercept for each individual, so it takes into account the different measures available for each of them, but differently from the previous model, it specifies $\beta_{0j} = b_0 + v_{0j}$, with $v_{0j} \sim$ Normal$(0, \sigma_{v_0}^2)$; on the log precision a noninformative logGamma prior is assumed. The graphical representation of the models using a DAG can be seen in Figure 5.11. Note that the hierarchical specification has a larger number of parameters than the other two models as for each individual it considers an intercept, and in addition it allows for the hyperparameter $\sigma_{v_0}^2$.

The three models are specified in R-INLA as follows:

```
> #Mod1: Pooled model
> formula.pooled <- y ~ 1 + drug + AIDS + Time
> CD4.1 <- inla(formula.pooled,family="gaussian", data=CD4,
               control.predictor=list(compute=TRUE),
               control.fixed=list(mean=list(0), prec=list(0.0001),
                           mean.intercept=0, prec.intercept=0.0001))
> CD4.1.summary <- CD4.1$summary.fixed
```

Note that since the mean and the precision specified for the priors of the fixed effects are the same, it is possible to simplify the code reported above using mean=0,prec=0.0001 instead of mean=list(0),prec=list(0.0001).

```
> #Mod2: Independent model
> formula.indep <- y ~ 1 + factor(id) + drug + AIDS + Time
> CD4.2 <- inla(formula.indep,family="gaussian", data=CD4,
               control.predictor=list(compute=TRUE),
               control.fixed=list(mean=0,prec=0.0001,
                           mean.intercept=0, prec.intercept=0.0001))
> CD4.2.summary <- CD4.2$summary.fixed
> #Mod3: Hierarchical model
> formula.hier <- y ~ 1 + drug + AIDS + Time +
                      f(id,model="iid",
                         hyper=list(prec=list(prior="loggamma",
                             param=c(1,0.0001))))
> CD4.3 <- inla(formula.hier,family="gaussian", data=CD4,
               control.predictor=list(compute=TRUE),
               control.fixed=list(mean=0,prec=0.0001,
                           mean.intercept=0, prec.intercept=0.0001))
```

Figure 5.12 shows the 95% credibility intervals (CI95) for the fixed effect β_{0j} in the independent model (top) and for the random effect $\beta_{0j} = b_0 + v_{0j}$ for the hierarchical model (bottom). The median for β_0 in the pooled model is represented by a vertical line. The code for computing β_{0j} is reported below and employs the rmarginal function for generating 1000 random values from the selected marginal distribution:

```
> b0 <- inla.rmarginal(1000,
             marg = CD4.3$marginals.fixed$'(Intercept)')
> v0 <- matrix(NA,1000,80)
> for(i in 1:80){
   v0[,i] <- inla.rmarginal(1000,
```

```
                marg = CD4.3$marginals.random$id[[i]])
  }
> beta0 <- b0 + v0
> #Compute quartiles for beta0
> beta0_quartiles <- t(apply(beta0, MARGIN=2,
          function(x) quantile( x, probs= c(0.025,0.5,0.975))))
> dim(beta0_quartiles)
[1] 80  3
```

The function `apply` returns a matrix of values obtained by applying a given function – `quantile` in this case – to the rows (`MARGIN=1`) or the columns (`MARGIN=2`) of a given array.

Note that an alternative for computing β_{0j} is through the `lincomb` option, which is described in Section 5.4.5.

In Figure 5.12, it can be seen that in the independent model the uncertainty is much larger than in the hierarchical one, as the CI95 estimates are based only on the four observations available for each patient. The widest interval ranges between -43 and 45, but in Figure 5.12 it is cut between -10 and 10 to make the plot readable. On the other hand, the hierarchical model shrinks the values of β_{0j} toward their mean, as they all are generated by a distribution characterized by the same precision. This means that they are similar, which has an impact in reducing the uncertainty on their estimates (resulting in narrower intervals), as they can *borrow strength* from each other. This is a characteristic of the hierarchical framework, known as global smoothing, which will be compared to the so-called local smoothing, arising for spatial structured models that we will see in Chapters 6 and 7.

5.4.5   Example: a hierarchical model for studying lip cancer in Scotland

Using the dataset described in Section 1.4.6, we specify a hierarchical model to study the association between working in an outdoor environment and the incidence of lip cancer in Scotland. The number of lip cancer cases is modeled following a Poisson distribution:

$$y_i \sim \text{Poisson}(\lambda_i); \qquad \log(\lambda_i) = \eta_i, \qquad (5.22)$$

with $i = 1, \ldots, 56$. On η_i we specify a linear regression with a random intercept and include the logarithm of the expected number of cases for each unit ($\log(E_i)$) as an offset, so that the parameters in η_i can be interpreted on the log relative risk scale:

$$\eta_i = b_0 + v_{0i} + \beta_1 x_i + \log(E_i). \qquad (5.23)$$

An exchangeable prior is specified on v_{0i}: $v_{0i} \sim \text{Normal}(0, \sigma_{v_0}^2)$.

In R-INLA the code for this model is the following:

```
> formula.inla <- O ~ 1 + X +
                    f(id,model="iid",
                        hyper=list(prec=list(prior="loggamma",
```

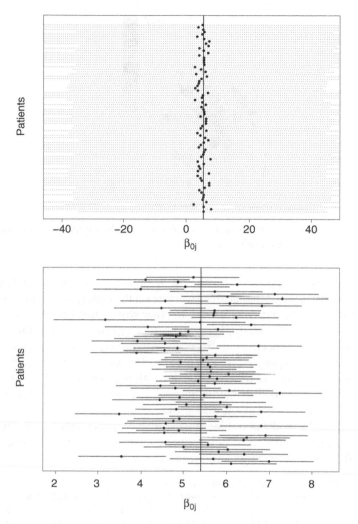

Figure 5.12 *CD4 example: 95% credibility intervals for the fixed effects β_{0j} in the independent model (top) and for the random effect β_{0j} for the hierarchical model (bottom); the dots identify the corresponding posterior medians. The vertical line represents the posterior median for the pooled model.*

```
                                param=c(1,0.00001))))
> lipcancer.poisson <- inla(formula.inla,family="poisson",
                    data=LipCancerData, offset=log(E),
                    control.predictor=list(compute=TRUE),
                    control.fixed=list(mean=0,prec=0.00001,
                                    mean.intercept=0,
                                    prec.intercept=0.00001))
```

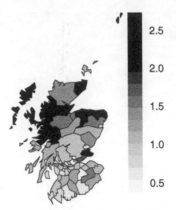

Figure 5.13   Map of the posterior mean for the random effects v_{0i} (on the natural scale) for the 56 Scottish counties.

where id represents the index for the 56 Scottish counties and f(id, model= "iid") identifies the exchangeable structure on the county intercepts and defines the distribution on the hyperparameter. In other words, this structure is equivalent to assume that id $\sim$ Normal$(0, 1/\sigma_{v_0}^2)$, where $\log(1/\sigma_{v_0}^2) \sim \log$Gamma$(1, 10^{-5})$. R-INLA allows for a specific number of hyperparameters for each latent structure, which can be seen typing ?inla.models. For instance, model="iid" has only one hyperparameter, which is the logarithm of the precision. Moreover, a noninformative Normal distribution is assumed on the fixed effects using the option control.fixed as showed above.

The output of the model is similar to what we have previously seen for regression models, except that now there is information also on the hyperparameter of the random effect (see summary(lipcancer.poisson)):

```
> round(lipcancer.poisson$summary.fixed,3)
              Mean    SD 0.025quant 0.5quant 0.975quant   mode kld
(Intercept) -0.489 0.156     -0.800   -0.488     -0.186 -0.485   0
X            0.068 0.014      0.041    0.068      0.096  0.068   0
> round(lipcancer.poisson$summary.hyperpar,3)
                   Mean    SD 0.025quant 0.5quant 0.975quant  mode
Precision for id  3.089 0.898      1.696    2.967      5.192 2.736
```

It is also possible to obtain marginal distributions for all the parameters, typing:

lipcancer.poisson$marginals.fixed	for fixed effects
lipcancer.poisson$marginals.random	for random effects
lipcancer.poisson$marginals.hyperpar	for hyperparameters

In addition, a summary of the random effects v_0 is available through lipcancer.poisson$summary.random, returning the mean, SD, and 95% CI for all the 56 random effects. As the parameters are on the logarithmic scale

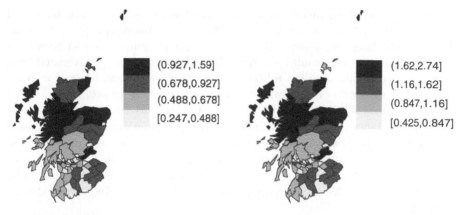

Figure 5.14   Map of the random effects β_{0i} (left) and β_{1i} (right) for the model with random intercept and slope in the 56 Scottish counties (posterior mean on the natural scale).

(see Eq. (5.23)), for the sake of interpretability it is advisable to report these on the natural scale using the same command presented in Section 5.3. Figure 5.13 reports the map of the random effects v_0 for this dataset on the natural scale, obtained through the following code:

```
> library(maptools)
> geobugs.map <- readSplus("LipCancer.map")
> post.mean.exp.v0 <- lapply(lipcancer.poisson$marginals.random$id,
                    function(x) inla.emarginal(exp,x))
> data.exp.v0 <- data.frame(ID=names(geobugs.map),
                        post.mean=unlist(post.mean.exp.v0))
> row.names(data.exp.v0) <- names(geobugs.map)
> wards <- SpatialPolygonsDataFrame(geobugs.map,data.exp.v0)
> spplot(obj=wards, zcol="post.mean",main="",
       col.regions=gray(99:0/99))
```

The R function `lapply(X, FUN, ...)` returns a list where each element is given by the result of applying FUN to the corresponding element of X. In the example under study, each element of the resulting list `post.mean.exp.v0` corresponds to the posterior mean (FUN=`inla.emarginal`) of the exponentiated random effect v_{0i} (thus `post.mean.exp.v0` is formed by 56 terms).

Note that to obtain the marginal posterior distribution for β_{0i} it is necessary to combine those of v_{0i} and b_0. This can be done through the INLA command `inla.make.lincombs`, which allows to build linear combinations of the parameters of interest. Assuming $\beta_0 = B\theta$, where θ is the latent field and B is a matrix of n rows (number of linear combinations to be created) and k columns (number of parameters in the latent field). There are two methods to deal with linear combinations in INLA. The first approach creates an enlarged latent field θ, e.g., adding β_0 and then using the INLA method as usual to fit the enlarged model. However, this leads to a slow computation as the number of parameters in the fitting part of the model increases substantially (e.g., in our case we would add 56 linear combinations to the latent field). Alternatively, it is possible to run INLA on the latent field not including the linear combinations and perform a post processing on the resulting output. Then $\beta_0 \mid \theta, \psi, y$ is approximated by a Gaussian distribution with the following parameters: the mean is equal to $B\mu^\star$, where $\mu^\star$ is the mean of the best marginal approximation for $p(\theta_i \mid \psi, y)$, which could be Gaussian, Simplified Gaussian or Laplace (as introduced in Section 4.7.1); the variance is $BQ^{\star^{-1}}B'$ with Q being the precision matrix of the Gaussian approximation $\tilde{p}(\theta_i \mid \psi, y)$, as described in Eq. (4.20). Then integrating out ψ returns the posterior marginal for β_0. In this case the computation of the posterior marginals for the linear combinations does not affect the graph of the latent field, leading to a much faster approximation, thus this is the default method used in INLA.

In practice to use `inla.make.lincombs` we need to define: (i) a matrix with ones on the diagonal (identity matrix), through `id=diag(56)`, which has dimension equal to the length of v_0, (ii) a vector of ones with v_0 length through `rep(1,56)`:

```
> lcs <- inla.make.lincombs(id = diag(56),"(Intercept)" = rep(1,56))
```

Including `lcs` into the `inla` command (through `lincomb=lcs`), we obtain the posterior distribution for β_0:

```
> lipcancer.poisson.int <- inla(formula.inla,family="poisson",
                    data=LipCancerData, offset=log(E),
                    control.predictor=list(compute=TRUE),
                    lincomb=lcs,
                    control.fixed=list(mean=0,prec=0.0001,
                                       mean.intercept=0,
                                       prec.intercept=0.00001))
```

Typing `lipcancer.poisson.int$summary.lincomb.derived` provides the summary statistics for the $\beta_{0i} = v_{0i} + b_0$ coefficients which can be used to obtain posterior mean and 95% CI or other summary indexes.

This model can be extended to include also a random slope so that the linear predictor becomes

$$\eta_i = b_0 + v_{0i} + (b_1 + v_{1i})x_i + \log(E_i). \tag{5.24}$$

The distribution of v_{0i} remains the same and an exchangeable prior is specified also on v_{1i}: $v_{1i} \sim \text{Normal}(0, \sigma^2_{v_1})$.

The R-INLA formula is the following:

```
> LipCancerData$id2 <- LipCancerData$id
> formula.inla2 <- O ~ 1 + X +
    f(id, model="iid",
      hyper = list(prec = list(prior="loggamma",param=c(1,0.00001)))) +
    f(id2, X, model="iid",
      hyper = list(prec = list(prior="loggamma",param=c(1,0.00001)))))
```

where `f(id2, X, model="iid",...)` identifies the random slope in terms of an interaction between the variable `X` and `id2` (the second argument in `f()` is an optional weight for the `f` term.). As before, we need to use the `inla.make.lincombs` for obtaining β_0 as well as $\beta_{1i} = b_1 + v_{1i}$:

```
> #beta0
> lcs1 <- inla.make.lincombs(id = diag(56),"(Intercept)" = rep(1,56))
> #beta1
> lcs2 <- inla.make.lincombs(id = diag(56), X = rep(1,56))
```

Note that `R-INLA` assigns the same names to each of the linear combinations, so we need to change these to avoid an error when we run `inla`

```
> names(lcs2) <- paste(names(lcs1),"X",sep="")
> all.lcs <- c(lcs1,lcs2)
```

The summary statistics provide information about both β_0 and β_1, which are reported in Figure 5.14 on the natural scale.

5.4.6   Example: studying stroke mortality in Sheffield (UK)

From Section 5.3, a pooled logistic regression model with a global intercept β_0 and slope β_1 was specified to assess the association between NOx (in quintiles) and stroke mortality rate in Sheffield, UK, considering enumeration districts as small area of analysis. Now we want to allow for an area-specific intercept ($\beta_{0i} = b_0 + v_{0i}$) which would assume that the baseline mortality rate is different for each enumeration district. An exchangeable structure is specified on v_0.

Similar to the previous example, the `R-INLA` formula changes including now `f(wbID,model='iid')` for the exchangeable structure. The model specification and the results for the fixed effects are the following:

```
> formula.inla.hier1 <- y ~ 1 + factor(NOx) + factor(Townsend) +
             offset(logit.adjusted.prob) + f(wbID,model="iid")
> model.logistic.hier1 <- inla(formula.inla.hier1,family="binomial",
                    Ntrials=Stroke$pop, data=Stroke)
> round(model.logistic.hier1$summary.fixed[,1:5], 3)
```

	Mean	SD	0.025quant	0.5quant	0.975quant
(Intercept)	-0.322	0.082	-0.485	-0.321	-0.161
factor(NOx)2	0.086	0.091	-0.093	0.086	0.263
factor(NOx)3	0.044	0.092	-0.137	0.044	0.225
factor(NOx)4	0.194	0.092	0.013	0.194	0.375
factor(NOx)5	0.278	0.098	0.086	0.278	0.470
factor(Townsend)2	0.018	0.093	-0.165	0.018	0.201
factor(Townsend)3	0.060	0.094	-0.124	0.060	0.244
factor(Townsend)4	-0.081	0.094	-0.266	-0.081	0.104
factor(Townsend)5	-0.022	0.099	-0.215	-0.022	0.172

which show some differences if compared with the ones from the pooled model described in Section 5.3; the effects for both NOx and deprivation become smaller, which is expected as part of these effects are now explained

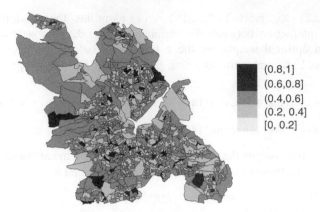

Figure 5.15   The figure maps for each ED in Sheffield the posterior mean of the baseline marginal probability of stroke mortality computed as $logit^{-1}(b_0 + v_{0i})$, *modeled using a random intercept model.*

by the area-specific intercepts. Figure 5.15 maps the marginal posterior probability of stroke for each enumeration district (ED) in Sheffield, calculated as $logit^{-1}(b_0 + v_{0j})$, and shows a high degree of variability, spanning from 0 to 1. Recall that from the pooled model, the baseline probability of stroke mortality for an area characterized by very low NOx and low deprivation (NOx and Townsend index are in the first category) was $logit^{-1}$ $(-0.181) = 0.455$.

5.5   Prediction

An important consequence of the concept of exchangeability is that we can also derive a predictive result on the variable Y. Suppose that $y^{\star}$ represents a future occurrence (or a value not yet observed in the current experiment) of the random phenomenon described by the information gathered by means of the sample y. If we assume exchangeability for the augmented dataset $y^{\circledR} = \{y, y^{\star}\}$, we then have

$$p(y^{\star} \mid y) = \frac{p(y, y^{\star})}{p(y)} \text{ from the conditional probability} \qquad (5.25)$$

$$= \frac{\int p(y^{\star} \mid \theta)p(y \mid \theta)p(\theta)\mathrm{d}\theta}{p(y)} \text{ by exchangeability}$$

$$= \frac{\int p(y^{\star} \mid \theta)p(\theta \mid y)p(y)\mathrm{d}\theta}{p(y)} \text{ applying Bayes' theorem}$$

$$= \int p(y^{\star} \mid \theta)p(\theta \mid y)\mathrm{d}\theta,$$

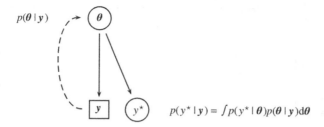

Figure 5.16   Graphical representation of the predictive distribution.

where, following the INLA notation presented in Section 4.7.1, θ identifies the vector of all the parameters. We assume that we are working with continuous variables, but note that the same calculation can be carried out for discrete variables swapping the integral with the sum.

Equation (5.25) is meaningful under the assumptions that the random variables Y and $Y^\star$ are exchangeable, i.e., that the new realization $y^\star$ is similar to the ones that have already been observed. Moreover, the quantity $p(y^\star \mid y)$, known as *predictive distribution*, is only meaningful within the Bayesian approach, since the posterior distribution for the θ parameters in Eq. (5.25) only exists if θ are random variables. Figure 5.16 shows the concept of predictive distribution in terms of a DAG. The variables Y and $Y^\star$ are generated by the same random process, which is governed by the parameters θ, associated with a suitable prior distribution, $p(\theta)$. Once Y is observed to the value y, the uncertainty about the parameter is updated into the posterior distribution $p(\theta \mid y)$, which in turns is used to infer about the future realization $y^\star$.

Going back to the logistic regression example on stroke mortality in Sheffield, suppose now that we want to predict the number of deaths for areas characterized by low NOx level (in the first quintile) and low deprivation (Townsend index in the first quintile). First, in the dataset `Stroke`, we substitute the y values for the areas that we want to predict with `NA`

```
> Stroke1 <- Stroke
> Stroke1$y[which(Stroke$Townsend==1 & Stroke$NOx==1)] <- NA
```

and we run the R-INLA model (named `model.logistic.hier.pred`) – as specified in Section 5.4.6 – and set the `control.predictor` option as `control.predictor=list(link=link)`. The object `link` is a vector of length given by the size of the response variable with values 1 if the corresponding data is missing and `NA` otherwise (so the prediction is computed only when `link=1`). With reference to the stroke example, we define the `link` object as follows:

```
> link <- rep(NA, length(Stroke1$y))
> link[which(is.na(Stroke1$y))] <- 1
```

and then run INLA through

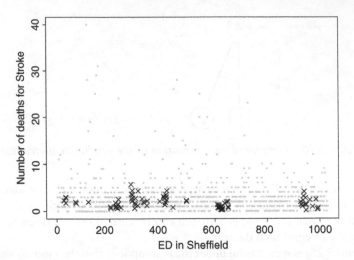

Figure 5.17   Posterior mean of the predictive distribution of stroke deaths in the 1030 ED in Sheffield. The grey dots are observed values, while the crosses identify the predicted values for the areas characterized by low NOx level and low deprivation.

```
> formula.inla.hier1 <- y ~ 1 + factor(NOx) + factor(Townsend) +
              f(wbID, model="iid") +  offset(logit.adjusted.prob)
> model.logistic.hier.pred <- inla(formula.inla.hier1, data=Stroke1,
              family="binomial", Ntrials=Stroke1$pop,
              control.predictor=list(link=link))
```

The summary statistics of the predicted values can be accessed by

```
> model.logistic.hier.pred$summary.fitted.values
> #partial output
```

	Mean	SD	0.025quant	0.5quant	0.975quant
fitted.predictor.0001	0.003	0.001	0.001	0.003	0.006
fitted.predictor.0002	0.002	0.001	0.001	0.002	0.005
fitted.predictor.0003	0.004	0.002	0.002	0.004	0.009

consisting of a matrix with 1030 rows (as the number of areas). Note that the predicted values are on the π scale (we are using the Binomial likelihood). To predict the mean number of deaths in each area we consider the corresponding population as follows:

```
> predicted.values.mean <- c()
> for(i in 1:nrow(Stroke1)){
   predicted.values.mean[i] <-
            inla.emarginal(function(x) x*Stroke1$pop[i],
            model.logistic.hier.pred$marginals.fitted.values[[i]])
 }
```

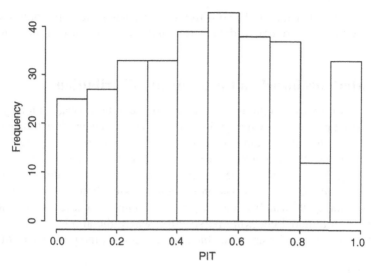

Figure 5.18   Histogram of the cross-validated PIT. Uniformly distributed PIT indicates that the predictive distribution matched the one for the data.

Figure 5.17 plots the number of deaths due to stroke: the observed values are identified by a small circle, while the predicted values for the areas characterized by low deprivation and low exposure to NOx are represented by a cross. It is visible how the predicted values are spread in the lower part of the plot, suggesting that under the model the probability of dying of stroke is lower for areas with low deprivation and low air pollution.

5.6   Model checking and selection

An important aspect of Bayesian modeling regards the assessment of its plausibility and fit. The first, also called *model criticism*, can be defined as the evaluation of which variables to include in the model, which assumptions to make on the parameters (e.g., exchangeability, independence, etc.) and on the likelihood (Normal, Student *t* distribution, etc.), which prior distribution to assign on parameters and hyperparameters. Are they plausible? Do they provide reasonable posterior inference? The second one, also called *model selection* focuses on finding the best fit for the data in hand, and compares model differing for the variables included, the assumptions on parameters and likelihood and the prior distribution on parameters and hyperparameters.

Sensitivity analysis is a concept which combines the two previous ones, as it tries to answer the basic question: how the posterior inference changes when the assumptions and/or distributions on parameters change. As Gelman *et al.* (2004) point out, in theory it would be possible to perform sensitivity analysis setting up a joint distribution which is a mixture of all models to be checked. However, in practice, this is infeasible and two different approaches are commonly used: the first is based on the predictive distribution and the second uses functions of the deviance.

5.6.1 Methods based on the predictive distribution

The idea behind these methods is to divide the sample of observations y in two groups, so that $y = (y_f, y_c)$, where y_f is used to fit the model and to estimate the posterior distribution of the parameters and y_c is used to perform model criticism. But how do we choose the two groups? Two ways are commonly used: (i) each observation belongs to only one of the two groups y_f and y_c, originating the so-called *cross-validation*; (ii) each observation is counted twice, both for fitting the model and for validating it, which is called *predictive checks*. These two methods are mostly used in a model checking perspective, where the aim is to evaluate if the assumptions on the model are plausible and to check for the presence of outliers.

Cross-validation

After splitting the data into the two groups, the model is run on y_f so that the posterior distribution for the parameters $p(\theta \mid y_f)$ is obtained; R-INLA runs the so-called *leave one out* cross-validation, which assumes that $y_f = y_{-i}$ and $y_c = y_i$. Two indices are used for evaluating the goodness of the model in this perspective:

1. the *conditional predictive ordinate* (Pettit, 1990): $\text{CPO}_i = p(y_i^\star \mid y_f)$;

2. the *probability integral transform (PIT)* (Dawid, 1984): $\text{PIT}_i = p(y_i^\star \leq y_i \mid y_f)$. This is valid if y come from a continuous distribution; for the discrete case an adjusted version of the PIT can be used (Czado *et al.*, 2009), as $\text{PIT}_i^{\text{adj}} = \text{PIT}_i + 0.5 \times p(y_i^\star = y_i \mid y_f)$ (even if this does not make so much sense for binary response or Poisson with very few counts).

As described by Rue *et al.* (2009) and Held *et al.* (2010), these quantities are computed in R-INLA routinely without rerunning the model, and can be controlled through the option `control.compute` of the `inla` command. Going back to the CD4 linear regression model presented in Section 5.4.4, we set `cpo` equal to TRUE and run the model as follows:

```
> CD4.3 <- inla(formula.hier,family="gaussian",data=CD4,
              control.predictor=list(compute=TRUE),
              control.fixed=list(mean=list(0),prec=list(0.0001),
                    mean.intercept=0,prec.intercept=0.0001),
              control.compute=list(cpo=TRUE))
```

Calling `names(CD4.3$cpo)` provides the cross-validation predictive ordinate (CPO) and the PIT for each of the 320 measurement of CD4. As highlighted by

Held *et al.* (2010), numerical problems may occur when the CPO and PIT indexes are computed. To this regards, R-INLA provides automatically a failure vector which contains a 0 or 1 value for each observation. In particular, a value equal to 1 indicates that for the corresponding observation the predictive measures are not reliable due to some problems in the calculation.[5] In our example no failures were detected:

```
> sum(CD4.3$cpo$failure)
[1] 0
```

As suggested by Gneiting *et al.* (2007), the empirical distribution of the PIT can be used to evaluate the predictive performance of the model: a Uniform distribution means that the predictive distribution is coherent with the data. The histogram of the PIT measure for our example

```
> hist(CD4.3$cpo$pit,breaks=10,main="",xlab="PIT")
```

is depicted in Figure 5.18 and it shows a distribution which tends to uniformity. Moreover, a summary measure of model fitting is given by the sum of the log of the CPO values (Carlin and Louis, 2008)

```
> sum(log(CD4.3$cpo$cpo))
[1] -465.0009
```

and it can be used to compare competitive models in terms of prediction performance (larger values denote a better fitting).

Posterior predictive check

The posterior predictive checks, introduced by Gelman *et al.* (1996), is based on the assumption that $y_c = y_f = y$, so all the observations are used for model estimate and checking. In particular two quantities are of interest:

1. the *posterior predictive distribution* $p(y_i^\star \mid y) = \int p(y_i^\star \mid \theta_i) p(\theta_i \mid y) \, d\theta_i$, which represents the likelihood of a replicate observation $y_i^\star$ having observed data y;

2. the *posterior predictive p-value* defined as $p(y_i^\star \leq y_i \mid y)$.

---

[5] Actually the failure value for each observation y_i is computed as the expected failure over the posterior distribution for the hyperparameters:

$$\text{failure}_i = \sum_j \text{failure}_{ij} p(\psi^{(j)} \mid y) \Delta_j,$$

where $\psi^{(j)}$ and Δ_j are the integration points and the corresponding weights (see Section 4.7.2).

Values of $p(y_i^\star \leq y_i \mid \boldsymbol{y})$ near 0 or 1 indicate that the model fails to fit the data and it should be reconsidered. Unusually small values of $p(y_i^\star \mid \boldsymbol{y})$ indicate observations that come from the tails of the assumed distribution and can be classified as outliers. If this happens for many values, this suggests that the model is not adequate for the data in hand.

In addition, summary indices can be obtained to globally evaluate the goodness of fit of the model. For instance, quantities commonly used in environmental and social sciences like mean square error (MSE) and R squared (R^2) can be calculated as

$$\text{MSE} = \frac{1}{n} \sum_{i=1}^{n} (y_i - y_i^\star)^2$$

and

$$R^2 = \frac{\sum_{i=1}^{n} (y_i^\star - \bar{y})^2}{\sum_i^n (y_i - \bar{y})^2}.$$

In R-INLA, the posterior predictive distribution can be obtained using the prediction procedure described in Section 5.5 while the posterior predictive p-value can be obtained using inla.pmarginal which returns the cumulative density function. For instance, going back to the lip cancer Poisson regression (see Section 5.4.5)

```
> lipcancer.poisson <- inla(formula.inla,family="poisson",
                   data=LipCancerData, offset=log(E),
                   control.predictor=list(link=1, compute=TRUE),
                   control.fixed=list(mean=0,prec=0.00001))
```

```
> predicted.p.value <- c()
> n <- length(LipCancerData[,1])
> for(i in (1:n)) {
   predicted.p.value[i] <- inla.pmarginal(q=LipCancerData$O[i],
          marginal=lipcancer.poisson$marginals.fitted.values[[i]])
   }
```

Figure 5.19 (top) shows the scatterplot of the posterior means for the predictive distributions versus the observed values, obtained with

```
> plot(LipCancerData$O,lipcancer.poisson$summary.fitted.values$mean,
      xlab="Observed Values",ylab="Mean Post. Pred. Distr.")
```

while the posterior p-value is represented in Figure 5.19 (bottom).

```
> hist(predicted.p.value,main="",xlab="Posterior predictive p-value")
```

It is clear that on average the prediction is very close to the observed values. Looking at the posterior p-value it seems that most of the areas have a p-value in the middle of the range, while very few show low or high p-values, suggesting that the model fits the data reasonably well.

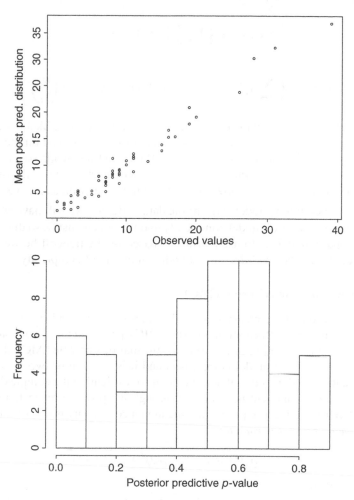

Figure 5.19   Scatterplot of the posterior mean for the predictive distributions against the observed values (top). Histogram of the posterior predictive p-value (bottom).

5.6.2   Methods based on the deviance

When the interest lays on the comparison between different models in terms of performance their deviance can be used. Given the data y with likelihood $p(y \mid \theta)$ the deviance of the model is defined as

$$D(\theta) = -2\log(p(y \mid \theta)),$$

where θ identifies the parameters of the likelihood. For instance, for a Bernoulli likelihood:

$$y_i \sim \text{Bernoulli}(\pi)$$

$$p(y \mid \pi) = \prod_{i=1}^{n} \binom{n_i}{y_i} \pi^{y_i}(1 - \pi)^{n_i-y_i}$$

$$D(\pi) = -2 \left(\sum_i y_i \log \pi + (n_i - y_i) \log(1 - \pi) + \log \binom{n_i}{y_i} \right).$$

The deviance of the model measures the variability linked to the likelihood, which is the probabilistic structure used for the observation (conditional on the parameters). This quantity is a random variable in the Bayesian framework, so it is possible to synthesize it through several indexes (mean, median, etc.). Typically, the posterior mean deviance $\overline{D} = E_{\theta|y}(D(\theta))$ is used as a measure of fit, as it is very robust. However more complex models will fit the data better and so will have smaller $\overline{D}$. This calls for measures of model complexity to trade-off against $\overline{D}$, so that a natural way to compare models is to use a criterion based on the tradeoff between the fit of the model to the data and the corresponding measure of complexity.

Deviance information criterion (DIC)

The most commonly used measure of model fit based on the deviance for Bayesian models is the deviance information criterion (DIC), proposed by Spiegelhalter *et al.* (2002). It is a generalization of the Akaike information criterion (AIC), developed especially for Bayesian model comparison and it is the sum of two components, one for quantifying the model fit and the other for evaluating the complexity of the model. The first component is measured through the posterior expectation of the deviance $D(\theta) = -2 \log(p(y \mid \theta))$ while the model complexity is measured through the *effective number of parameters*:

$$p_D = E_{\theta|y}(D(\theta)) - D(E_{\theta|y}(\theta)) = \overline{D} - D(\overline{\theta}),$$

so that the DIC is

$$\text{DIC} = \overline{D} + p_D. \tag{5.26}$$

Analogously to the AIC, models with smaller DIC are better supported by the data.

The option `control.compute=list(dic=TRUE)` specified inside the `inla` function is used to compute the DIC. It also returns the different components: the posterior mean of the deviance $\overline{D}$ (`mean.deviance`), the deviance of the posterior mean of the parameters $D(\overline{\theta})$ (`deviance.mean`) and the effective number of parameters p_D (`p.eff`). Note that INLA, instead of evaluating the deviance at the posterior mean of all parameters, evaluates the deviance at the posterior mean of the latent field θ and at the posterior mode of the hyperparameters ψ. The reason is that the posterior marginals for some hyperparameters (especially the precisions) might be highly skewed, so that the posterior expectation is not a good representation of the distribution and the mode is preferred.

We calculate the DIC for the pooled and hierarchical models specified on the CD4 example which we presented in Section 5.4.4 using the following code:

```
> CD4.1$dic$dic
[1] 1112.531
> CD4.3$dic$dic
[1] 920.1855
```

It shows how adding the hierarchical structure improves the fitting of the model despite the added complexity due to the increased number of parameters. We can also look at the separate components of the DIC:

```
> #Mean Deviance
> CD4.1.deviance <- CD4.1$dic$mean.deviance
> CD4.1.deviance
[1] 1107.881
> CD4.3.deviance <- CD4.3$dic$mean.deviance
> CD4.3.deviance
[1] 851.9963
> #pD
> CD4.1.pD <- CD4.1$dic$p.eff
> CD4.1.pD
[1] 4.649632
> CD4.3.pD <- CD4.3$dic$p.eff
> CD4.3.pD
[1] 68.18922
```

and then calculate the DIC manually:

```
> CD4.1.deviance + CD4.1.pD
[1] 1112.531
> CD4.3.deviance + CD4.3.pD
[1] 920.1855
```

obtaining the same values.

References

Aldous, D. (1981). Representations for partially exchangeable arrays of random variables. *Journal of Multivariate Analysis*, **11**(4), 581–598.

Carlin, B. and Louis, T. (2008). *Bayesian Methods for Data Analysis*. Chapman & Hall.

Casella, G. and Berger, R. (2002). *Statistical Inference*. Duxbury, Thompson Learning.

Congdon, P. (2007). *Bayesian Statistical Modelling*. John Wiley and Sons, Ltd.

Czado, C., Gneiting, T., and Held, L. (2009). Predictive model assessment for count data. *Biometrics*, **65**(4), 1254–1261.

Dawid, A. (1984). Statistical theory: The prequential approach. *Journal of the Royal Statistical Society, Series A*, **147**, 278–292.

De Finetti, B. (1974). *Probability, Induction and Statistics*. Wiley, New York.

Dellaportas, P. and Smith, A. (1993). Bayesian inference for generalized linear and proportional hazards models via Gibbs sampling. *Journal of the Royal Statistical Society, Series C*, **42**(3), 443–459.

Edwards, D. (2000). *Introduction to Graphical Modelling*, 2nd edition. Springer Verlag.

Feller, W. (1968). *An Introduction to Probability Theory and its Applications (Volume 1)*. John Wiley and Sons.

Galton, F. (1886). Regression towards mediocrity in hereditary stature. *Journal of the Anthropological Institute*, **15**, 246–263.

Gelman, A., Bois, F., and Jiang, J. (1996). Physiological pharmacokinetic analysis using population modeling and informative prior distributions. *Journal of the American Statistical Association*, **91**, 1400–1412.

Gelman, A., Carlin, J., Stern, H., and Rubin, D. (2004). *Bayesian Data Analysis*. Chapman & Hall/CRC.

Gilks, W. and Spiegelhalter, D. (1996). *Markov Chain Monte Carlo in Practice*. Chapman & Hall/CRC.

Gneiting, T., Balabdaoui, F., and Raftery, A. E. (2007). Probabilistic forecasts, calibration and sharpness. *Journal of the Royal Statistical Society, Series B (Statistical Methodology)*, **69**(2), 243–268.

Held, L., Schrödle, B., and Rue, H. (2010). Posterior and Cross-validatory Predictive Checks: A comparison of MCMC and INLA. In T. Kneib and G. Tutz, editors, *Statistical Modelling and Regression Structures*, pages 91–110. Physica-Verlag HD.

Ibrahim, J. and Purushottam, W. (1991). On Bayesian analysis of generalized linear models using Jeffreys's prior. *Journal of the American Statistical Association*, **86**(416), 981–986.

Kingman, J. (1978). Uses of exchangeability. *Annals of Probability*, **6**(2), 183–197.

Maheswaran, R., Haining, R., Pearson, T., Law, J., Brindley, P., and Best, N. (2006). Outdoor NOx and stroke mortality: Adjusting for small area level smoking prevalence using a Bayesian approach. *Statistical Methods in Medical Research*, **15**(5), 499–516.

McCullagh, P. and Nelder, J. (1989). *Generalized Linear Models, Second Edition*. Chapman & Hall.

Nelder, J. and Wedderburn, R. (1972). Generalized linear models. *Journal of the Royal Statistical Society, Series A*, **135**(3), 370–384.

Pettit, L. (1990). The conditional predictive ordinate for the Normal distribution. *Journal of the Royal Statistical Society, Series B*, **56**, 3–48.

Rue, H., Martino, S., and Chopin, N. (2009). Approximate Bayesian inference for latent Gaussian model by using integrated nested Laplace approximations (with discussion). *Journal of the Royal Statistical Society, Series B*, **71**, 319–392.

Spiegelhalter, D. J., Best, N. G., Carlin, B. P., and Van Der Linde, A. (2002). Bayesian measures of model complexity and fit. *Journal of the Royal Statistical Society, Series B (Statistical Methodology)*, **64**(4), 583–639.

Townsend, P. (1987). Deprivation. *Journal of Social Policy*, **16**, 125–146.

Whittaker, J. (1990). *Graphical Models in Applied Multivariate Statistics*. John Wiley and Sons.

Zellner, A. (1971). *An Introduction to Bayesian Inference in Econometrics*. John Wiley and Sons, Ltd.

6

Spatial modeling

In many applications researchers analyze data which are geographically referenced, e.g., their location in space is known. These are also called *spatial data* and are defined as realizations of a stochastic process indexed by space

$$Y(s) \equiv \{y(s), s \in \mathcal{D}\},$$

where $\mathcal{D}$ is a (fixed) subset of $\mathbb{R}^d$.

Following the distinction presented by Cressie (1993), Banerjee *et al.* (2004) and Gelfand *et al.* (2010), we can specify three types of spatial data:

1. *Area or lattice data*, where $y(s)$ is a random aggregate value over an areal unit s with well-defined boundaries in $\mathcal{D}$, which is defined as a countable collection of d-dimensional spatial units. The difference between area and lattice is that the first is typically irregular and based on administrative boundaries (e.g., districts, regions, counties, etc.), while the latter is regular. Figure 6.1 displays the proportion of children with respiratory illness (left) and the standardized morbidity ratio of lung cancer in the 44 London wards (right) and represents two realizations of an areal process, defined on a regular grid and irregularly shaped areas, respectively. In these cases, we are often interested in smoothing or mapping an outcome over $\mathcal{D}$. This type of data will be treated in Sections 6.1–6.3.

2. *Point-referenced (or geostatistical) data*, where $y(s)$ is a random outcome at a specific location and the spatial index s can vary continuously in the fixed domain $\mathcal{D}$. The location s is typically a two-dimensional vector with latitude and longitude but may also include altitude. The actual data are represented by a collection of observations $y = (y(s_1), \ldots, y(s_n))$, where the set $(s_1, \ldots, s_n)$ indicates the locations at which the measurements are taken. For instance, the zinc measurements shown in Figure 6.2 are an example of geostatistical data.

Spatial and Spatio-temporal Bayesian Models with R-INLA, First Edition.
Marta Blangiardo and Michela Cameletti.
© 2015 John Wiley & Sons, Ltd. Published 2015 by John Wiley & Sons, Ltd.

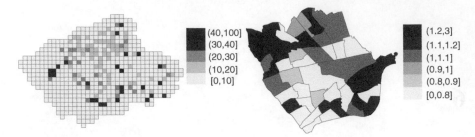

Figure 6.1   Proportion of children with respiratory illness in England (left) and standardized morbidity ratio of lung cancer in 44 London wards (right).

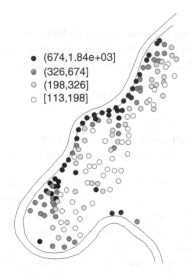

Figure 6.2   Zinc measurements (ppm) at 155 locations near the Meuse river.

In this context, we are interested in predicting the outcome at unobserved locations in $\mathcal{D}$. This type of data will be treated from Section 6.4 onward.

3. *Spatial point patterns*, where $y(s)$ represents the occurrence or not of an event and the locations themselves are random. The spatial domain $\mathcal{D}$ is a set of points in $\mathbb{R}^d$ at which some events happened. For example, we might be interested in the locations of trees of a species in a forest or addresses of persons with a particular disease. In this case, while locations $s \in \mathbb{R}^d$ are random, the measurement $y(s)$ takes 0 or 1 values, i.e., the event has occurred or not. If some additional covariate information is available, we talk about *marked* point pattern process. In this case, we are often interested in evaluating possible clustering or inhibition behavior between observations. As an example of spatial point pattern, we consider the foot and mouth disease data provided in the `fmd` dataset in the `stpp` package (Diggle *et al.*, 2005). Figure 6.3

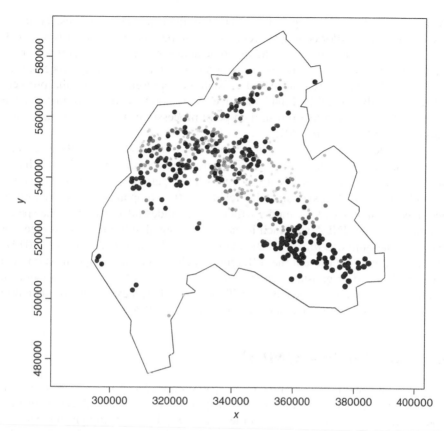

Figure 6.3   Locations of the 648 cases of foot and mouth disease in the North Cumbria region (UK) in 2001, marked by time (in light gray the oldest events and in dark gray the more recent ones). The data are part of the fmd *dataset in the* stpp *package.*

shows the marked locations of cases of foot and mouth diseases in the North Cumbria region (UK) in 2001. Light gray identifies the oldest events, while in dark gray the more recent ones are showed. We are not discussing methods to analyze this type of data here and we refer the readers to Gelfand *et al.*, 2010, Chap. 21.

When working with spatial data their spatial trend needs to be taken into account in the inferential process: this additional information can provide insight knowledge and dismissing it could lead to biases in the estimates. Under these circumstances, the Bayesian approach is generally particularly effective (Dunson, 2001) and has been used in several epidemiological applications, from ecology (Clark, 2005) to environmental studies (Wikle, 2003; Clark and Gelfand, 2006), to infectious disease (Jewell *et al.*, 2009). If the data are available at the area level and consist of aggregated counts of outcomes and covariates, typically disease mapping and/or ecological regression can be specified (Richardson, 2003; Lawson, 2009). Alternatively, if the outcome and/or risk factors data are observed at point locations and are a realizations of a continuous underlying process, then geostatistical models are considered as suitable representations of the problem (Diggle and Ribeiro, 2007). Finally, if the data are point locations, for instance the exact locations of trees in a forest, then point processes can be used to study their spatial pattern (Illian *et al.*, 2012).

These models can be specified in a Bayesian framework by simply extending the concept of hierarchical structure, allowing us to account for similarities based on the neighborhood or on the distance. However, particularly in these cases, the main challenge in Bayesian statistics resides in the computational aspects, given the added complexity of the model which also includes information on the spatial structure; thus the INLA approach is particularly suitable in this context (see, for instance, Blangiardo *et al.*, 2013, Bivand *et al.*, 2015, Gómez-Rubio *et al.*, 2014)

In this chapter, we present the different models which can be specified on area or lattice data and on geostatistical data, and describe how to apply such models in R-INLA, while we refer the reader to Illian (2015) for an exhaustive presentation of point processes theory and applications using R-INLA.

6.1   Areal data – GMRF

When working with area level data, the spatial dependency is taken into account through the neighborhood structure. Simplifying the notation introduced in the previous section so that $(s_1, \ldots, s_n)$ becomes $(1, \ldots, n)$, then typically given the area i, its neighbors $\mathcal{N}(i)$ are defined as the areas which share borders with it (first-order neighbors, Figure 6.4, left) or which share borders with it and with its first-order neighbors (second-order neighbors, Figure 6.4, right).

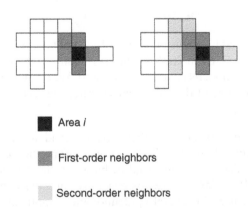

Area i

First-order neighbors

Second-order neighbors

Figure 6.4   Neighboring structure: first-order neighbors (left), first- and second-order neighbors (right).

Under the Markovian property that the parameter θ_i for the ith area is indepen-dent of all the other parameters, given the set of its neighbors $\mathcal{N}(i)$ (local Markov property), then

$$\theta_i \perp\!\!\!\perp \theta_{-i} | \theta_{\mathcal{N}(i)},$$

where θ_{-i} indicates all the elements in θ but the ith. The point is that the preci-sion matrix Q of θ is sparse, which produces great computational benefits. In other words, for any pair of elements (i, j) in θ

$$\theta_i \perp\!\!\!\perp \theta_j | \theta_{-ij} \iff Q_{ij} = 0,$$

i.e., the nonzero pattern in the precision matrix is given by the neighborhood struc-ture of the process (pairwise Markov property). Thus, $Q_{ij} \neq 0$ only if $j \in \{i, \mathcal{N}(i)\}$. This specification is again a *GMRF* (Rue and Held, 2005), as presented in Section 4.7.1. The important difference is that now the independence of θ_i from θ_j is not only conditional to the hyperparameters as described in Section 4.7.1, but also to the set of neighbors. We can specify the precision matrix as a function of the so-called *structure matrix* R:

$$Q = \tau R$$

where

$$R_{ij} = \begin{cases} \mathcal{N}_i^r & \text{if } i = j \\ 1 & \text{if } i \sim j \\ 0 & \text{otherwise} \end{cases} \tag{6.1}$$

with $i \sim j$ denoting that areas i and j are neighbors.

6.1.1 Disease mapping

Disease mapping is commonly used with areal data to assess the spatial pattern of a particular disease and to identify areas characterized by unusually high or low relative risk (Pascutto *et al.*, 2000; Lawson, 2009). The data in this case are dis-crete in nature, as they are counts of diseases or deaths in each area. A simplistic approach to this type of data might consider the calculation of the standardized mortality (or morbidity) ratio (also called SMR), which is simply the ratio between the number of observed cases y_i and the number of expected cases E_i in the ith area $(i = 1, \ldots, n)$, typically calculated using age and sex standardized reference rates r_j $(j = 1, \ldots, J$ combinations of age and sex categories) and census population counts Pop_{ij} as follows:

$$r_j = \frac{\sum_{i=1}^{n} y_{ij}}{\sum_{i=1}^{n} \text{Pop}_{ij}} \tag{6.2}$$

$$E_i = \sum_{j=1}^{J} \text{Pop}_{ij} \times r_j. \tag{6.3}$$

Throughout the book, we assume that the expected counts are already available and calculated using the procedure above, but we refer the reader to Elliott *et al.* (2000) or Lesaffre and Lawson (2012) for more information about alternative ways of obtaining E_i.

Such simplistic approach does not take into account the spatial dependence amongst the areas, meaning that essentially, we are throwing away a piece of important information, as described in the previous section. To take this into account, we go back to the Poisson model described in Section 5.3, and for each area we assume

$$y_i \sim \text{Poisson}(\lambda_i) \qquad \lambda_i = E_i \rho_i \qquad \log(\rho_i) = \eta_i, \tag{6.4}$$

so that the mean λ_i is defined in terms of a rate ρ_i and of the expected number of cases E_i, as already presented in Section 5.4.5. Then a log linear model is specified on the linear predictor η_i:

$$\eta_i = b_0 + u_i + v_i, \tag{6.5}$$

where b_0 is the intercept, quantifying the average outcome rate in the entire study region, while v_i is the area-specific effect modeled as exchangeable. In addition, we have u_i, another area-specific effect, which we now model as spatially structured.

Several structures can be specified on $\boldsymbol{u} = \{u_1, \dots, u_n\}$. We will focus here on the conditional autoregressive one (Besag, 1974), which is implemented in R-INLA. Considering n areas, each characterized by a set of neighbors $\mathcal{N}(i)$, let us assume that u_i is the following random variable:

$$u_i | \boldsymbol{u}_{-i} \sim \text{Normal}\left(\mu_i + \sum_{j=1}^{n} r_{ij}(u_j - \mu_j), s_i^2 \right),$$

where μ_i is the mean for the area i and $s_i^2 = \sigma_u^2 / \mathcal{N}_i$ is the variance for the same area, which depends on its number of neighbors ($\mathcal{N}_i = \#\mathcal{N}(i)$), e.g., if an area has many neighbors then its variance will be smaller. This variance structure recognizes the fact that in the presence of strong spatial correlation, the more neighbors an area has the more information there is in the data about the value of its random effect, while the variance parameter σ_u^2 controls the amount of variation between the spatially structured random effects. The quantity r_{ij} indicates the spatial proximity and can be calculated as $\phi \times W_{ij}$, where $W_{ij} = a_{ij}/\mathcal{N}_i$, a_{ij} is 1 if areas i and j are neighbors and 0 otherwise (note that a_{ii} is set to 0, thus W_{ii} and r_{ii} are 0 as well); finally, the parameter ϕ controls the properness of the distribution.

Considering W as the matrix of generic elements W_{ij} and $S = \text{diag}(s_1, \dots, s_n)$, to ensure that the distribution for the spatially structured random effect is proper, the covariance matrix $(I - \phi W)^{-1} S^2$ must be positive definite; thus the values of ϕ must be between $1/\min_{i=1,\dots,n}\kappa_i$ and $1/\max_{i=1,\dots,n}\kappa_i$, with κ_i being the generic eigenvalues of W (Cressie, 1993). Then the proper conditional autoregressive specification (CAR) $\boldsymbol{u}$ is a multivariate Normal random variable:

$$\boldsymbol{u} \sim \text{MVNormal}\,(\boldsymbol{\mu}, (I - \phi W)^{-1} S^2),$$

where $\mu = \{\mu_1, \ldots, \mu_n\}$ is the mean vector, I is the identity matrix and S^2 is defined above. Thus the conditional distribution of $u_i|u_{-i}$ is

$$u_i|u_{-i} \sim \text{Normal}\left(\mu_i + \phi\frac{1}{\mathcal{N}_i}\sum_{j=1}^{n}a_{ij}(u_j - \mu_j), s_i^2\right)$$

and the correlation between areas i and j depends only on ϕ and W (see Assuncao and Krainski, 2009) and is given by

$$\frac{\sqrt{\mathcal{N}_i}}{\mathcal{N}_j}\frac{(I - \phi W)_{ij}^{-1}}{\sqrt{(I - \phi W)_{ii}^{-1}(I - \phi W)_{jj}^{-1}}}.$$

This specification is not greatly used in disease mapping studies as the ϕ parameter can prove hard to estimate. A simplified version of the formulation above can be obtained fixing $\phi = 1$, meaning that the covariance matrix is not positive definite; this leads to the following conditional distribution for u_i:

$$u_i|u_{-i} \sim \text{Normal}\left(\mu_i + \frac{1}{\mathcal{N}_i}\sum_{j=1}^{n}a_{ij}(u_j - \mu_j), s_i^2\right).$$

Such specification is called intrinsic conditional autoregressive (iCAR) and coupled with the exchangeable random effect presented in Eq. (6.5) originates the so-called *Besag–York–Molliè* (BYM) model presented by Besag *et al.* (1991). However, due to the nonpositive definition of the covariance matrix, there is no proper joint distribution for u, as it would be possible to add any constant to each u_i without changing the distribution.[1] This issue can be rectified fixing a constraint such as $\sum_{i=1}^{n} u_i = 0$.

If we assume $\mu_i = 0$ for each i the conditional distribution is now in the form typically presented in the literature on disease mapping (see, for instance, Besag *et al.*, 1991, Best *et al.*, 2005, Lawson, 2009, Lee, 2011):

$$u_i|u_{-i} \sim \text{Normal}\left(\frac{1}{\mathcal{N}_i}\sum_{j=1}^{n}a_{ij}u_j, s_i^2\right). \tag{6.6}$$

6.1.2 BYM model: suicides in London

To show how R-INLA can be used to perform disease mapping with a BYM model we use the dataset presented by Congdon (2007) to investigate suicide mortality in $n = 32$ London boroughs in the period 1989–1993 and described in Section 1.4.7.

---

[1] Being an improper prior and lacking a joint distribution, the iCAR can only be used as prior for the random effects and not as a distribution of the observations.

For the ith area, the number of suicides y_i is modeled as

$$y_i \sim \text{Poisson}(E_i \rho_i),$$

$$\eta_i = \log(\rho_i) = b_0 + u_i + v_i$$

with b_0 quantifying the average suicide rate in all the 32 boroughs. E_i is the number of expected cases of suicides for each areas, which acts as an offset (see Section 5.3); u_i is the spatially structured residual, modeled using the iCAR specification given in Eq. (6.6), and v_i is the unstructured residual modeled using exchangeability among the 32 boroughs such that

$$v_i \sim \text{Normal}(0, \sigma_v^2).$$

Before running this model, we need to specify a graph which assigns the set of neighbors for each borough. In R-INLA this can be done in the following three ways.

ASCII or binary file

This is probably the simplest way of defining the graphical structure if the number of areas is not too large and consists in creating an ASCII file with a number of rows equal to the number of areas (n) plus 1.

The first row contains n. The next n rows specify: (i) the area label indexed as $1, 2, \ldots, n$, (ii) its number of neighbors, and (iii) the label of the neighboring areas. In our example, $n = 32$ and the graph would look like the following:

```
32
1 4 19 20 21 22
2 4 3 11 19 21
3 6 2 11 12 13 14 15
4 4 5 7 20 23
. . .
```

so for the first area there are four neighbors which are areas number 19, 20, 21, and 22 and a similar reasoning applies to the other areas. Note that there must be symmetry in the neighboring structure, so for instance if area 1 is neighbor with area 19, it must also be true that area 19 is neighbor with area 1.

Instead of saving the graph specification in a .dat file, it can also be specified as a character string. Using the following toy example assuming $n = 4$, the first area being neighbor with the third and fourth and the second area having no neighbors (remember that for symmetry the third and fourth areas must be neighbors with the first) the neighborhood structure can be written as follows:

```
"4 1 2 3 4  2 0 3 1 1 4 1 1"
```

Matrix specification

Another way of defining the model graph is through a symmetric adjacency matrix H, so that $H_{ij} \neq 0$ if and only if i and j areas are neighbors. For instance, the simple structure created above using a character string can be re-written using the matrix specification as follows:

```
> H <- matrix(c(1,0,1,1,0,1,0,0,1,0,1,0,1,0,0,1),
            ncol=4,nrow=4,byrow=TRUE)
> H
     [,1] [,2] [,3] [,4]
[1,]    1    0    1    1
[2,]    0    1    0    0
[3,]    1    0    1    0
[4,]    1    0    0    1
```

However, for large matrices doing this by hand could be rather time consuming and a good alternative is to use the sparseMatrix R function, available when the R-INLA package is loaded:

```
> H <- sparseMatrix(i=c(1,1,1,2,3,4),j=c(1,3,4,2,3,4),
                symmetric=TRUE)
```

where i identifies the row numbers and j the column numbers for the nonzero elements. Specifying symmetric=TRUE means that only the upper (or lower) triangular needs to be provided and the rest is filled automatically. Note that it is not important what value is put on the diagonal as R-INLA does not consider it (an area cannot be a neighbor of itself).

Using inla.graph

An alternative method to the previous ones produces the graph from a shape file with information on all the area boundaries and uses a combination of functions from different R packages. First, we need to upload the shape file, through the function readShapePoly of the maptools package, e.g., for the London boroughs:

```
> library(maptools)
> london.gen <- readShapePoly("LDNSuicides")
```

Then, we use the poly2nb and nb2INLA functions from the spdep package to transform the shape file into an adjacency matrix and to make it compatible with the R-INLA format

```
> library(spdep)
> temp <- poly2nb(london.gen)
> nb2INLA("LDN.graph", temp)
> LDN.adj <- paste(getwd(),"/LDN.graph",sep="")
```

Now we have a file called LDN.graph stored in the current working directory which is in the right format to be read by R-INLA. The last command creates an object (LDN.adj) with the location of the graph.

A graph can be imported in R-INLA using the inla.read.graph function and from this the adjacency matrix can also be obtained through

```
> H <- inla.read.graph(filename="LDN.graph")
> image(inla.graph2matrix(H),xlab="",ylab="")
```

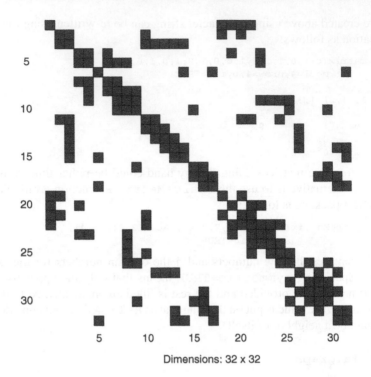

Dimensions: 32 x 32

*Figure 6.5   Adjacency matrix for the London suicides example: rows and columns
identify areas; squares identify neighbors.*

which is shown in Figure 6.5 for the 32 London boroughs of our example. Looking
at it we can see the pattern in the neighborhood structure and identify more isolated
or more central areas. For instance, the 6th borough has three neighboring ones,
while the 9th borough has seven neighbors (black squares).

After having defined the neighborhood structure, we need to specify the formula
for the model, through

```
> formula <- y ~ 1 + f(ID, model="bym",graph=LDN.adj)
```

where ID represents the identifiers for the boroughs and through the graph option
we include the name of the object containing the neighborhood structure. Note that
with f(ID, model="bym", ...) R-INLA parameterizes $\xi_i = u_i + v_i$ and u_i.[2]

By default, minimally informative priors are specified on: (i) the log of the
unstructured effect precision $\log(\tau_v) \sim \log\text{Gamma}(1, 0.0005)$, and (ii) the log
of the structured effect precision $\log(\tau_u) \sim \log\text{Gamma}(1, 0.0005)$. However, for

---

[2] Alternatively it is possible to specify the two BYM components separately using f(ID,
model="besag") for the spatial structured one (iCAR) and f(ID2, model="iid") for the
unstructured one (exchangeable). In this case, the ID needs to be duplicated (ID2=ID) as it is not
allowed to define two effects with f() on the same index variable.

intrinsic models such as iCAR (and random walks which we will see extensively in Chapter 7), the precision matrix Q is equal to τR, where τ is a random parameter and R is the neighboring structure (see Eq. (6.1)); thus even assuming the same distribution on τ leads to marginal variances/precisions which are different depending on the neighboring structure R.

As reported by Sørbye and Rue (2014), to make the precision parameters of models with different intrinsic gaussian random field comparable, it is possible to compute the generalized variance of the vector θ fixing $\tau = 1$ as

$$\sigma_{GV}^2(\theta) = \exp\left(\frac{1}{n}\sum_{i=1}^{n}\log(\sigma_{\tau=1}^2(\theta_i))\right)$$

and then scale it so that $\sigma_{GV}^2 = 1$. This process can be done in a simple way in R-INLA using the option scale.model=TRUE within the formula specification.

Recall also that different priors can be specified through the option hyper, for instance

```
> formula <- y ~ 1 + f(ID, model="bym",graph=LDN.adj,
                     scale.model=TRUE,
                     hyper=list(prec.unstruct=
                     list(prior="loggamma",param=c(1,0.001)),
                     prec.spatial=list(
                     prior="loggamma",param=c(1,0.001)))))
```

Of course, as in any Bayesian analysis, the choice of the prior may have a considerable impact on the results. Thus, it is necessary to think carefully about its choice and perform sensitivity analyses to assess how the prior influences the estimations. Finally, the model can be run using the inla function:

```
> mod.suicides <- inla(formula,family="poisson",
             data=data.suicides,E=E,
             control.compute=list(dic=TRUE))
```

In this case, the parameters estimated by R-INLA are represented by $\theta = \{b_0, \xi, u\}$ and the hyperparameters are given by the precisions $\psi = \{\tau_u, \tau_v\}$. Summary information (e.g., the posterior mean and standard deviation, together with a 95% credibility interval) can be obtained for each component of θ and ψ. In particular, for the so-called fixed effects (b_0, in this case) and for the random effects (i.e. ξ and u) this can be obtained typing

```
> round(mod.suicides$summary.fixed,3)
              mean     sd 0.025quant 0.5quant 0.975quant  mode kld
(Intercept) 0.045  0.019      0.006    0.045      0.082 0.045   0
> round(head(mod.suicides$summary.random$ID),3) #partial output
  ID    mean     sd 0.025quant 0.5quant 0.975quant   mode kld
1  1   0.465  0.063      0.340    0.466      0.588  0.467   0
2  2   0.012  0.072     -0.132    0.013      0.153  0.015   0
3  3  -0.137  0.073     -0.284   -0.136      0.005 -0.135   0
```

4	4	0.310	0.079	0.153	0.311	0.463	0.312	0
5	5	-0.135	0.079	-0.293	-0.134	0.017	-0.131	0
6	6	-0.422	0.095	-0.613	-0.420	-0.240	-0.417	0

The latter is a dataframe formed by $2n$ rows: the first n rows include information on the area-specific residuals ξ_i, which are the primary interest in a disease mapping study, while the remaining present information on the spatially structured residual u_i only. Recall that all these parameters are on the logarithmic scale; for the sake of interpretability it would be more convenient to transform them back to the natural scale.

To compute the posterior mean and 95% credibility interval for the fixed effect b_0 on the original scale, we type

```
> exp.b0.mean <- inla.emarginal(exp,mod.suicides$marginals.fixed[[1]])
> exp.b0.mean
[1] 1.045792
> exp.b0.95CI <- inla.qmarginal(c(0.025,0.975),
              inla.tmarginal(exp,mod.suicides$marginals.fixed[[1]]))
> exp.b0.95CI
[1] 1.006715 1.085415
```

The posterior mean of the exponentiated intercept b_0 implies a 4.6% suicide rate across London, with a 95% credibility interval ranging from 0.7% to 8.5%. The computation of the posterior mean for the random effects ξ is performed in two steps as we have more than one parameter:

```
> csi <- mod.suicides$marginals.random$ID[1:Nareas]
> zeta <- lapply(csi,function(x) inla.emarginal(exp,x))
```

First, we extract the marginal posterior distribution for each element of ξ and then apply the exponential transformation and calculate the posterior mean for each of them using the lapply function.

Figure 6.6 (left) shows the map of the posterior mean for the borough-specific relative risks of suicides $\zeta = \exp(\xi)$, compared to the whole of London. The code to obtain the map is the following:

```
> #Define the cutoff for zeta
> zeta.cutoff <- c(0.6, 0.9, 1.0, 1.1, 1.8)
> #Transform zeta in categorical variable
> cat.zeta <- cut(unlist(zeta),breaks=zeta.cutoff,
                include.lowest=TRUE)
> #Create a dataframe with all the information needed for the map
> maps.cat.zeta <- data.frame(ID=data.suicides$ID, cat.zeta=cat.zeta)

> #Add the categorized zeta to the spatial polygon
> data.boroughs <- attr(london.gen, "data")
> attr(london.gen, "data") <- merge(data.boroughs, maps.cat.zeta,
                        by="ID")

> #Map zeta
> spplot(obj=london.gen, zcol= "cat.zeta",
      col.regions=gray(seq(0.9,0.1,length=4)), asp=1)
```

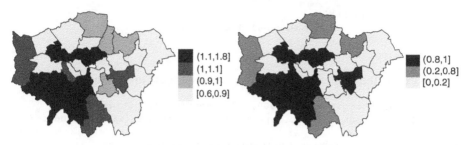

	(1.1,1.8]			(0.8,1]
	(1,1.1]			(0.2,0.8]
	(0.9,1]			[0,0.2]
	[0.6,0.9]			

Figure 6.6   Posterior mean for the borough-specific relative risks $\zeta = \exp(\xi)$ compared with the whole of London (left) and posterior probability $p(\zeta_i > 1|y)$.

The uncertainty associated with the posterior means can also be mapped and provide useful information (Richardson *et al.*, 2004). In particular, as the interest lays on the excess risk, we can visualize $p(\zeta_i > 1|y)$ (or equivalently $p(\xi_i > 0|y)$) which is easier to obtain) using the built-in function `inla.pmarginal`:

```
> a <- 0
> prob.csi <- lapply(csi, function(x) {1 - inla.pmarginal(a, x)})
```

The resulting map – obtained using the same procedure described before for ζ – is presented in Figure 6.6 (right).

Finally, it could be interesting to evaluate the proportion of variance explained by the structured spatial component. The quantity σ_u^2 is the variance of the conditional autoregressive specification, while σ_v^2 is the variance of the marginal unstructured component. Thus, the two are not directly comparable. Nevertheless, it is possible to obtain empirically an estimate of the posterior marginal variance for the structured effect through

$$s_u^2 = \frac{\sum_{i=1}^n (u_i - \bar{u})^2}{n-1},$$

where $\bar{u}$ is the average of u, and then compare it to the posterior marginal variance for the unstructured effect, provided by σ_v^2, as

$$\text{frac}_{\text{spatial}} = s_u^2 / (s_u^2 + \sigma_v^2).$$

To obtain this in R-INLA, we adopt a simulation-based approach through the `inla.rmarginal` function: for each area we extract a large enough number of values (e.g., 100 000) from the corresponding marginal posterior distribution of v_i and save the simulated values in a matrix with rows equal to the number of areas and 100 000 columns. Then we calculate the empirical variance (over column).

```
> mat.marg <- matrix(NA, nrow=Nareas, ncol=100000)
> m <- mod.suicides$marginals.random$ID
> for (i in 1:Nareas){
    #Remember that the first Nareas values of the random effects
    #are u+v, while u values are stored in the (Nareas+1) to
    #(2*Nareas) elements.
```

```
  u <- m[[Nareas+i]]
  mat.marg[i,] <- inla.rmarginal(100000, u)
}
> var.u <- apply(mat.marg, 2, var)
```

We also extract the expected value of the variance for the unstructured component

```
> var.v <- inla.rmarginal(100000,inla.tmarginal(function(x) 1/x,
      mod.suicides$marginals.hyper$"Precision for ID (iid component)"))
```

and finally we compute the spatial fractional variance frac$_{spatial}$ as

```
> perc.var.u <- mean(var.u/(var.u+var.v))
> perc.var.u
[1] 0.9418849
```

In the current example, the proportion of spatial variance is about 0.94 suggesting that a large part of the variability is explained by the spatial structure.

Note that when the option scale.model is set equal to TRUE in the f() environment, we can sample directly from the marginal posterior of τ_u and τ_v using inla.hyperpar.sample, which returns a matrix with the number of rows equal to the size of the sample and number of columns equal to the number of hyperparameters (2 in our case).

```
> marg.hyper <- inla.hyperpar.sample(100000,mod.suicides)
```

Then we can obtain the posterior distribution of the proportion of variance explained by the spatial component as follows:

```
> perc.var.u1 <- mean(marg.hyper[,1] / (marg.hyper[,1]+marg.hyper[,2]))
```

which in this case is 0.92. Note that the two methods returns marginally different results due to sampling variability, as in both cases we sample from the posterior distributions.

6.2   Ecological regression

When risk factors are available and the aim of the study is to evaluate their effect on the risk of disease (or death), ecological regression models can be specified, simply extending the procedure described in the previous section for the disease mapping. For instance, going back to the London boroughs suicides example, for each of the 32 boroughs the values of an index of social deprivation and an index of social fragmentation (describing lack of social connections and of sense of community) are known and stored respectively in the variables x_1 and x_2. To evaluate their impact on the risk of suicides, the model in Eq. (6.5) can be reformulated as

$$\eta_i = b_0 + \beta_1 x_{1i} + \beta_2 x_{2i} + u_i + v_i,$$

which can be coded in R-INLA using the formula

Table 6.1   Summary statistics: posterior mean,
posterior standard deviation (SD) and posterior 95%
credibility interval for the fixed effects of the ecological
regression model.

	Mean	SD	2.5%	50%	97.5%
b_0	0.059	0.017	0.025	0.059	0.093
β_1	0.090	0.024	0.042	0.091	0.136
β_2	0.180	0.022	0.137	0.180	0.224

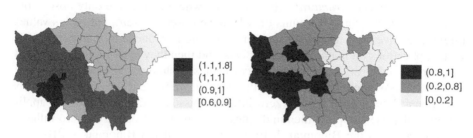

*Figure 6.7   Ecological regression: posterior mean for the borough-specific rel-
ative risks $\zeta = \exp(\xi)$ compared with the whole of London (left) and posterior
probability $p(\zeta_i > 1|y)$ (right).*

```
> formula.eco.reg <- y ~ 1 + x1 + x2 + f(ID,model="bym",
                                    graph=LDN.adj)
> mod.eco.reg <- inla(formula.eco.reg,family="poisson",
                  data=data.suicides,E=E,
                  control.compute=list(dic=TRUE))
```

The fixed effects $\{b_0, \beta_1, \beta_2\}$ estimated by R-INLA are presented in Table 6.1. If
reported on the natural scale, they can be interpreted as relative risks: an increase
of 1 unit in the deprivation index and in the social fragmentation index is associated respectively with an increase of around 9% and around 18% in the risk of
suicides.

The maps of the borough-specific relative risks ζ (recall that $\zeta_i = \exp(u_i + v_i)$)
and their posterior probability of exceeding 1 are shown in Figure 6.7; note that
now they are interpreted as the residual relative risk for each area (compared to the
whole of London) after the risk factors x_1 and x_2 are taken into account.

Using the DIC presented in Chapter 5, as a tool for evaluating the fit of a model,
suggests that the ecological regression is better suited for the data (with a DIC of
259.76 vs 273.81 obtained for the disease mapping). This means that the variables
on social deprivation and social fragmentation explain part of the variability in the
risk of suicides in London. This is also confirmed if we look at the proportion
of variance explained by the spatially structured component, which goes down to
0.704 from 0.922, registered for the disease mapping model, suggesting that some

of the spatial patterns in the risk of suicides can be explained by the two covariates included in the regression.

6.3   Zero-inflated models

In some applications the specification of Poisson or Binomial models for counts data might be inappropriate due to the excess of zeros in the data compared with what expected from the model (overdispersion). To overcome this issue the so-called *zero-inflated* models can be specified. These are a mixture of two components: a point mass at zero and a count distribution. In this way, such models distinguish between *structural* zeros, for units where zero is the only observable value, and *sample* zeros, for units on which we observe a zero, but others values might also have been recorded. Such models were introduced by Lambert (1992) with applications on manufacturing defects, and then they were rapidly embraced by a large number of areas, from medical studies (Bohning, 1998) to econometric applications (Winkelmann, 2003). In this section, we present zero-inflated models based on a Poisson distribution (zero-inflated Poisson – ZIP) and show an application on disease mapping; then in the next section, we introduce the zero-inflated models based on the Binomial distribution (zero-inflated Binomial – ZIB) and describe an application in the framework of ecological regression.

6.3.1   Zero-inflated Poisson model: brain cancer in Navarra

As we have seen in the previous sections, the Poisson distribution is commonly used with counts data and it is the reference model for disease mapping studies. However, being characterized by a single parameter for mean and variance, such a model can suffer from overdispersion. Allowing for a hierarchical and/or spatial structure can help model some of the heterogeneity in the data, but when the overdispersion is caused by an excessive number of zeros, combining the spatial or hierarchical structure with a ZIP helps address this issue, as shown in Agarwal *et al.* (2002) and in Gschlobl and Gzado (2008).

Given n areas, the probability function for y_i ($i = 1, \ldots, n$) is as follows:

$$p(y_i|\lambda_i, \pi_0) = \pi_0 I(y_i = 0) + (1 - \pi_0)\frac{\exp(-\lambda_i)\lambda_i^{y_i}}{y_i!}, \quad (6.7)$$

where $I(y_i = 0)$ is the indicator variable. The probability of observing a zero in the ith area is $\pi_0 + (1 - \pi_0)\exp(-\lambda_i)$, and the mean and variance are the following:

$$E(y_i) = (1 - \pi_0)\lambda_i \quad (6.8)$$

$$\text{Var}(y_i) = (1 - \pi_0)\lambda_i + \frac{\pi_0}{1 + \pi_0}((1 - \pi_0)\lambda_i). \quad (6.9)$$

To illustrate how to implement this model in R-INLA, we use the example on brain cancer incidence in Navarra, presented in Section 1.4.8. The number of brain cancer cases reported in each of the 40 health districts in the Navarra region is modeled following Eq. (6.7). Then conditional on y_i not being a structural zero, the logarithmic transformation of λ_i is modeled as

$$\log(\lambda_i) = b_0 + v_i + v_i + \log(E_i),$$

allowing for a global intercept and a BYM specification ($u_i + v_i$) as done previously with the simpler Poisson model.

In R-INLA this can be done easily specifying the zero-inflated distribution into the inla function:

```
> data.navarra <- data.frame(ZBS=brainnav$ZBS,
                       Y=brainnav$OBSERVED,E=brainnav$EXPECTED)
> formula.zip <- Y ~ 1 + f(ZBS,  model="bym", graph=navarra.graph,
           hyper=list(prec.unstruct=list(prior="gaussian",param=c(0,1)),
                    prec.spatial=list(prior="gaussian",param=c(0,1))))
> mod.zip1 <- inla(formula.zip,family="zeroinflatedpoisson1",
                 data=data.navarra, offset = log(E),
                 control.predictor=list(compute=TRUE))
```

where ZBS identifies the health districts and Navarra.graph is the graph specifying the neighborhood structure. The formula environment remains exactly the same as with the standard disease mapping model as it is only the likelihood that is affected and not the latent part of the model. Note that in this specification there is the additional hyperparameter π_0 on which a prior distribution needs to be set. R-INLA parameterizes the inverse logit transformation, defined as $\frac{\exp(\pi_0)}{1+\exp(\pi_0)}$, and by default it specifies a Normal(-2, 1) distribution on it.

Another type of ZIP model is also available in R-INLA, assuming that only structural zeros are present in the data, which means that Eq. (6.7) changes to

$$p(y_i|\lambda_i, \pi_0) = \pi_0 I(y_i = 0) + (1 - \pi_0)I(y_i > 0)\frac{\exp(-\lambda_i)\lambda_i^{y_i}}{y_i!}. \qquad (6.10)$$

This alternative model can be accessed typing zeroinflatedpoisson0 in the likelihood specification.

```
> mod.zip0 <- inla(formula.zip,family="zeroinflatedpoisson0",
                 data=data.navarra, E = E,
                 control.predictor=list(compute=TRUE))
```

The output of the two models returns (as seen before) the precision for the spatially structured and unstructured effect and information about the posterior distribution for the π_0 parameter, which governs the probability of observing a zero. In our case we obtain that using the model specified in Eq. (6.7) provides a lower value for π_0 as some of the observed zeros come from the Poisson distribution (they are sample zeros). On the other hand, if we assume that there are only structural zeros, as in the model specified in Eq. (6.10), then the probability π_0 is much higher (see Table 6.2).

Figure 6.8 maps the posterior relative risk of disease ζ_i for the 40 health districts using the BYM model with zero inflation allowing for structural and sample zeros

Table 6.2   Posterior estimates for the hyperparameters in
the two zero-inflated models, with structural and sample
zeros (ZIP1) and with structural zeros only (ZIP0).

	ZIP0		ZIP1	
	Mean	SD	Mean	SD
π_0	0.324	0.072	0.065	0.052
τ_v	7.136	5.312	4.441	2.270
τ_u	5.047	3.918	4.257	2.370

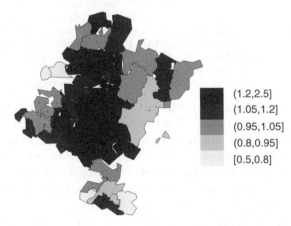

(1.2,2.5]
(1.05,1.2]
(0.95,1.05]
(0.8,0.95]
[0.5,0.8]

*Figure 6.8   Health district specific posterior relative risks with a zero-inflated
Poisson disease mapping models allowing for structural and sample zeros (ZIP1).*

(ZIP1). A similar picture is obtained using the model which allows for structural
zeros only (ZIP0).

6.3.2   Zero-inflated binomial model: air pollution and respiratory hospital admissions

So far we have focused on the Poisson distribution and its use in disease mapping
which is justified as an approximation of a Binomial model when the disease is rare
(i.e., the Binomial probability is small), generally the case in most applications on
social and noncommunicable epidemiological data. Despite this, Binomial models
can also be used in a spatial setting, either when the assumption of a rare disease
does not hold (which, for instance, may be the case for some infectious diseases)
or when the interest of the study lies on the prevalence rate (cases/total population
at risk), as specified by Staunbach *et al.* (2002). For instance, if we are interested in
the mortality prevalence in n areas, we know that $y_1, \dots, y_n$ is the number of deaths
for each area and $n_1, \dots, n_n$ is the total number of individuals living in each area,

then the natural distribution of y_i is

$$y_i \sim \text{Binomial}(\pi_i, n_i)$$

and the spatial random effects (e.g., iCAR) are specified on the logistic transformation of π_i together with any covariate:

$$\text{logit}(\pi_i) = b_0 + u_i + v_i + x_i\beta.$$

Then the inverse logit transformation of π_i will return the posterior area-specific prevalence, while $\exp(u_i + v_i)$ provides the residual odds ratio for each area.

The Binomial distribution has the same overdispersion issues as seen with the Poisson, since it is essentially ruled by a single parameter π_i for each area. To overcome this, Hall (2000) presented the ZIB model. Given n areas, the density function for y_i is the following:

$$p(y_i | \pi_i, \pi_0) = \pi_0 I(y_i = 0) + (1 - \pi_0) \binom{n_i}{y_i} \pi_i^{y_i} (1 - \pi_i)^{n_i - y_i}. \tag{6.11}$$

The probability of observing a zero is $\pi_0 + (1 - \pi_0)(1 - \pi_i)^{n_i}$, and the mean and variance are the following:

$$E(y_i) = (1 - \pi_0)n_i\pi_i \tag{6.12}$$

$$\text{Var}(y_i) = (1 - \pi_0)n_i\pi_i(1 - \pi_i(1 - \pi_0 n_i)). \tag{6.13}$$

Similar to what we have presented for the Poisson case, this model allows for structural and sample zeros and can be accessed in R-INLA setting zeroinflatedbinomial1 as the likelihood in the model specification. Alternatively the model which considers only the structural zeros can also be implemented in R-INLA typing zeroinflatedbinomial0.

To illustrate how to implement this model in R-INLA, we use the example on air pollution level (PM$_{10}$) and hospital admissions for respiratory causes in the Turin province, presented in Section 1.4.9. The number of hospitalizations in 2004 in each of the 315 municipalities in the province is modeled as presented in Eq. (6.11). Then conditionally on y_i not being a structural zero, the logistic transformation of π_i is modeled as follows:

$$\text{logit}(\pi_i) = b_0 + v_i + v_i + \beta_1 \text{PM}_{10i}$$

allowing for a global intercept b_0, a BYM specification as done above with the Poisson models and, in addition, including the annual average concentration of PM$_{10}$ obtained through monitoring sites. We run this model in R-INLA using

```
> formula.inla <- RESP ~ PM10 + f(ID.MUNICIPALITY,
                           model="besag",graph=torino.adj)
> mod.zib <- inla(formula.inla,family= "zeroinflated.binomial.0",
              Ntrials=TotalPop,data=data,
              control.compute=list(dic=TRUE))
```

and present the results in Table 6.3 and Figure 6.9.

Table 6.3   Posterior estimates for the hyperparameters and the fixed effect β_1 in the zero-inflated model with structural zeros only (ZIB0). β_1 quantifies the effect of a change in 10 µg/m^3 of PM$_{10}$ on the odds ratio of respiratory hospital admission.

	ZIB0				
	Mean	SD	2.5%	50%	97.5%
π_0	0.548	0.0280	0.493	0.549	0.603
τ_v	2.207	0.3620	1.580	2.177	3.001
β_1	4e−04	0.0162	−0.031	5e−04	0.032

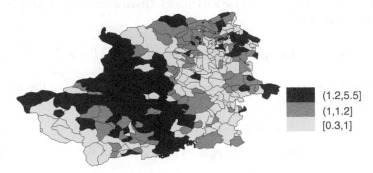

Figure 6.9   Posterior mean of the residual spatial relative risk for the communalities in the Turin province using the zero-inflated model with structural zeros only (ZIB0).

In this modelization PM$_{10}$ is included through a fixed effect, which shows a slight increase in the odds ratio of hospitalization when the air polllution concentration level increases of 10 µg/m^3. However it might be plausible to investigate the fitting of the model with a random slope, implying that the effect of air pollution on the odds ratio of admissions is different for each municipality with an exchangeable structure. To do so we simply set

```
> formula.inla1 <- RESP ~ f(ID.PM10,  PM10, model = "iid",
        graph=torino.adj, constr=TRUE,
        hyper=list(prec = list(prior="gaussian",param=c(0,1)))) +
    f(ID.MUNICIPALITY, model="besag",graph=torino.adj)
```

which in practice puts an exchangeable structure on the municipalities identifiers weighted by the value of the PM$_{10}$.

```
> mod.zib1 <- inla(formula.inla1, family= "zeroinflated.binomial.0",
            Ntrials=TotalPop, data=data,
            control.compute=list(dic=TRUE))
```

Table 6.4 shows the summary statistics for the hyperparameters. Note that the probability of observing a zero does not change when we include the random slope for

Table 6.4 Posterior estimates for the hyperparameters in the zero-inflated model with structural zeros only (ZIB0) and exchangeable structure on the effect of PM_{10}.

	ZIB0	
	Mean	SD
π_0	0.548	0.028
$\tau_{PM_{10}}$	62745.345	12578.390
τ_v	30.071	27.870

PM_{10}; the precisions for the spatially structured intercept increases slightly, but the one for the random slope become extremely large, suggesting that there is no variability amongst the municipalities in the effect of PM_{10} on hospitalizations. Comparing the DIC it emerges that the model with random intercept only has the same fit (1458.09 vs 1457.66 observed for the one with random intercept and slope), suggesting that in this case the simpler model should be used.

6.4 Geostatistical data

Geostatistical or point-referenced data are realizations of a spatial process (or random field) $\{y(s), s \in D\}$ characterized by a spatial index s which varies continuously in the fixed domain D. The spatial process is a Gaussian field (GF) if for any $n \geq 1$ and for each set of locations $(s_1, \ldots, s_n)$, the vector $(y(s_1), \ldots, y(s_n))$ follows a multivariate Normal distribution with mean $\boldsymbol{\mu} = (\mu(s_1), \ldots, \mu(s_n))$ and spatially structured covariance matrix $\boldsymbol{\Sigma}$. The generic element of $\boldsymbol{\Sigma}$ is defined by a covariance function $C(\cdot, \cdot)$ such that $\Sigma_{ij} = \mathrm{Cov}(y(s_i), y(s_j)) = C(y(s_i), y(s_j))$. The spatial process is *second-order stationary* if the mean function is constant in space, i.e., $\mu(s_i) = \mu$ for each i, and the spatial covariance function depends only on the distance vector $(s_i - s_j) \in \mathbb{R}^2$, i.e., $\mathrm{Cov}(y(s_i), y(s_j)) = C(s_i - s_j)$. Moreover, if the covariance function does not depend on the direction but just on the Euclidean distance $\|s_i - s_j\| \in \mathbb{R}$, then the process is said to be *isotropic*.

The first step in defining a model for a random field in a hierarchical framework is to identify a probability distribution for the observations available at n spatial locations and represented by the vector $y = (y(s_1), \ldots, y(s_n)) = (y_1, \ldots, y_n)$ (recall that, as we have seen before, we simplify the notation and use the index i for denoting the generic spatial point s_i). At the first level of the hierarchy, we usually select a distribution from the exponential family, indexed by a set of parameters θ which also includes a latent GF denoted by $\xi(s)$ which accounts for the spatial correlation through the covariance function $C(\cdot, \cdot)$. The last stage of the hierarchical model includes the specification of the prior distributions $p(\psi)$ for the hyperparameters.

The disadvantage of the modeling approach involving the spatial covariance function is known as "big n problem" (Banerjee *et al.*, 2004; Jona Lasinio *et al.*, 2013) and concerns the computational costs required for algebra operations with dense covariance matrices (such as Σ). In particular dense matrix operations scale cubically with the matrix size, given by the number of locations where the process is observed. A computationally effective alternative is given by the stochastic partial differential equation (SPDE) approach (Lindgren *et al.*, 2011) and consists in performing the computations using a GMRF representation of the GF, thus allowing us to adopt the INLA approach. In fact, as introduced in Section 6.1, GMRFs are characterized by sparse precision matrices and this feature allows us to implement computationally efficient numerical methods, especially for fast matrix factorization (Rue and Held, 2005). Note, for example, that for a GMRF in $\mathbb{R}^2$ the computational cost is typically of the order $n^{3/2}$, which is a significant speed up compared to the cubic complexity of the GF with a dense covariance matrix.

Applications of SPDE for geostatistical data can be found, for example, in Simpson *et al.* (2011), Bolin (2012), Simpson *et al.* (2012a,b), Cameletti *et al.* (2013), Ingebrigtsen *et al.* (2013), and Musenge *et al.* (2013).

6.5   The stochastic partial differential equation approach

The SPDE approach proposed by Lindgren *et al.* (2011) consists in representing a continuous spatial process (i.e., a GF) using a discretely indexed spatial random process (i.e., a GMRF). The starting point is the linear fractional stochastic partial differential equation (SPDE)

$$(\kappa^2 - \Delta)^{\alpha/2}(\tau \xi(s)) = \mathcal{W}(s), \qquad (6.14)$$

where $s \in \mathbb{R}^d$, Δ is the Laplacian, α controls the smoothness, $\kappa > 0$ is the scale parameter, τ controls the variance, and $\mathcal{W}(s)$ is a Gaussian spatial white noise process. The exact and stationary solution to this SPDE is the stationary GF $\xi(s)$ with Matèrn covariance function given by

$$\text{Cov}(\xi(s_i), \xi(s_j)) = \text{Cov}(\xi_i, \xi_j) = \frac{\sigma^2}{\Gamma(\lambda)2^{\lambda-1}}(\kappa \|s_i - s_j\|)^\lambda K_\lambda(\kappa \|s_i - s_j\|), \quad (6.15)$$

where $\|s_i - s_j\|$ is the Euclidean distance between two generic locations $s_i, s_j \in \mathbb{R}^d$ and σ^2 is the marginal variance. The term K_λ denotes the modified Bessel function of the second kind and order $\lambda > 0$ (Abramowitz and Stegun, 1972), which measures the degree of smoothness of the process and is usually kept fixed due to poor identifiability. Conversely, $\kappa > 0$ is a scaling parameter related to the range r, i.e. the distance at which the spatial correlation becomes almost null. Typically, the empirically derived definition for the range is $r = \frac{\sqrt{8\lambda}}{\kappa}$ (see Section 2 in Lindgren

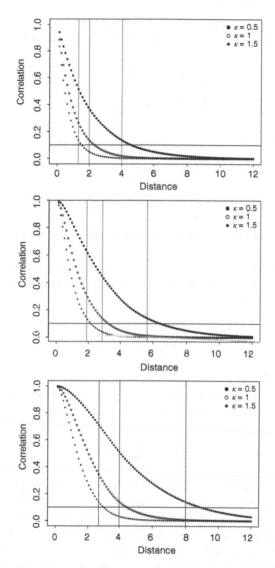

Figure 6.10   Matérn correlation function for different values of κ and distance values: $\lambda = 0.5$ *(top),* $\lambda = 1$ *(center),* $\lambda = 2$ *(bottom). The vertical dashed lines denote the value of the range given by* $r = \sqrt{8\lambda}/\kappa$ *and represent the distance at which the correlation is close to 0.1 (value highlighted by a solid horizontal line).*

et al., 2011), with r corresponding to the distance at which the spatial correlation is close to 0.1, for each $\lambda \geq 1/2$. To assess the appropriateness of this empirical range definition, Figure 6.10 displays the decay of the Matérn correlation function with distance for different values of λ and κ and includes vertical lines for denoting the values of the empirical range r.

The link between the SPDE in Eq. (6.14) and the Matérn parameters is given by the following equations involving the smoothness parameter λ and the marginal variance σ^2:

$$\begin{cases} \lambda = \alpha - d/2 \\ \sigma^2 = \dfrac{\Gamma(\lambda)}{\Gamma(\alpha)(4\pi)^{d/2}\kappa^{2\lambda}\tau^2} \end{cases}.$$

As we consider the case of $s \in \mathbb{R}^2$ ($d = 2$), it follows that

$$\begin{cases} \lambda = \alpha - 1 \\ \sigma^2 = \dfrac{\Gamma(\lambda)}{\Gamma(\alpha)(4\pi)\kappa^{2\lambda}\tau^2} \end{cases}.$$

In R-INLA the default value for the smoothness parameter is $\alpha = 2$ (corresponding to $\lambda = 1$), but the values $0 \leq \alpha < 2$ are also available even if not fully tested (for noninteger values of α the approximation method described in the authors' discussion response in Lindgren *et al.* (2011) is used). Note that with $\alpha = 2$ the range r and the variance σ^2 are given by

$$r = \sqrt{8}/\kappa \qquad\qquad (6.16)$$

$$\sigma^2 = 1/(4\pi\kappa^2\tau^2). \qquad\qquad (6.17)$$

The solution to the SPDE – represented by the stationary and isotropic Matérn GF $\xi(s)$ – can be approximated using the finite element method through a basis function representation defined on a triangulation[3] of the domain $\mathcal{D}$:

$$\xi(s) = \sum_{g=1}^{G} \varphi_g(s)\tilde{\xi}_g. \qquad\qquad (6.18)$$

Here G is the total number of vertices of the triangulation, $\{\varphi_g\}$ is the set of (deterministic) basis functions, and $\{\tilde{\xi}_g\}$ are zero mean Gaussian distributed weights. In order to obtain a Markov structure, the basis functions are chosen to have a local support and to be piecewise linear in each triangle, i.e., φ_g is 1 at vertex g and 0 at all other vertices. Using Neumann boundary conditions, it follows that (for the case $\alpha = 2$) the precision matrix Q for the Gaussian weight vector $\tilde{\xi} = \{\tilde{\xi}_1, \dots, \tilde{\xi}_G\}$ is given by

$$Q = \tau^2(\kappa^4 C + 2\kappa^2 G + GC^{-1}G), \qquad\qquad (6.19)$$

where the generic element of the diagonal matrix C is $C_{ii} = \int \varphi_i(s)\mathrm{d}s$ and the one of the sparse matrix G is $G_{ij} = \int \nabla\varphi_i(s)\nabla\varphi_j(s)\mathrm{d}s$ (∇ denotes the gradient). The precision matrix Q, whose elements depend on τ and κ, is sparse and consequently ξ is a GMRF with distribution Normal$(0, Q^{-1})$ and it represents the approximated solution to the SPDE (in a stochastically weak sense).

---

[3] Through a triangulation the spatial domain is subdivided into a set of nonintersecting triangles, where any two triangles meet in at most a common edge or corner. As an example, see Figure 6.12.

An illustration of the SPDE approach is given in Figure 4 of Blangiardo *et al.* (2013), which displays a continuously indexed spatial random field and the corresponding finite element representation with piecewise linear basis functions over a triangulated mesh. The height of each triangle (the value of the spatial field at each triangle vertex) is given by the weight φ_g and the values in the interior of the triangle are determined by linear interpolation.

In R-INLA the default internal representation for the SPDE parameters is $\log(\tau) = \theta_1$ and $\log(\kappa) = \theta_2$, with θ_1 and θ_2 being given a joint Normal prior distribution (by default independent). See Section 6.9 for more details about prior specification.

6.5.1   Nonstationary Gaussian field

When modeling some environmental phenomena, the stationarity assumption may not be suitable. For example, in the case of atmospheric phenomena it may be inappropriate to assume that the spatial correlation is the same throughout the domain as topographical variables (e.g., altitude, river, lakes, etc.) might influence the spatial dependence structure. In such cases, it may be more suitable to consider a nonstationary spatial process (see Chapter 9 in Gelfand *et al.*, 2010 for a short review).

In the framework of the SPDE approach, it is possible to extend the stationary case described in Section 6.5 to the nonstationary version (Lindgren *et al.*, 2011; Bolin and Lindgren, 2011; Ingebrigtsen *et al.*, 2013) by specifying spatially varying parameters $\kappa(s)$ and $\tau(s)$. In this case, the SPDE in Eq. (6.14) is simply rewritten as

$$(\kappa^2(s) - \Delta)^{\alpha/2}(\tau(s)\xi(s)) = \mathcal{W}(s) \tag{6.20}$$

with $s \in \mathbb{R}^2$, and the precision matrix Q is a modified version of the stationary one given in Eq. (6.19):

$$Q = T(K^2CK^2 + K^2G + GK^2 + GC^{-1}G)T,$$

where $T = \text{diag}(\tau(s_i))$ and $K = \text{diag}(\kappa(s_i))$, with locations s_i being part of the mesh vertices.

For the nonstationary case the link between the SPDE and Matérn parameters given in Eqs. (6.16) and (6.17) is not valid. However, it is possibile to obtain nominal approximations to the variance and to the range if the spatial correlation interaction between the nonstationary parameter fields is disregarded; for $\alpha = 2$ (the case implemented in the current version of R-INLA) the approximations are the following:

$$\sigma^2(s) \approx \frac{1}{4\pi\kappa(s)^2\tau(s)^2} \tag{6.21}$$

$$r(s) \approx \frac{\sqrt{8}}{\kappa(s)}. \tag{6.22}$$

Note that these approximations are valid when the parameters κ and τ vary slowly with s. This requirement is met by the internal representation in R-INLA for the nonstationary model, based on the following linear combination of basis functions for $\log(\tau(s))$ and $\log(\kappa(s))$:

$$\log(\tau(s)) = b_0^\tau(s) + \sum_{k=1}^{N} b_k^\tau(s)\theta_k \tag{6.23}$$

$$\log(\kappa(s)) = b_0^\kappa(s) + \sum_{k=1}^{N} b_k^\kappa(s)\theta_k, \tag{6.24}$$

where $b_k^\tau(\cdot)$ and $b_k^\kappa(\cdot)$ are deterministic spatial basis functions (they can be possibly equal to zero for some values of k) and $\{\theta_1, \ldots, \theta_N\}$ is a set of internal parameters for which priors are specified (see Section 6.12 for more details about priors).

6.6   SPDE within R-INLA

As described in the previous chapters, in R-INLA the linear predictor η_i is defined using the formula which includes f() terms for nonlinear effects of covariates or random effects. In the same way, the Matérn GF will be included in the formula using a proper specification for f(). For making the connection between the linear predictor η_i and the formula more explicit, it is convenient to follow Lindgren and Rue (2015) and to rewrite the linear predictor introduced in Eq. (4.12) as

$$\eta_i = \sum_k h_k(z_i^k), \tag{6.25}$$

where k denotes the kth term of the formula, z_i^k represents the covariate value for a fixed/nonlinear effect or, in the case of a random effect, the index of a second-order unit (e.g., area or point ID). The mapping function $h_k(\cdot)$ links z_i^k to the actual value of the latent field for the kth formula component.

As an example consider the case where the linear predictor η_i includes a fixed effect of a covariate (named z1 in R), a nonlinear effect (e.g., RW2) of the variable time (given by a sequence of time points), and a random effect with iid components indexed by the variable index.random. Thus the corresponding R-INLA formula is

```
> formula <- -1 + z1 + f(time, model="rw2") +
                   f(index.random, model="iid")
```

The default intercept is not included as we specify -1 in the formula. With the new linear predictor specification of Eq. (6.25), we have that $h_1(z_i^1)$ is equal to $z_i^1\beta$, $h_2(z_i^2)$ is the smooth effect evaluated at z_i^2 (the ith element of vector time), and $h_3(z_i^3)$ is the random effect component with index equal to z_i^3 (the ith element of index.random). As usual, the latent field θ is the joint vector of all the latent Gaussian variables included in the linear predictor.

The formulation in Eq. (6.25) only allows each observation to directly depend on a single element z_i^k from each effect $h_k(\cdot)$ and this does not cover the case when a random effect is defined as a linear combination of temporal or areal values, such as the SPDE representation given in Eq. (6.18). In such cases each observation y_i depends on a linear combination of the elements of $\boldsymbol{\theta}$ and the observation distribution will be defined as

$$y_i|\boldsymbol{\theta},\boldsymbol{\psi} \sim p\left(y_i \Big| \sum_j A_{ij}\theta_j, \boldsymbol{\psi}\right)$$

instead of $y_i|\theta_i,\boldsymbol{\psi} \sim p(y_i|\theta_i,\boldsymbol{\psi})$ as in Eq. (4.13). The term A_{ij} is the generic element of the matrix A, referred to as the *observation or projector matrix*. In Sections 6.7.2 and 6.7.3, we will show how to create the A matrix using the helper function `inla.spde.matrix.A` and how to include it in the `inla` call through the `control.predictor` option. The A matrix defines a mapping between the spatial latent field (defined on the mesh) and the observations (defined in a set of locations) and this allows the SPDE models to be treated as standard indexed random effects (the mapping is done by placing appropriate $\varphi_g(s)$ values in the A matrix, see Eq. (6.18)). Internally, R-INLA creates a new linear predictor $\boldsymbol{\eta}^\star$ defined as a linear combination of the original one $\boldsymbol{\eta}$:

$$\boldsymbol{\eta}^\star = A\boldsymbol{\eta}$$

and in this case the likelihood is linked to the latent field through $\eta_i^\star$ instead of η_i

$$p(\boldsymbol{y}|\boldsymbol{\theta},\boldsymbol{\psi}) = \prod_{i=1}^n p(y_i|\eta_i^\star,\boldsymbol{\psi}).$$

6.7   SPDE toy example with simulated data

In this section, we consider a simple example with simulated data in order to show the functions available in R-INLA for the SPDE approach. To this regard, we use the SPDEtoy dataset included in the R-INLA package

```
> data(SPDEtoy)
> dim(SPDEtoy)
[1] 200    3
> head(SPDEtoy, n=3)
          s1         s2          y
1 0.08265625 0.05640625 11.521206
2 0.61230625 0.91680625  5.277960
3 0.16200625 0.35700625  6.902959
```

The dataset consists of 200 simulated values for the variable y which refer to as many randomly sampled locations in the unit square area delimited by the points $(0, 0)$ and $(1, 1)$ and with coordinates given by s1 and s2. The data are displayed in Figure 6.11.

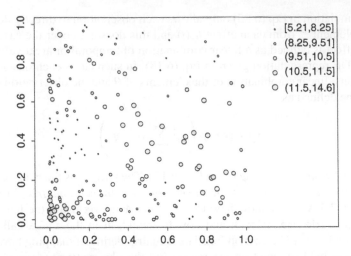

Figure 6.11   Locations of the 200 spatial points included in the SPDEtoy *dataset. The size of the points is determined by the values of the simulated variable y.*

The model used for simulating the SPDEtoy data assumes that the distribution of the observation y_i is

$$y_i \sim \text{Normal}(\eta_i, \sigma_e^2) \qquad i = 1, \dots, 200,$$

where σ_e^2 is the variance of the zero mean measurement error e_i which is supposed to be normally distributed and independent of e_j for each $i \neq j$. The response mean, which coincides with the linear predictor, is defined as

$$\eta_i = b_0 + \xi_i \tag{6.26}$$

and includes the intercept b_0 and a random effect represented by ξ_i, which is the realization of the latent GF $\xi(s) \sim \text{MVNormal}(\mathbf{0}, \mathbf{\Sigma})$. The covariance matrix $\mathbf{\Sigma}$ is defined by the Matérn spatial covariance function of Eq. (6.15). The parameter values chosen for simulating the data are: $b_0 = 10$, $\sigma_e^2 = 0.3$, $\sigma^2 = 5$, $\kappa = 7$, and $\lambda = 1$. For more details about the simulation, see Krainski and Lindgren (2013).

6.7.1   Mesh construction

As introduced in Section 6.1, the SPDE approach is based on a triangulation of the spatial domain. Note that in practice the definition of the mesh is a trade-off between the accuracy of the GMRF representation and computational costs, both depending on the number of vertices used in the triangulation: the bigger the number of mesh triangles, the finer the GF approximation but the higher the computational costs.

In R-INLA, we make use of the helper function inla.mesh.2d. This function requires as input some information about the spatial domain, given either by some relevant spatial points (not necessarily the points where observations are available) or by the domain extent, to be specified using the `loc` or `loc.domain` arguments, respectively. Another nonoptional argument is `max.edge` which represents the largest allowed triangle edge length. If a vector of two values is provided, the spatial domain is divided into an inner and an outer area whose triangle resolution is specified by `max.edge` (the higher the value for `max.edge` the lower the resolution and the accuracy). This extension of the original domain can be useful in order to avoid the boundary effects related to the SPDE approach (the Neumann boundary conditions used in `R-INLA` have as a drawback an increase of the variance near the boundary). As suggested by Lindgren and Rue (2015), to avoid the boundary effect the domain should be extended by a distance at least equal to the range r.

The following code creates three different triangulations for the `SPDEtoy` dataset: in all three cases the data locations (represented by the `coords` object) are included as triangle vertices, by means of the `loc` argument, and different values for `max.edge` are chosen:

```
> coords <- as.matrix(SPDEtoy[,1:2])
> mesh0 <- inla.mesh.2d(loc=coords, max.edge=0.1)
> mesh1 <- inla.mesh.2d(loc=coords, max.edge=c(0.1, 0.1))
> mesh2 <- inla.mesh.2d(loc=coords, max.edge=c(0.1, 0.2))
```

The graphical representation of a mesh is very simple, e.g.

```
> plot(mesh0, main="")
> #Include data locations:
> points(coords, pch=21, bg=1, col="white", cex=1.8)
```

and the three resulting meshes are reported in Figure 6.12. It can be seen that mesh0, for which just one `max.edge` value is specified, is not characterized by an outer extension of the domain. Moreover, the difference between mesh1 and mesh2, which instead are both extended outside, is that for mesh2 a bigger `max.edge` value is chosen giving rise to an outer domain characterized by larger triangles (i.e., lower accuracy). In this way, it is possible to extend the original spatial domain, for avoiding boundary effects, without increasing too much the computational costs.

The optional argument `offset` of the `inla.mesh.2d` function can be used to define how much the domain should be extended in the inner and outer part. The default values used for mesh1 and mesh2 are `offset = c(-0.05, -0.15)`. The following triangulations, which are represented in Figure 6.13, are characterized by two different choices for the `offset` option:

```
> mesh3 <- inla.mesh.2d(loc=coords, max.edge=c(0.1, 0.2),
    offset=c(0.4,0.1))
> mesh4 <- inla.mesh.2d(loc=coords, max.edge=c(0.1, 0.2),
    offset=c(0.1,0.4))
```

For mesh3 the inner domain is more extended than the outer one, whereas the opposite holds for mesh4. It is worth mentioning that for the `SPDEtoy` dataset, the range is approximately equal to $r = \sqrt{8}/\kappa = \sqrt{8}/7 = 0.4$ and, with respect to

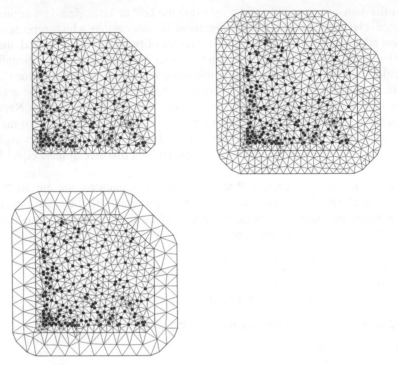

Figure 6.12   Three triangulations for the SPDEtoy *dataset with different values for* max.edge: mesh0 *(top left),* mesh1 *(top right), and* mesh2 *(bottom). Black points denote the observation locations.*

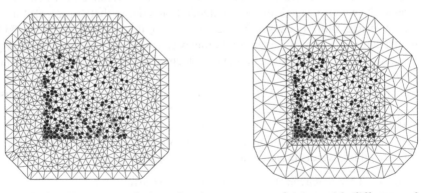

Figure 6.13   Two triangulations for the SPDEtoy *dataset with different values for the* offset *option:* mesh3 *(left) and* mesh4 *(right). Black points denote the observation locations.*

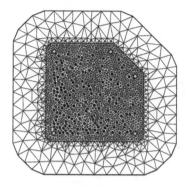 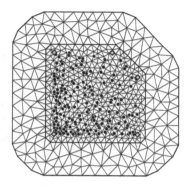

Figure 6.14   Two triangulations for the SPDEtoy *dataset with different values for the* cutoff *option:* mesh5 *(left) and* mesh6 *(right). Black points and gray diamonds denote the observation locations and the boundary points, respectively.*

the boundary effect, mesh4 is preferrable than mesh3 as it extends the spatial domain with a lower triangle resolution for the outer part.

As said previously, it is not required to include the observation locations in the mesh. As an alternative, it is possible to provide, through the loc.domain option, a matrix of point locations used to determine the domain extent. Another optional argument of the inla.mesh.2d function is cutoff which can be used to avoid building too many small triangles around clustered data locations (the default value is equal to 0). In the following, we create two new meshes by specifying a domain and by replacing points with distance less than 0.015 and 0.05 by a single vertex (the offset and max.edge specifications are the same as for mesh4):

```
> domain <- matrix(cbind(c(0,1,1,0.7,0), c(0,0,0.7,1,1)),ncol=2)
> mesh5 <- inla.mesh.2d(loc.domain=domain,
   max.edge=c(0.04, 0.2), cutoff=0.015, offset = c(0.1, 0.4))
> mesh6 <- inla.mesh.2d(loc.domain=domain,
   max.edge=c(0.04, 0.2), cutoff=0.05, offset = c(0.1, 0.4))
```

The resulting meshes are represented in Figure 6.14: note that the observation locations are not placed on triangle vertices.

The number of vertices of a mesh is stored in the n.spde component of the output of the inla.spde2.matern function which will be introduced later in Section 6.7.3. For example for mesh0, we type

```
> inla.spde2.matern(mesh0,alpha=2)$n.spde
[1] 503
```

To retrieve the number of vertices for all the meshes created so far the following code is run:

```
> vertices <- c()
> for(i in 0:6){
```

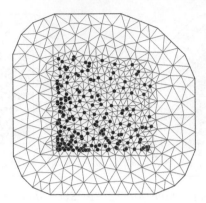

Figure 6.15   Triangulations for the SPDEtoy *dataset given by* mesh7. *Black points denote the observation locations, while the internal line represents the boundary obtained as nonconvex hull.*

```
vertices[i+1] <- inla.spde2.matern(get(paste("mesh",i,sep="")),
                                   alpha=2)$n.spde
}
> vertices
[1]    503   801   593 1008   700 2419   549
```

where the function `get` is used to call an R object (in this case a mesh) using a character string.

A feature in R-INLA named `inla.nonconvex.hull` makes it possible to include a nonconvex hull as boundary in the mesh construction.[4] We include below an example whose resulting mesh is reported in Figure 6.15.

```
> bnd <- inla.nonconvex.hull(as.matrix(coords),convex=0.07)
> mesh7 <- inla.mesh.2d(loc=coords, boundary=bnd,
  max.edge=c(0.04, 0.2), cutoff=0.05, offset = c(0.1, 0.4))
```

6.7.2   The observation or projector matrix

Given the basis function representation of Eq. (6.18), the linear predictor in Eq. (6.26) can be rewritten as

$$\eta_i = b_0 + \sum_{g=1}^{G} \varphi_g(s_i)\tilde{\xi}_g, \tag{6.27}$$

---

[4] If the boundary is nonconvex not all the line segments connecting any generic couple of points s_i and s_j are inside the boundary.

where $\varphi_g(s_i)$ is the value of the gth basis function evaluated in s_i. More generally it is possible to express the linear predictor as

$$\eta_i = b_0 + \sum_{g=1}^{G} A_{ig}\tilde{\xi}_g,$$

with $A_{ig} = \varphi_g(s_i)$ being the generic element of the sparse matrix A which maps the GMRF $\tilde{\xi}$ from the G triangulation vertices to the n observation locations. The R-INLA function `inla.spde.make.A` creates the sparse weight matrix A by identifying the data locations in the mesh and organizing the corresponding values of the basis functions. As an example, the following code is used to create the A matrix for `mesh1` and `mesh6` (characterized by 801 and 549 vertices, respectively):

```
> A.est1 <- inla.spde.make.A(mesh=mesh1, loc=coords)
> dim(A.est1)
[1] 200 801
> A.est6 <- inla.spde.make.A(mesh=mesh6, loc=coords)
> dim(A.est6)
[1] 200 549
```

The dimension of the resulting A matrix is given by the number of data locations times the number of mesh nodes. Since `mesh1` was created by including observation locations as mesh vertices, the projector matrix `A.est1` has one nonzero value (equal to 1) for each row (check with `apply(A.est1,1,nnzero)`, where the `nnzero` function is part of the `Matrix` package and returns the number of nonzero values). Conversely, for `mesh6` it happens that each spatial location is placed inside a triangle which is delimited by three vertices; for this reason `A.est6` is characterized by three nonzero elements for each row whose sum is equal to 1 (i.e., $\sum_{g=1}^{G} A_{ig} = 1$). The code

```
> table(apply(A.est6,1,nnzero))
  3
200
```

verifies that for all the 200 rows of the `A.est6` matrix three elements are different from zero; moreover, the sum by row is always equal to 1:

```
> table(apply(A.est6,1,sum))
  1
200
```

In addition, there are some columns with zero values corresponding to vertices not connected to points; to compute the number of columns of `A.est6` whose sum is equal to zero (TRUE) or bigger than zero (FALSE), we use

```
> table(apply(A.est6,2,sum) > 0)
FALSE   TRUE
  313    236
```

and obtain that 313 columns of A.est6 contain only null values. For A.est1 this computation is easier as the data locations are included as triangle vertices and the observation matrix contains only zeros and ones. Thus, we just compute the sum by column

```
> table(apply(A.est1,2,sum))
  0   1
601 200
```

and check that, as expected, it is is equal to 1 for 200 columns (corresponding to the 200 data locations).

6.7.3   Model fitting

According to the notation introduced in Section 4.8, in this toy example, the vector of parameters is defined as $\theta = \{\tilde{\xi}, b_0\}$ with hyperparameters vector $\psi = (\sigma_e^2, \kappa, \sigma^2)$, where κ and σ^2 are the Matérn covariance function parameters.

We show now how to estimate the model parameters using the mesh6 triangulation and the projector matrix A.est6 created previously and choosing the default prior specifications for the SPDE parameters; see Section 6.9 for more details about how to change priors. First of all, we need to create a Matérn SPDE object through

```
> spde <- inla.spde2.matern(mesh=mesh6, alpha=2)
```

Then we define the linear predictor through the formula

```
> formula <- y ~ -1 + intercept + f(spatial.field, model=spde)
```

removing the default intercept (with the code spefication -1) and including an explicit one named intercept. The spatial random effect is included with the f() term where spatial.field is a proper index variable and spde is the model created previously with inla.spde2.matern. As usual the model is fitted by means of the inla function:

```
> output6 <- inla(formula,
    data = list(y=SPDEtoy$y, intercept=rep(1,spde$n.spde),
                spatial.field=1:spde$n.spde),
                control.predictor=list(A=A.est6,compute=TRUE))
```

Note that the data list also includes the spatial.field variable for the random effect, defined as the sequence of integers from 1 to the number of mesh vertices. Moreover, the projector matrix is provided through the control.predictor option by setting compute=TRUE for obtaining the posterior marginals for the linear predictor.

The posterior summaries of the intercept and of the precision for the Gaussian observations can be retrieved with the following commands:

```
> round(output6$summary.fixed,3)
            mean      sd 0.025quant  0.5quant  0.975quant  mode kld
intercept  9.505  0.696     8.036     9.524     10.865   9.555   0
> round(output6$summary.hyperpar[1,],3)
    mean         sd 0.025quant   0.5quant  0.975quant          mode
   2.859      0.467      2.041      2.826       3.870         2.765
```

If the interest is on the variance σ_e^2 (and not on the precision), it is possible to compute the mean of the transformed posterior marginal through

```
> inla.emarginal(function(x) 1/x, output6$marginals.hyper[[1]])
[1] 0.3591352
```

The posterior summaries of the spatial parameters can be obtained from the `inla` output by means of the `inla.spde2.result` function which extracts all the relevant bits of information from the list `output6`. Moreover, the function transforms the results from internal parameter scales and provides the posterior distributions for the nominal variance σ^2 and the nominal range r, in addition to the internal results regarding $\theta_1 = \log(\tau)$ and $\theta_2 = \log(\kappa)$. In the code

```
> output6.field <- inla.spde2.result(inla=output6,
                name="spatial.field", spde=spde, do.transf=TRUE)
```

`name` denotes the name of the SPDE effect used in the `formula` (in this case `spatial.field`) and `spde` is the result of the call to `inla.spde2.matern`. The option `do.transf=TRUE` is used to compute marginals of the parameters on the transformed scale. See `names(output6.field)` for exploring the elements of the resulting list. The posterior mean of κ, σ^2 and the range r can be obtained by typing

```
> inla.emarginal(function(x) x, output6.field$marginals.kappa[[1]])
[1] 8.27741
> inla.emarginal(function(x) x,
                output6.field$marginals.variance.nominal[[1]])
[1] 4.025953
> inla.emarginal(function(x) x,
                output6.field$marginals.range.nominal[[1]])
[1] 0.3609755
```

The corresponding 95% highest probability density intervals are

```
> inla.hpdmarginal(0.95, output6.field$marginals.kappa[[1]])
                 low       high
level:0.95 4.699922 12.10546
> inla.hpdmarginal(0.95, output6.field$marginals.variance.nominal[[1]])
                 low       high
level:0.95 1.941526 6.494604
> inla.hpdmarginal(0.95, output6.field$marginals.range.nominal[[1]])
                 low       high
level:0.95 0.2089423 0.5370679
```

which contain the true parameter values.

6.8 More advanced operations through the `inla.stack` function

When the model complexity increases, e.g., many random effects are included in the linear predictor or more likelihoods are involved, matrix and vector manipulation of SPDE objects can be tedious and lead to errors. To avoid this kind of complications for the users, a function named `inla.stack` has been introduced in R-INLA for an optimal and easy management of the SPDE objects. Here below, using the same notation as in Lindgren and Rue (2015), we introduce the operations which can be dealt with `inla.stack`, first from an abstract point of view and then through some examples.

We collect all the z_i^k terms of the linear predictor in Eq. (6.25) using a compact matrix-like notation

$$Z = [z^1 \ \ldots \ z^K].$$

It follows that the linear predictor with K effects and for all the observations can be written as

$$\eta = H(Z) = \sum_{k=1}^{K} h_k(z^k),$$

while R-INLA creates internally a new linear predictor $\eta^\star = AH(Z)$ defined as linear combination of the elements in η by means of the projector matrix A.

In case of more complex models it may be useful to define the *sum* of linear predictors as

$$\eta^\star = \eta_1^\star + \eta_2^\star + \cdots = A_1 H(Z_1) + A_2 H(Z_2) + \cdots = \tilde{A} H(\tilde{Z}),$$

where $\tilde{A} = [A_1 \ A_2 \ \ldots \ ]$ and $\tilde{Z} = \begin{bmatrix} Z_1 \\ Z_2 \\ \vdots \end{bmatrix}$. The `inla.stack` syntax for implementing the *sum* of linear predictors is the following:

```
stack <-  inla.stack(data = list(...),
   A = list(A1, A2, ...),
   effects = list( list(...), list(...), ...),
   tag = "...")
```

where each A matrix is associated with an effect specified by a `list` containing the covariate values or the random effect indexes related to the corresponding term in Z. The `data` list contains the response variable and should be of the same length of the predictor.

Another possibility is to *join* predictors previously created using the `inla.stack` function and characterized by different specifications in the `tag` argument. For example, considering the case of two or more components, we have

$$\eta_1^\star = A_1 H(Z_1), \ \eta_2^\star = A_2 H(Z_2), \ \ldots$$

and the joint predictor is defined as

$$\tilde{\eta}^{\star} = \begin{bmatrix} \eta_1^{\star} \\ \eta_2^{\star} \\ \vdots \end{bmatrix} = \tilde{A}H(\tilde{Z})$$

with

$$\tilde{A} = \begin{bmatrix} A_1 & 0 & \cdots \\ 0 & A_2 & \ddots \\ \vdots & \ddots & \ddots \end{bmatrix}$$

and

$$\tilde{Z} = \begin{bmatrix} Z_1 \\ Z_2 \\ \vdots \end{bmatrix}.$$

The syntax for the join operation is simply

```
stack <-  inla.stack(stack1, stack2, ...)
```

where `stack1` and `stack2` are the output of a call to `inla.stack` each with a different Lag specification. This kind of joining operation is useful for example when, besides parameter estimation, we are interested in spatial prediction.

By default for both the sum and join operation, the new matrices $\tilde{Z}$ and $\tilde{A}$ are analyzed in order to detect any duplicate row in $\tilde{Z}$ or any all-zero columns in $\tilde{A}$ and those are by default removed in order to minimize the internal size of the model representation.

We now consider the simple `SPDEtoy` example discussed in the previous section, and show how to obtain the same parameter estimates but with the new `inla.stack` function (this is alternative to the procedure described in Section 6.7.3). Due to the internal definition of `inla.stack`, an automatic intercept is not included and has to be specified explicitly; here we consider the intercept, rather than a constant covariate, as part of the spatial effect (i.e., like a spatial effect which is constant over all the spatial domain).

We also introduce a new function named `inla.spde.make.index` which takes care of creating all the required indexes for the SPDE model and which is particularly useful when replicates or groups are involved in the model specification:

```
> s.index <- inla.spde.make.index(name="spatial.field",
                          n.spde=spde$n.spde)
```

Here name represents the name of the effect which will then be used in the `formula`. The output returned by `inla.spde.make.index` is composed of a list with the following components:

```
> names(s.index)
[1] "spatial.field"        "spatial.field.group" "spatial.field.repl"
```

and, in this simple example with no replicates or groups, the three vectors are defined as

```
s.index$spatial.field = seq(1,spde$n.spde)
s.index$spatial.field.group = rep(1,spde$n.spde)
s.index$spatial.field.repl = rep(1,spde$n.spde)
```

The call to inla.stack is the following

```
> stack.est <- inla.stack(data=list(y=SPDEtoy$y),
    A=list(A.est6),
    effects=list(c(s.index, list(intercept=1))),
    tag="est") #Estimation
```

where the A matrix A.est6 has an associated list of effects including both the intercept and the indexes of the spatial random field contained in s.index. Note that in the effects specification we do not use list(...) for s.index as it is already a list (check with class(s.index)). Then the final call is

```
> output6.stack <- inla(formula,
    data=inla.stack.data(stack.est, spde=spde),
    family="gaussian",
    control.predictor=list(A=inla.stack.A(stack.est),
    compute=TRUE))
```

Here the functions inla.stack.data and inla.stack.A are used for extracting the data and the projector matrix from the stack.est object. As expected, the results in output6.stack are the same as the ones in output6 (see Section 6.7.3).

It is possible to reproduce the estimation procedure described above using other mesh specifications. Figure 6.16 displays the marginal posterior distributions of the SPDEtoy parameters obtained considering the eight meshes defined in Section 6.7.1. The posterior distributions of the intercept b_0 and of the spatial variance σ^2 are almost the same for the different mesh specifications, if we exclude the case of σ^2 estimated using mesh0. Recall that mesh0 is a triangulation which would not be used in practical applications since it is not extended externally and estimation may be influenced by the boundary effects.

6.8.1   Spatial prediction

In geostatistical applications, the main interest resides in the spatial prediction of the spatial latent field or of the response variable in new locations. To describe how to perform spatial prediction with R-INLA, we create a regular grid of 50×50 points in the same spatial domain of the SPDEtoy dataset:

```
> grid.x <- 50
> grid.y <- 50
> pred.grid <- expand.grid(x = seq(0, 1, length.out = grid.x),
          y = seq(0, 1, length.out = grid.y))
```

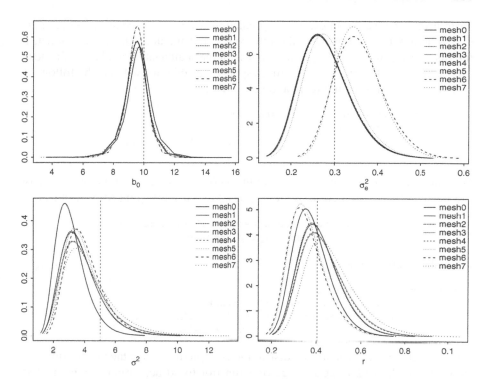

Figure 6.16   Marginal posterior distributions of the parameters of the SPDEtoy dataset with different specifications for the mesh: intercept b_0 (top left), measurement error variance σ_e^2 (top right), spatial variance σ^2 (bottom left), and range r (top right). The vertical dashed line indicates the true parameter values.

```
> dim(pred.grid)
[1] 2500    2
```

In R-INLA, the simplest way for performing spatial prediction is by joining linear predictors (one for parameter estimation and one for prediction) through the inla.stack function, as described in the previous section. To do this, first of all a new projector matrix for the 2500 grid locations has to be created:

```
> A.pred6 <- inla.spde.make.A(mesh=mesh6, loc=as.matrix(pred.grid))
> dim(A.pred6)
[1] 2500  549
```

and then the inla.stack object is built using a proper tag (pred.latent):

```
> stack.pred.latent <- inla.stack(data=list(xi=NA),
        A=list(A.pred6),
        effects=list(s.index),
        tag="pred.latent")
```

Note that, since we are interested in prediction, we need to specify xi=NA in the data argument; moreover, as the intercept is not included in the effects list, it means we are computing the prediction just for the spatial latent field $\xi(s)$. If instead the interest is in the prediction of the response variable, we will use the following call which includes the intercept and sets y=NA:

```
> stack.pred.response <- inla.stack(data=list(y=NA),
          A=list(A.pred6),
          effects=list(c(s.index, list(intercept=1))),
          tag="pred.response")
```

We join all together the three linear predictors (parameter estimation, prediction of the latent field and prediction of the response) into a single joint stack object:

```
> join.stack <- inla.stack(stack.est, stack.pred.latent,
                      stack.pred.response)
```

and call the inla function

```
> join.output <- inla(formula,
          data=inla.stack.data(join.stack),
          control.predictor=list(A=inla.stack.A(join.stack),
                      compute=TRUE))
```

To access the posterior marginal distributions of predictions at the target grid locations, we use the inla.stack.index function to extract the corresponding data indexes from the full stack object using the corresponding tags:

```
> index.pred.latent <- inla.stack.index(join.stack,
                      tag="pred.latent")$data
> index.pred.response <- inla.stack.index(join.stack,
                      tag="pred.response")$data
```

A summary of the posterior summaries for the spatial latent field can be obtained with one of the following commands:

```
> round(head(
    join.output$summary.linear.predictor[index.pred.latent,1:5],n=3),3)
                mean     sd 0.025quant 0.5quant 0.975quant
Apredictor.0201 2.743 0.733      1.339    2.719      4.290
Apredictor.0202 2.702 0.725      1.291    2.684      4.219
Apredictor.0203 2.610 0.756      1.135    2.597      4.168
> round(head(
    join.output$summary.fitted.values[index.pred.latent,1:5],n=3),3)
                        mean     sd 0.025quant 0.5quant 0.975quant
fitted.Apredictor.0201 2.743 0.733      1.339    2.719      4.290
fitted.Apredictor.0202 2.702 0.725      1.291    2.684      4.219
fitted.Apredictor.0203 2.610 0.756      1.135    2.597      4.168
```

which are equivalent because in the case of Gaussian likelihood the linear predictor values coincide with the fitted values (the link function is the identity function). The latent field posterior mean can be extracted with

```
> post.mean.pred.latent <-
    join.output$summary.linear.predictor[index.pred.latent,"mean"]
```

and the corresponding plot is reported in Figure 6.17. The same procedure can be used for the standard deviation (use `"sd"` instead of `"mean"`) and for the response posterior summaries (use `"index.pred.response"` instead of `"index.pred.latent"`). As expected, in Figure 6.17, the posterior mean of the latent field and that of the response differ only for the intercept value and not for the spatial pattern. For the standard deviation, it seems that the latent field is more uncertain (higher variability) than the response and this may be explained by a negative correlation between the intercept and the spatial field. This makes sense considering that the larger the spatial range, the stronger the intercept and the spatial field can only be identified in terms of their sum (thus giving rise to negative correlation). One way to deal with this is to simply not look at either of them individually, but to consider the posterior distribution of their sum (which in this case corresponds to the linear predictor).

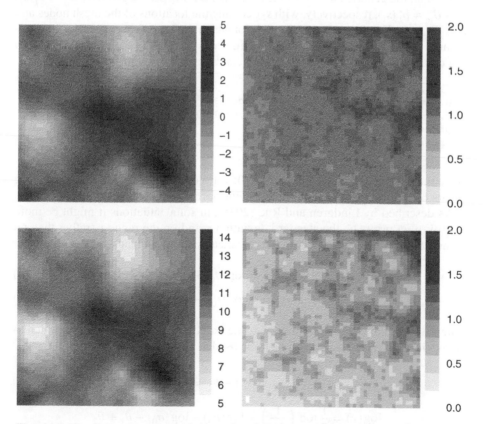

Figure 6.17   Posterior mean (left) and standard deviation (right) of the spatial latent field (top) and of the response variable (bottom) predicted at the grid level.

Note that if the marginal distributions of the spatial random effect and of the linear predictor are not required, it is possible to disable their computation (saving computing time) with the option in the `inla` function `control.results=list(return.marginals.random=FALSE)`, `return.marginals.predictor=FALSE)`.

6.9 Prior specification for the stationary case

The most general parameterization for the SPDE parameters is given by Eqs. (6.23) and (6.24). Note that setting $N = 2$, $b_0^\tau(s) = b_2^\tau(s) = 0$, and $b_1^\tau(s) = 1$ for each s in Eq. (6.23), we obtain the simplest representation $\log(\tau(s)) = \log(\tau) = \theta_1$, which is the default option for the stationary model. In the same way, by fixing $b_0^\kappa(s) = b_1^\kappa(s) = 0$ and $b_2^\kappa(s) = 1$ in Eq. (6.24), we get $\log(\kappa(s)) = \log(\kappa) = \theta_2$.

In R-INLA the basis function values $b_k^\tau(\cdot)$ and $b_k^\kappa(\cdot)$ are specified in the B.tau and B.kappa matrices as arguments of the `inla.spde2.matern` function. In particular, the generic elements of B.tau and B.kappa are given by $B_{ik}^\tau = b_k^\tau(s_i)$ and $B_{ik}^\kappa = b_k^\kappa(s_i)$, respectively, with s_i denoting the locations of the mesh nodes and $k = 0, \dots, N$. For the stationary model, for which the basis function values are constant in space, only the first row of B.tau and B.kappa has to be specified, as in the default setting of the `inla.spde2.matern` function reported below:

```
inla.spde2.matern(...,
  B.tau = matrix(c(0,1,0),nrow=1,ncol=3)
  B.kappa = matrix(c(0,0,1),nrow=1,ncol=3),
  prior.tau = c(...),
  prior.kappa = c(...),
  ...)
```

Note that the `prior.tau` and `prior.kappa` options can be used for specifying priors on θ_1 and θ_2 (by default independent Normal(0, 1) priors are used).

As described by Lindgren and Rue (2015), in some situations it might be more useful to set priors on the standard deviation σ and on the range r (rather than on θ_1 and θ_2); in this case the following parameterization can be used:

$$\log(\sigma) = \log(\sigma_0) + \theta_1 \tag{6.28}$$

$$\log(r) = \log(r_0) + \theta_2, \tag{6.29}$$

where $\log(\sigma_0)$ and $\log(r_0)$ represent some baseline values. Some simple calculations yield the following equations to be used in the internal representation:

$$\log(\kappa) = \frac{\log(8)}{2} - \log(r_0) - \theta_2 = \log(\kappa_0) - \theta_2 \tag{6.30}$$

$$\log(\tau) = \frac{1}{2}\log\left(\frac{1}{4\pi}\right) - \log(\kappa_0) - \log(\sigma_0) - \theta_1 + \theta_2$$

$$= \log(\tau_0) - \theta_1 + \theta_2 \tag{6.31}$$

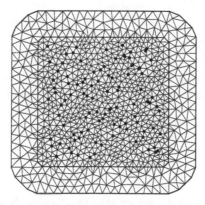

Figure 6.18   Mesh for the simulated data example. Black points denote the 100 simulated locations.

leading to $b_0^\kappa = \log(\kappa_0)$, $b_1^\kappa = 0$, $b_2^\kappa = +1$, $b_0^\tau = \log(\tau_0)$, $b_1^\tau = -1$, and $b_2^\tau = +1$. This setting can be specified in R-INLA using the following code:

```
inla.spde2.matern(...,
  B.tau = matrix(c(log(tau0),-1,+1),nrow=1,ncol=3)
  B.kappa = matrix(c(log(kappa0),0,-1),nrow=1,ncol=3),
  prior.tau = c(...),
  prior.kappa = c(...),
  ...)
```

6.9.1   Example with simulated data

We present here a simple example in order to show how to simulate data for a given GMRF in $\mathbb{R}^2$ and how to set priors for the SPDE parameters of a stationary GF. The area used for the simulation is a square domain with bottom-left and top-right limits given by the points $(0, 0)$ and $(1, 1)$. The following code generates $n = 100$ locations in the given domain and defines the mesh:

```
> limits <- cbind(c(0,1,1,0,0), c(0,0,1,1,0))
> n.loc <- 100
> set.seed(1653)
> locations <- cbind(s1=sample(1:n.loc / n.loc),
                     s2=sample(1:n.loc / n.loc))
> mesh <- inla.mesh.2d(loc=locations,loc.domain= limits,
                       cutoff=0.03, max.edge=c(0.07,.12))
```

The obtained mesh together with the simulated locations is displayed in Figure 6.18.

To simulate the values of the spatial field, we set the standard deviation $\sigma_0 = 1$ and the range $r_0 = 0.3$. Moreover, we consider the parameterization given in Eqs. (6.30) and (6.31) with $\theta_1 = \theta_2 = 0$. With the following code, we set the values for the known parameters and compute κ and τ (see Eqs. (6.16) and (6.17)):

```
> range0 <- 0.3
> sigma0 <- 1
> kappa0 <- sqrt(8)/range0
> tau0 <- 1/(sqrt(4*pi)*kappa0*sigma0)
```

We define the SPDE object by means of the `inla.spde2.matern` function using the specification for B.tau and B.kappa as given in Eqs. (6.30) and (6.31):

```
> spde_stat <- inla.spde2.matern(mesh,
                    B.tau=matrix(c(log(tau0), -1, +1),nrow=1,ncol=3),
                    B.kappa=matrix(c(log(kappa0), 0, -1),nrow=1,ncol=3),
                    theta.prior.mean=c(0, 0),
                    theta.prior.prec=c(0.1, 0.1))
```

As regards priors for θ_1 and θ_2, we set zero mean vague Normal independent distributions with precisions equal to 0.1. This results in a Normal($\log(\kappa_0), 0.1$) prior for $\log(k)$ and a Normal($\log(\tau_0), 0.2$) prior for $\log(\tau)$.

The next step consists in computing the precision matrix Q of the SPDE object `spde_stat`. This is done using the `inla.spde2.precision` function:

```
> Q_stat <- inla.spde2.precision(spde=spde_stat, theta=c(0,0))
```

where we set `theta=c(0,0)` as we are assuming $\theta_1 = \theta_2 = 0$. Finally, the `inla.qsample` function is run in order to generate one sample from a GMRF with precision matrix given by `Q_stat` (which is the approximation of the stationary Matérn field):

```
> sample_stat <- as.vector(inla.qsample(n=1, Q=Q_stat, seed=1434))
> length(sample_stat)
[1] 949
```

Note that the length of the simulated spatial process is given by the number of the mesh vertices.

Before proceeding with the simulation of the observations (including also the covariate and the measurement error) and the estimation step, we point out that the approach described above for obtaining `sample_stat` is equivalent to the following one, which is based on the simplest internal parameterization with $\log(\tau) = \theta_1$ and $\log(\kappa) = \theta_2$:

```
> spde_stat_v2 <- inla.spde2.matern(mesh,
                    B.tau=matrix(c(0, 1, 0),nrow=1,ncol=3),
                    B.kappa=matrix(c(0, 0, 1),nrow=1,ncol=3),
                    theta.prior.mean=c(0, 0),
                    theta.prior.prec=c(0.1, 0.1))
> Q_stat_v2 <- inla.spde2.precision(spde_stat_v2,
                        theta=c(log(tau0),log(kappa0)))
> sample_stat_v2 <- as.vector(inla.qsample(n=1, Q=Q_stat_v2,
                        seed=1434))
> #Check that the simulated values of the GMRF are the same:
> sum(sample_stat - sample_stat_v2)
[1] 0
```

We now simulate the observations y_i by assuming the following distribution:

$$y_i \sim \text{Normal}(\eta_i, \sigma_e^2) \qquad i = 1, \ldots, 100,$$

where

$$\eta_i = b_0 + \beta_1 x_i + \xi_i$$

with $b_0 = 10$, $\beta_1 = 3$, $\sigma_e^2 = 0.25$, and x_i denoting the values of a covariate simulated from a Normal$(0, 1)$ distribution. The term ξ_i is the realization of the stationary GF $\xi(s)$ and it is given by the values stored in the vector `sample_stat`.

```
> #Simulate the covariate values
> set.seed(344)
> covariate <- rnorm(n.loc,mean=0,sd=1)
> #Compute the observation matrix
> A <- inla.spde.make.A(mesh, loc=locations)
> dim(A)
[1] 100 949
> #Simulate the observations y
> set.seed(545)
> y <- 10 + 3*covariate + as.vector(A %*% sample_stat) +
      rnorm(n.loc,mean=0,sd=sqrt(0.25))
```

We now follow the procedures described in Section 6.7.3 for estimating the model parameters:

```
> mesh.index <- inla.spde.make.index(name="field",
                          n.spde=spde_stat$n.spde)
> stack.est <- inla.stack(data=list(y=y),
                    A=list(A,1),
                    effects=list(c(mesh.index,list(intercept=1)),
                            list(x=covariate)), tag="est")
> formula <- y ~ -1 + intercept + x + f(field,model=spde_stat)
> output_stat <- inla(formula,
                    data=inla.stack.data(stack.est,spde=spde_stat),
                    family="normal",
                    control.predictor=list(A=inla.stack.A(stack.est),
                            compute=TRUE) )
> spde.result <- inla.spde2.result(inla=output_stat,name="field",
                            spde=spde_stat)
```

The posterior distributions of the parameters b_0, β_1, σ^2, and r are reported in Figure 6.19 (they all contain the corresponding true values).

6.10   SPDE for Gaussian response: Swiss rainfall data

In this section, we consider rainfall measurements (in 10th of mm) taken on the 8th of May 1986 at 467 locations in Switzerland. As described in Section 1.4.11, the rainfall data are part of the `sic` dataset in the `geoR` library (Ribeiro and Diggle, 2001). In particular, we employ the SPDE approach in order to estimate the parameters of the spatial model and to predict rainfall values both at some validation stations and for a set of points placed on a regular grid covering Switzerland.

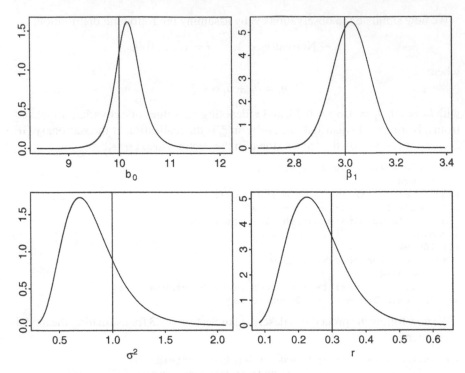

Figure 6.19   Posterior distributions of the parameters for the example with simulated data from a stationary spatial field: intercept b_0 (top left), covariate coefficient β_1 (top right), spatial variance σ^2 (bottom left), and range r (bottom right). Vertical lines denote the values used for the simulation.

Data preparation

For mapping convenience, we center the coordinates with respect to the mean of the Switzerland borders:

```
> sic.all$coords[,1] <- (sic.all$coords[,1] -
                         apply(sic.borders,2,mean)[1])
> sic.all$coords[,2] <- (sic.all$coords[,2] -
                         apply(sic.borders,2,mean)[2])
> sic.borders <- apply(sic.borders, 2, scale, scale=F)
```

In order to make the distribution of the rainfall data approximately Normal, we use a square root transformation. Moreover, following the guidelines described by Dubois (1998), we use the 100 locations included in the `sic.100 geodata` object for estimation purposes and we retain the remaining 367 stations for model validation (i.e., we predict rainfall at the validation sites and evaluate the model

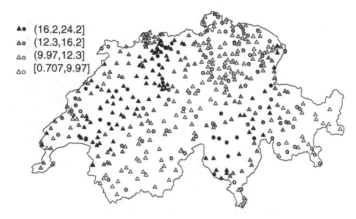

Figure 6.20   Locations of the 467 spatial points in Switzerland included in the SIC *dataset. Bullets denote the 100 stations used for estimation, while triangles denote the 367 stations retained for model validation. Colors are determined by the rainfall values on the square root scale.*

predictive performance). The data are selected and arranged through the following code:

```
> #Find in sic.all the 100 locations
> #given in sic.100 and used for estimation
> index.est <- which(as.numeric(rownames(sic.all$coords))
                       %in% as.numeric(rownames(sic.100$coords)))
> #Prepare data for estimation (100 locations)
> est.coord <- sic.all$coords[index.est,]
> est.data <-  sqrt(sic.all$data[index.est])
> est.elevation <- sic.all$altitude[index.est]/1000
> #Prepare data for validation (367 locations)
> val.coord <- sic.all$coords[-index.est,]
> val.data <- sqrt(sic.all$data[-index.est])
> val.elevation <- sic.all$altitude[-index.est]/1000
```

The rainfall values for estimation and validation stations are plotted in Figure 6.20.

For the same spatial domain, elevation is available in the sic97 dataset of the gstat package (Pebesma, 2004) as a SpatialGridDataFrame object named demstd:

```
> library(gstat)
> data(sic97)
```

We perform some transformations with the demstd object in order to obtain an elevation matrix (named elevation.grid) of dimensions 376 × 253 which will be used for spatial prediction:

```
> x.res <- demstd@grid@cells.dim[1]   #376
> y.res <- demstd@grid@cells.dim[2]   #253
```

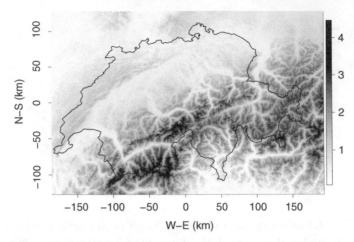

Figure 6.21   Map of elevation (in km) defined on a 376 × 253 regular grid covering Switzerland.

```
> pred.elevation <- as.matrix(demstd@data)
> elevation.grid <- matrix(pred.elevation, nrow=x.res,ncol=y.res,
                           byrow=F)
> #Set the right orientation for the grid
> elevation.grid <- elevation.grid[,y.res:1]/1000
> dim(elevation.grid)
[1] 376 253
```

The resulting elevation map is represented in Figure 6.21 (note that the original scale was in meters and we divide it by 1000 for obtaining kilometers). Moreover, we create a regular grid of points named `pred.grid`, where rainfall prediction will be computed, with the same resolution of the elevation matrix:

```
> seq.x.grid <- seq(from=demstd@coords[1,1],to=demstd@coords[2,1],
                    length=x.res)/1000
> seq.y.grid <- seq(from=demstd@coords[1,2],to=demstd@coords[2,2],
                    length=y.res)/1000
> pred.grid <- as.matrix(expand.grid(x=seq.x.grid,y=seq.y.grid))
```

Model fitting and spatial prediction at the validation stations

The model we specify for the Swiss rainfall data assumes normally distributed observations

$$y_i \sim \text{Normal}(\eta_i, \sigma_e^2),$$

where the mean

$$\eta_i = b_0 + x_i\beta + \xi_i$$

includes an intercept b_0, a linear effect of the site specific covariate x_i (i.e., elevation) and a spatial random effect ξ_i which is a priori a Matérn GF.

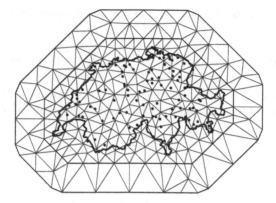

Figure 6.22   The Switzerland triangulation with 237 vertices. Black dots denote the 100 stations used for parameter model estimation.

As described in Section 6.7, the first step required for model fitting through SPDE is the triangulation of the considered spatial domain. We use the `inla.mesh.2d` function and specify the region borders (`sic.borders`) to define the outer domain:

```
> Swiss.mesh <- inla.mesh.2d(loc.domain=sic.borders,
                             max.edge=c(35,100))
```

The resulting mesh is composed of 237 vertices and is displayed in Figure 6.22. Note that rainfall stations are not included as triangle vertices. Given the mesh, we create the `spde` model object (using default priors)

```
> Swiss.spde <- inla.spde2.matern(mesh=Swiss.mesh,alpha=2)
```

and the projector matrices A for the estimation and validation steps

```
> A.est <- inla.spde.make.A(mesh=Swiss.mesh, loc=est.coord)
> A.val <- inla.spde.make.A(mesh=Swiss.mesh, loc=val.coord)
```

The required indexes for the spatial field are obtained through

```
> s.index <- inla.spde.make.index(name="spatial.field",
                             n.spde=Swiss.spde$n.spde)
```

where `s.index` is a list whose first component is named `spatial.field` and contains the mesh vertex indexes (i.e., the sequence of integer numbers from 1 to $G = 237$).

As introduced in Section 6.6, `R-INLA` creates a new linear predictor $\eta^\star$ defined as a linear combination of the original linear predictor η with weights given in the observation matrix A such that

$$\eta_e^\star = A_e \eta_e,$$

where in this case the subscript e stands for estimation. It follows that now $y \sim$ MVNormal($\eta_e^\star, \sigma_e^2 I$). If we separate the effect of the covariate x from the spatial random effect, represented by the Matérn GF ξ and the constant in space intercept b_0, we obtain

$$\eta_e^\star = A_e \eta_e = [A \; I] \begin{bmatrix} \xi + 1b_0 \\ x\beta \end{bmatrix} = A(\xi + 1b_0) + x\beta.$$

Thanks to the `inla.stack` function we need not take care of the creation and management of the objects A_e and η_e. The required syntax is simply

```
> stack.est <- inla.stack(data = list(rain=est.data),
  A = list(A.est, 1),
  effects = list(c(s.index, list(Intercept=1)),
    list(Elevation=est.elevation)),
  tag="est")
```

The correspondence between matrix and R-INLA objects is made explicit below:

$$A \; : \; \text{A.est}$$

$$I \; : \; 1 \text{ (identity matrix is abbreviated to scalar)}$$

$$\xi + 1b_0 \; : \; \text{list(c(s.index, list(Intercept=1))}$$

$$x\beta \; : \; \text{list(Elevation=est.elevation)}.$$

Similarly, we create the corresponding object `stack.val` for the 367 validation stations with the only difference that, since we are interested in prediction, we specify `data=list(rain=NA)` in the `inla.stack` function:

```
> stack.val <- inla.stack(data = list(rain=NA),
  A = list(A.val,1),
  effects = list(c(s.index, list(Intercept=1)),
            list(Elevation=val.elevation)),
  tag="val")
```

Finally, we join all the stack objects with

```
> join.stack <- inla.stack(stack.est, stack.val)
```

In this case, we deal with two linear predictors: $\eta_e^\star$ for estimation and $\eta_p^\star$ for prediction in the validation stations, where $\eta_p^\star = A_p \eta_p$. The `inla.stack` function defines a new joint linear predictor $\eta_{\text{join}}^\star$ through the following matrix operations:

$$\eta_{\text{join}}^\star = \begin{bmatrix} A_e & 0 \\ 0 & A_p \end{bmatrix} \begin{bmatrix} \eta_e \\ \eta_p \end{bmatrix}$$

$$= \begin{bmatrix} A_{n \times G} & I & 0 & 0 \\ 0 & 0 & A_{m \times G} & I \end{bmatrix} \begin{bmatrix} \xi + 1b_0 \\ x_{1:n}\beta \\ \xi + 1b_0 \\ x_{1:m}\beta \end{bmatrix}$$

$$= \begin{bmatrix} A_{n \times G} & I & 0 \\ A_{m \times G} & 0 & I \end{bmatrix} \begin{bmatrix} \xi + 1b_0 \\ x_{1:n}\beta \\ x_{1:m}\beta \end{bmatrix} = A_{\text{join}} \eta_{\text{join}},$$

where m is used to denote the number of locations where spatial prediction is required, $A_{n \times G}$ denotes that the observation matrix is of dimensions $n \times G$ and the notation $x_{1:m}$ is used for example to indicate the m values of the covariate in the new locations. Here, as already introduced in Section 6.8, we do not perform any matrix construction and leave the object management to `inla.stack` which keeps track of removing duplicated or unused effects.

After the `formula` specification, which includes all the fixed and random effects,

```
> formula <- rain ~ -1 + Intercept + Elevation +
            f(spatial.field, model=spde)
```

we call the `inla` function

```
> Swiss.output <-  inla(formula,
    data=inla.stack.data(join.stack, spde=Swiss.spde),
    family="gaussian",
    control.predictor=list(A=inla.stack.A(join.stack), compute=TRUE),
    control.compute=list(cpo=TRUE, dic=TRUE))
```

The posterior summary statistics of the parameters are retrieved using the procedure described in Section 6.7.3, and all the relevant posterior estimates are reported in the upper part of Table 6.5. As the elevation parameter β is not significant, we also implement the model without elevation (the code to obtain `Swiss.output.noelev` is not shown here) and use the DIC as a model selection criterion. The DIC values reported in Table 6.5 are almost identical, so we select the model without elevation (note that the posterior estimates for the other parameters do not change considerably between the two models).

Table 6.5   Posterior estimates (mean, standard deviation (SD) and quantiles) and DIC for the Swiss rainfall model with and without elevation as covariate.

Parameter	Mean	SD	2.5%	50%	97.5%
		With elevation DIC $= 431.076$			
b_0	11.707	2.013	7.292	11.839	15.372
β	−0.100	0.779	−1.643	−0.097	1.421
σ_e^2	2.566	0.638	1.554	2.480	4.052
σ^2	28.060	8.845	14.820	26.611	49.338
r	71.185	21.174	38.905	67.909	121.608
		Without elevation DIC $= 428.845$			
b_0	11.609	1.871	7.450	11.740	15.047
σ_e^2	2.511	0.623	1.528	2.425	3.964
σ^2	28.312	8.701	15.018	26.988	48.992
r	71.587	21.768	39.042	67.978	124.017

We now focus on the prediction in the 367 validation stations (this case was previously identified with the string `tag="val"`). We first type

```
> index.val <- inla.stack.index(join.stack,"val")$data
```

in order to retrieve, from the full `stack` object, the indexes identifying the validation stations. Then the posterior summaries (mean and standard deviation) for the linear prediction η (on the square root scale) can be obtained from the `Swiss.output.noelev` object through

```
> post.mean.val <-
  Swiss.output.noelev$summary.linear.predictor[index.val,"mean"]
> post.sd.val <-
  Swiss.output.noelev$summary.linear.predictor[index.val,"sd"]
```

It is then straightforward to compare observed and predicted values (represented by the posterior mean `post.mean.val`) and to compute predictive performance statistics. For example, the root mean square error is equal to 2.28 and the Pearson correlation coefficient is 0.85, which denotes a good correlation between observed and predicted values.

Spatial prediction at the grid locations

Prediction on the regular grid regards the 95 128 locations included in the `pred.grid` object defined previously. Following the usual approach, we use the code

```
> A.pred <- inla.spde.make.A(mesh=Swiss.mesh, loc=pred.grid)
> stack.pred <- inla.stack(data = list(rain=NA),
    A = list(A.pred,1),
    effects = list(c(s.index, list(Intercept=1)),
      list(Elevation=pred.elevation)),
    tag="pred")
> join.stack.noelev <- inla.stack(stack.est.noelev, stack.pred)
> Swiss.output.noelev.pred <-  inla(formula,
    data=inla.stack.data(join.stack.noelev, spde=Swiss.spde),
    family="gaussian",
    control.predictor=list(A=inla.stack.A(join.stack.noelev),
    compute=TRUE))
```

which is a computationally expensive task due to the high number of locations involved in the prediction step at the grid level. If the linear predictor marginal distributions are not necessary, a less computationally heavy solution consists in projecting the latent field – estimated at the mesh vertices – onto the grid locations. To follow this approach, a new projection matrix is created

```
> A.pred <- inla.spde.make.A(mesh=Swiss.mesh)
```

without specifying the `loc` argument (by default it is NULL). This gives rise to a diagonal matrix A with dimension G. Then as usual we use the `inla.stack` function

```
> stack.pred <- inla.stack(data = list(rain=NA),
    A = list(A.pred),
    effects = list(c(s.index, list(Intercept=1))),
    tag="pred")
> join.stack.noelev <- inla.stack(stack.est.noelev, stack.pred)
```

and then run

```
> Swiss.output.noelev <-  inla(formula,
    data=inla.stack.data(join.stack.noelev, spde=Swiss.spde),
    family="gaussian",
    control.predictor=list(A=inla.stack.A(join.stack.noelev),
    compute=TRUE))
```

We extract information about the posterior mean and standard deviation of the latent field in the mesh vertices with

```
> index.pred <-
    inla.stack.index(join.stack.noelev,"pred")$data
> post.mean.pred <-
    Swiss.output.noelev$summary.linear.predictor[index.pred,  "mean"]
> post.sd.pred <-
    Swiss.output.noelev$summary.linear.predictor[index.pred,  "sd"]
```

The procedure now requires to create a linkage between the mesh and the grid using the `inla.mesh.projector` command:

```
> proj.grid <- inla.mesh.projector(Swiss.mesh,
                xlim=range(pred.grid[,1]), ylim=range(pred.grid[,2]),
                    dims=c(x.res,y.res))
```

and then project the linear predictor from the mesh to the grid using the `inla.mesh.project` function

```
> post.mean.pred.grid <- inla.mesh.project(proj.grid, post.mean.pred)
> post.sd.pred.grid <- inla.mesh.project(proj.grid, post.sd.pred)
```

The map of the rainfall posterior mean (on the square root scale) and standard deviation at the grid level are shown in Figure 6.23.

6.11   SPDE with nonnormal outcome: malaria in the Gambia

In this section, we consider the `gambia` dataset which is included in the `geoR` package and regards malaria prevalence in 2035 children at 65 villages in the Gambia, Africa. The dataset was introduced in Section 1.4.10. Here the aim consists in implementing a model to describe the spatial variation in the prevalence of malaria using data coming from a sample of villages in the Gambia. In this framework, the prevalence of malaria can be considered as a continuous spatial phenomenon and a Matérn GF appears as an appropriate stochastic framework for this application.

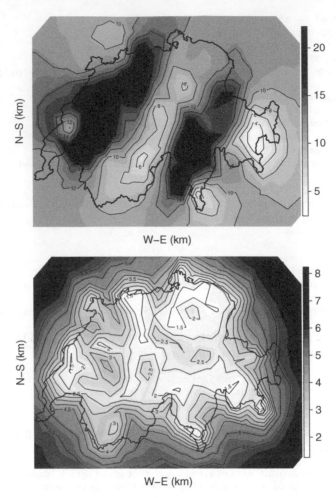

Figure 6.23   Map of the rainfall posterior mean and standard deviation at the grid level.

Together with the child and village covariates described in Section 1.4.10, for each child the village coordinates are available and saved in a separate object

```
> coords <-  as.matrix(gambia[,1:2])/1000 #in km
```

We perform some data manipulation (not shown here) in order to create an index at the village level (`village.index`), i.e., a sequence of integer numbers from 1 to 65.

We assume the following Binomial distribution for the generic binary observation y_{ij} referred to child i ($i = 1, \ldots, 2035$) in village j ($j = 1, \ldots, 65$):

$$y_{ij} \sim \text{Binomial}(\pi_{ij}, n_{ij} = 1).$$

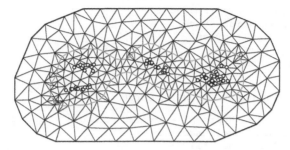

Figure 6.24   Triangulation for Gambia with black points denoting the village locations where information about child is available. The internal line defines the nonconvex hull.

The linear predictor η_{ij} is defined as the logit transformation of the probability π_{ij} that the ith child in the jth village has a positive blood test result:

$$\eta_{ij} = \text{logit}(\pi_{ij}) = b_0 + x_i \beta_{\text{child}} + x_j \beta_{\text{village}} + u_i + \xi_i$$

and it includes an intercept b_0, linear effects β for the child covariates x_i (age, netuse and treated) and for the village level covariates x_j (green and phc), and separate components for the residual spatial and nonspatial effects. In particular, ξ_i is supposed to be distributed as a Matérn GF, while u_i is the unstructured residual term with mean equal to zero and variance equal to σ_u^2.

To estimate this model with the SPDE approach, we first create the mesh using a nonconvex hull as described in Section 6.7.1:

```
> bnd <- inla.nonconvex.hull(coords,convex=-0.1)
> gambia.mesh <- inla.mesh.2d(boundary = bnd,
    offset=c(30, 60), max.edge=c(20,40))
```

and the resulting mesh with 330 vertices is displayed in Figure 6.24.

As usual, we create the SPDE object

```
> gambia.spde <- inla.spde2.matern(mesh=gambia.mesh, alpha=2)
```

the projector matrix

```
> A.est <- inla.spde.make.A(mesh=gambia.mesh, loc=coords)
```

and the list of indexes for the spatial effect

```
> s.index <- inla.spde.make.index(name="spatial.field",
            n.spde=gambia.spde$n.spde)
```

Finally, we stack all the relevant pieces together

```
> gambia.stack.est <- inla.stack(data=list(y=gambia$pos),
    A=list(A.est, 1, 1, 1, 1, 1, 1),
    effects=list(c(s.index, list(Intercept=1)),
      list(age=gambia$age/365),
```

```
    list(treated=gambia$treated),
    list(netuse=gambia$netuse),
    list(green=gambia$green),
    list(phc=gambia$phc),
    list(village.index=gambia$village.index)),
  tag="est")
```

and define the formula including all the effects

```
> formula <- y ~ -1 + Intercept + treated + netuse + age + green + phc +
    f(spatial.field, model=gambia.spde) +
    f(village.index, model="iid")
```

Then the `inla` function with Binomial likelihood is run

```
> gambia.output <- inla(formula,
    data=inla.stack.data(gambia.stack.est, spde=gambia.spde),
    family="binomial",Ntrials=1,
    control.predictor=list(A=inla.stack.A(gambia.stack.est),
                           compute=TRUE),
    control.compute=list(dic=TRUE))
```

All the posterior estimates are reported in Table 6.6. The results confirm the progressive increase in prevalence with age, and the protective effects of bed nets. In particular, the variation in the probability π_{ij} when bed net is used can be computed through the antilogit transformation:

```
> inla.emarginal(function(x) exp(x)/(1+exp(x)),
    gambia.output$marginals.fixed[["netuse"]])
[1] 0.4096611
```

Note that the previous code can be simplified using the INLA antilogit function named `inla.link.invlogit` (see `?inla.link`):

```
> inla.emarginal(inla.link.invlogit,
    gambia.output$marginals.fixed[["netuse"]])
[1] 0.4096611
```

Table 6.6   Posterior estimates (mean, standard deviation (SD) and quantiles) for the Gambia model.

Parameter	Mean	SD	2.5%	50%	97.5%
b_0	−1.169	1.296	−3.635	−1.201	1.462
β_{treated}	−0.361	0.202	−0.759	−0.361	0.033
β_{netuse}	−0.368	0.158	−0.678	−0.368	−0.057
β_{age}	0.246	0.044	0.159	0.246	0.333
β_{green}	0.009	0.026	−0.044	0.009	0.058
β_{phc}	−0.323	0.231	−0.781	−0.323	0.129
σ_u^2	0.263	0.119	0.098	0.241	0.557
σ^2	1.145	0.818	0.221	0.932	3.318
r	0.042	0.047	0.006	0.027	0.173

Neither inclusion in the primary health care system nor the greenness of the surrounding space appeared to affect significantly the prevalence of malaria.

To test the significance of the spatial effect, we have implemented the same model but removed the ξ_i component in the linear predictor. For this new model the DIC is equal to 2334.13, a value which is slightly bigger with respect to the one obtained for the original model (2326.44). Thus, it is possible to conclude that the data support the presence of a spatial effect.

6.12   Prior specification for the nonstationary case

For the nonstationary extension introduced in Section 6.5.1, it is possible to adopt the following parameterization (similarly to what has been done for the stationary case, see Eqs. (6.28) and (6.29)):

$$\log(\sigma(s)) = b_0^\sigma(s) + \sum_{k=1}^{N} b_k^\sigma(s)\theta_k$$

$$\log(r(s)) = b_0^r(s) + \sum_{k=1}^{N} b_k^r(s)\theta_k,$$

where $\sigma(s)$ and $r(s)$ are the nominal standard deviation and range, $b_0^\sigma(s)$ and $b_0^r(s)$ are the offsets and $b_k^\sigma(s)$ and $b_k^r(s)$ are the values of the basis functions (possibly equal to 0 for some values of k). As shown in Lindgren and Rue (2015), this parameterization, after some simple calculations, yields the following representation used internally in R-INLA:

$$b_0^\kappa(s) = \frac{\log(8)}{2} - b_0^r(s)$$

$$b_k^\kappa(s) = -b_k^r(s)$$

$$b_0^\tau(s) = \frac{1}{2}\log\left(\frac{1}{4\pi}\right) - b_0^\kappa(s) - b_0^\sigma(s)$$

$$b_k^\tau(s) = -b_k^\kappa(s) - b_k^\sigma(s).$$

The resulting values of $b_k^\kappa(s)$ and $b_k^\tau(s)$ (for $k = 0, \dots, N$) are specified in the B.tau and B.kappa matrices.

6.12.1   Example with simulated data

We consider as an example of nonstationarity a spatial process with spatially varying variance $\sigma^2(s)$. Given the nominal variance introduced in Eq. (6.21), here we assume that $\tau(s)$ depends on a function of the first spatial coordinate (e.g., longitude) – denoted by $h(s)$ – as follows:

$$\log(\tau(s)) = \theta_1 + \sin(\pi h(s))\theta_3. \tag{6.32}$$

We suppose that the range is constant in space so that $\log(\kappa(s)) = \log(\kappa) = \theta_2$.

With respect to the representation given in Eqs. (6.23) and (6.24), in this example, we have that $N = 3$, $b_0^\tau(s) = b_2^\tau(s) = 0$, $b_1^\tau(s) = 1$ for each s and $b_3^\tau(s) = \sin(\pi h(s))$. Moreover, $b_1^\kappa(s) = b_1^\kappa(s) = b_3^\kappa(s) = 0$ and $b_2^\kappa(s) = 1$ for each s. This setting is specified in R-INLA through the following code:

```
> spde_nstat <- inla.spde2.matern(mesh,
            B.tau=matrix(cbind(0, 1, 0, sin(pi*mesh$loc[,1])),ncol=4),
            B.kappa=matrix(c(0, 0, 1, 0),nrow=1,ncol=4),
            theta.prior.mean=c(0, 0, 0),
            theta.prior.prec=c(0.1, 0.1, 0.1))
```

We choose a vague distribution with zero mean and unit variance as prior specification on θ_i with $i = 1, \ldots, 3$.

For the simulation, we use the same set of locations and the mesh defined in Section 6.9.1 for the stationary case. Moreover, for generating the values of the nonstationary spatial process, we fix the values of the parameters $\theta_1, \theta_2, \theta_3$ as follows[5]

```
> theta <- c(-1, 2, -1)
```

By substituting the values of theta in Eq. (6.32), we get $\log(\tau(s)) = -1 - \sin(\pi h(s))$ while the value of $\log(\kappa)$ is equal to 2. The resulting precision matrix Q can be obtained through

```
> Q_nstat <- inla.spde2.precision(spde=spde_nstat, theta=theta)
```

It is now possible to generate realizations of the nonstationary field defined previously

```
> sample_nstat <- as.vector(inla.qsample(n=1, Q=Q_nstat, seed=1))
```

and to simulate observations y_i according to the same model as used in Section 6.9.1:

```
> set.seed(5514)
> y_nstat <- 10 + 3*covariate + as.vector(A %*% sample_nstat) +
  rnorm(n,mean=0,sd=sqrt(0.25))
```

The last step requires the creation of the stack object, of the formula and the run of the inla function:

```
> mesh.index_nstat <- inla.spde.make.index(name="field",
                          n.spde=spde_nstat$n.spde)
> stack.est_nstat = inla.stack(data=list(y=y_nstat),
              A=list(A,1),
              effects=list(c(mesh.index_nstat,list(intercept=1)),
                          list(x=covariate)),
              tag="est")
> formula_nstat <- y ~ -1+ intercept + x + f(field,model=spde_nstat)
```

---

[5] Differently to the example described in Section 6.9.1, where we set the values of the variance and of the range and use the parameterization given by Eqs. (6.30) and (6.31), here we adopt the standard specification as in Eqs. (6.23) and (6.24), and fix the values of θ_1, θ_2 and θ_3.

```
> output_nstat <- inla(formula_nstat,
          data=inla.stack.data(stack.est_nstat,spde=spde_nstat),
          family="normal",
          control.predictor=list(A=inla.stack.A(stack.est_nstat),
                                  compute=TRUE))
```

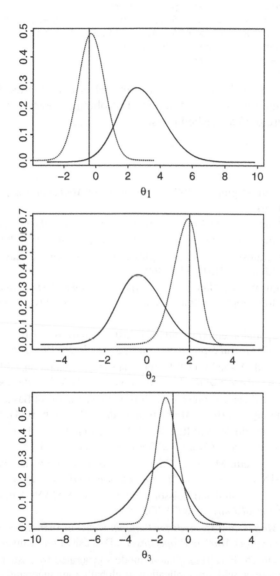

Figure 6.25   Posterior distributions of the parameters θ_1, θ_2 and θ_3 with two different prior specifications for θ_2: Normal(0, 0.1) (solid lines) and Normal(2, 0.1) (dashed lines). Vertical lines denote the true values used for simulating the nonstationary spatial process.

The posterior distribution of the parameters θ_1, θ_2, and θ_3 are displayed in Figure 6.25 with solid lines. To assess how a change in the prior specification affects the posterior distritutions, we adopt a more informative prior for θ_2 (with a mean equal to 2 instead of 0):

```
> spde_nstat_prior2 <- inla.spde2.matern(mesh,
            B.tau=matrix(cbind(0, 1, 0, sin(pi*mesh$loc[,1])),ncol=4),
            B.kappa=matrix(c(0, 0, 1, 0),nrow=1,ncol=4),
            theta.prior.mean=c(0, 2, 0),
            theta.prior.prec=c(1,1,1))
```

The code for running the corresponding model is not reported because it does not differ from the one presented before. The obtained posterior distributions are reported in Figure 6.25 as dashed lines.

References

Abramowitz, M. and Stegun, I. (1972). *Handbook of Mathematical Functions*. Courier Dover Publications.

Agarwal, D., Gelfand, A., and Citron-Pousty, S. (2002). Zero-inflated models with application to spatial count data. *Environmental and Ecological Statistics*, **9**(4), 341–355.

Assuncao, R. and Krainski, E. (2009). Neighborhood dependence in Bayesian spatial models. *Biometrical Journal*, **5**(51), 851–869.

Banerjee, S., Carlin, B., and Gelfand, A. (2004). *Hierarchical Modeling and Analysis for Spatial Data*. Monographs on Statistics and Applied Probability. Chapman & Hall, New York.

Besag, J. (1974). Spatial interaction and the statistical analysis of lattice systems (with discussion). *Journal of Royal Statistical Society, Series B*, **36**, 192–236.

Besag, J., York, J., and Mollie, A. (1991). Bayesian image restoration, with two applications in spatial statistics. *Annals of the Institute of Statistical Mathematics*, **43**, 1–59.

Best, N., Richardson, S., and Thomson, A. (2005). A comparison of Bayesian spatial models for disease mapping. *Statistical Methods in Medical Research*, **1**(14), 35–59.

Bivand, R., Gómez-Rubio, V., and Rue, H. (2015). Spatial data analysis with R-INLA with some extensions. *Journal of Statistical Software*, **63**(20), 1–31.

Blangiardo, M., Cameletti, M., Baio, G., and Rue, H. (2013). Spatial and spatio-temporal models with R-INLA. *Spatial and Spatio-temporal Epidemiology*, **4**, 33–49.

Bohning, D. (1998). Zero-inflated Poisson models and C.A.MAN: A tutorial collection of evidence. *Biometrical Journal*, **40**(7), 833–843.

Bolin, D. (2012). *Models and Methods for Random Fields in Spatial Statistics with Computational Efficiency from Markov Properties*. Ph.D. thesis, Lund University.

Bolin, D. and Lindgren, F. (2011). Spatial models generated by nested stochastic partial differential equations, with an application to global ozone mapping. *Annals of Applied Statistics*, **5**(1), 523–550.

Cameletti, M., Lindgren, F., Simpson, D., and Rue, H. (2013). Spatio-temporal modeling of particulate matter concentration through the SPDE approach. *Advances in Statistical Analysis*, **97**(2), 109–131.

Clark, J. (2005). Why environmental scientists are becoming Bayesians. *Ecology Letters*, **8**(1), 2–14.

Clark, J. and Gelfand, A., editors (2006). *Hierarchical Modeling for the Environmental Sciences. Statistical Methods and Applications*. Oxford University Press, New York.

Congdon, P. (2007). *Bayesian Statistical Modelling*. John Wiley and Sons, Ltd.

Cressie, N. (1993). *Statistics for Spatial Data*. Wiley.

Diggle, P. and Ribeiro, J. (2007). *Model-Based Geostatistics*. Springer.

Diggle, P., Rowlingson, B., and Su, T. (2005). Point process methodology for on-line spatio-temporal disease surveillance. *Environmetrics*, **16**, 423–434.

Dubois, G. (1998). Spatial interpolation comparison 97: Foreword and introduction. *Journal of Geographic Information and Decision Analysis*, **2**, 1–10.

Dunson, D. (2001). Commentary: Practical advantages of Bayesian analysis of epidemiologic data. *American Journal of Epidemiology*, **153**(12), 1222–1226.

Elliott, P., Wakefield, J., Best, N., and Briggs, D., editors (2000). *Spatial Epidemiology: Methods and Applications*. Oxford University Press.

Gelfand, A., Diggle, P., Fuentes, M., and Guttorp, P., editors (2010). *Handbook of Spatial Statistics*. Chapman & Hall.

Gómez-Rubio, V., Bivand, R., and Rue, H. (2014). Spatial models using Laplace Approximation methods. In: Handbook of Regional Science. Springer 2014. pp. 1401–1417 `http://link.springer.com/referenceworkentry/10.1007%2F978-3-642-23430-9_104`.

Gschlobl, S. and Gzado, C. (2008). Modelling count data with overdispersion and spatial effects. *Statistical Papers*, **49**, 531–552.

Hall, D. (2000). Zero-inflated poisson and binomial regression with random effects: A case study. *Biometrics*, **56**(4), 1030–1039.

Illian, J., Sørbye, S., and Rue, H. (2012). A toolbox for fitting complex spatial point process models using integrated nested Laplace approximation (INLA). *Annals of Applied Statistics*, **6**(4), 1499–1530.

Illian, J. (2015). *Fitting Statistical Models to Spatial Data with INLA – A Case Study Approach*. CRC, to be published.

Ingebrigtsen, R., Lindgren, F., and Steinsland, I. (2013). Spatial models with explanatory variables in the dependence structure. *Spatial Statistics*, **8**, 20–38.

Jewell, C., Kypraios, T., Neal, P., and Roberts, G. (2009). Bayesian analysis for emerging infectious diseases. *Bayesian Analysis*, **4**(3), 465–496.

Jona Lasinio, G., Mastrantonio, G., and Pollice, A. (2013). Discussing the "big n problem". *Statistical Methods & Applications*, **22**(1), 97–112.

Krainski, E. and Lindgren, F. (2013). The R-INLA tutorial: SPDE models. Available at `http://www.math.ntnu.no/inla/r-inla.org/tutorials/spde/spde-tutorial.pdf`.

Lambert, D. (1992). Zero-inflated Poisson regression, with an application to defects in manufacturing. *Technometrics*, **34**, 1–14.

Lawson, A. (2009). *Bayesian Disease Mapping. Hierarchical Modeling in Spatial Epidemiology*. CRC Press.

Lee, D. (2011). A comparison of conditional autoregressive models used in Bayesian disease mapping. *Spatial and Spatio-Temporal Epidemiology*, **2**(2), 79–89.

Lesaffre, E. and Lawson, A. (2012). *Bayesian Biostatistics*. Wiley–Blackwell.

Lindgren, F. and Rue, H. (2015). Bayesian spatial modelling with R-INLA. *Journal of Statistical Software*, **63**(29), 1–25. http://www.jstatsoft.org/v63/i19/paper.

Lindgren, F., Rue, H., and Lindström, J. (2011). An explicit link between Gaussian fields and Gaussian Markov random fields: The stochastic partial differential equation approach (with discussion). *Journal of Royal Statistical Society Series B*, **73**(4), 423–498.

Musenge, E., Chirwa, T. F., Kahn, K., and Vounatsou, P. (2013). Bayesian analysis of zero inflated spatio-temporal hIV/TB child mortality data through the {INLA} and {SPDE} approaches: Applied to data observed between 1992 and 2010 in rural northeast South Africa. *International Journal of Applied Earth Observation and Geoinformation*, **22**(0), 86–98.

Pascutto, C., Wakefield, J., Best, N., Richardson, S., Bernardinelli, L., Staines, A., and Elliott, P. (2000). Statistical issues in the analysis of disease mapping data. *Statistics in Medicine*, **19**(17-18), 2493–2519.

Pebesma, E. (2004). Multivariable geostatistics in S: The gstat package. *Computers and Geosciences*, **30**, 683–691.

Ribeiro, J. and Diggle, P. (2001). geoR: A package for geostatistical analysis. *R-NEWS*, **1**(2). http://cran.r-project.org/doc/Rnews.

Richardson, S. (2003). Spatial models in epidemiological applications. In P. Green, N. Hjort, and S. Richardson, editors, *Highly Structured Stochastic Systems.*, pp. 237–259. Oxford Statistical Science Series.

Richardson, S., Thomson, A., Best, N., and Elliott, P. (2004). Interpreting posterior relative risk estimates in disease-mapping studies. *Environmental Health Perspectives*, **112**(9), 1016–1025.

Rue, H. and Held, L. (2005). *Gaussian Markov Random Fields. Theory and Applications*. Chapman & Hall.

Simpson, D., Illian, J., Lindgren, F., Sørbye, S., and Rue, H. (2011). Going off grid: Computationally efficient inference for log-Gaussian Cox processes. *(http://arxiv.org/abs/1111.0641v2)*.

Simpson, D., Lindgren, F., and Rue, H. (2012a). In order to make spatial statistics computationally feasible, we need to forget about the covariance function. *Environmetrics*, **23**(1), 65–74.

Simpson, D., Lindgren, F., and Rue, H. (2012b). Think continuous: Markovian Gaussian models in spatial statistics. *Spatial Statistics*, **1**, 16–29.

Sørbye, S. H. and Rue, H. (2014). Scaling intrinsic Gaussian Markov random field priors in spatial modelling. *Spatial Statistics*, **8**, 39–51.

Staunbach, C., Schmid, V., Knorr-Held, L., and Ziller, M. (2002). A Bayesian model for spatial wildlife disease prevalence data. *Preventive Veterinary Medicine*, **56**, 75–87.

Wikle, C. (2003). Hierarchical models in environmental science. *International Statistical Review*, **71**(2), 181–199.

Winkelmann, R. (2003). *Econometric Analysis of Count Data*. Springer-Verlag.

7

Spatio-temporal models

Investigating only the spatial pattern of diseases or exposures as introduced in the previous chapter does not allow us to say anything about their temporal variation which could be equally important and interesting. For instance, let us assume we are interested in evaluating the spatial pattern of stroke mortality across London for the years 2000–2009, but we analyze only the data aggregated over the 10 years. Specifying a disease mapping similar to what was presented in Section 6.1.1 only allows us to identify areas with low or high risk compared to the whole of London. However, we are not able to say anything about the temporal trend of risk. Typically two situations can occur as presented in Abellan *et al.* (2008): the rate is constant across time and only varies spatially or it changes with time across all or some of the areas. The same situations can arise when we estimate a spatially varying phenomenon, for example the amount of rain in a particular period, e.g., a year; if we consider the data aggregated over time we can only model the spatial pattern, but if we disaggregate the data by day, we can now investigate a temporal trend and allow for it to be the same across all the areas or different for some of them.

In the above cases, the spatial process introduced in the previous chapter can be easily extended to the spatio-temporal case including a time dimension; the data are now defined by a process indexed by space and time

$$Y(s, t) \equiv \{y(s, t), (s, t) \in \mathcal{D} \subset \mathbb{R}^2 \times \mathbb{R}\}$$

and are observed at n spatial locations or areas and at T time points. When spatio-temporal geostatistical data are considered (Gelfand *et al.*, 2010, Chapter 23), we need to define a valid nonseparable spatio-temporal covariance function given by $\text{Cov}(y(s_i, t), y(s_j, u)) = C(y_{it}, y_{ju})$. If we assume stationarity in space and time, it can be written as a function of the spatial Euclidean distance $\Delta_{ij} = \|s_i - s_j\|$ and of the temporal lag $\Lambda_{tu} = |t - u|$, i.e., $\text{Cov}(y_{it}, y_{ju}) = C(\Delta_{ij}; \Lambda_{tu})$; several

---

Spatial and Spatio-temporal Bayesian Models with R-INLA, First Edition.
Marta Blangiardo and Michela Cameletti.
© 2015 John Wiley & Sons, Ltd. Published 2015 by John Wiley & Sons, Ltd.

examples of valid nonseparable space–time covariance functions are reported by
Cressie and Huang (1999) and Gneiting (2002).

In practice, to overcome the computational complexity of nonseparable models,
some simplifications are introduced. For example, we could simply assume sep-
arability so that the space–time covariance function is decomposed into the sum
(or the product) of a purely spatial and a purely temporal term, e.g., $\text{Cov}(y_{it}, y_{ju}) =$
$C_1(\Delta_{ij})C_2(\Lambda_{tu})$, as described by Gneiting *et al.* (2006). Alternatively, it is possible
to assume that the spatial correlation is constant in time, giving rise to a space–time
covariance function that is purely spatial when $t = u$, i.e., $\text{Cov}(y_{it}, y_{ju}) = C(\Delta_{ij})$, and
is zero otherwise. In this case, the temporal evolution could be introduced assum-
ing that the spatial process evolves in time following an autoregressive dynamics
(see, e.g., Harvill, 2010).

Similar reasoning can be applied to area level data; the GMRF framework can be
extended to include a precision matrix defined also in terms of time, assuming again
a neighborhood structure. If a space–time interaction is included, its precision can
be obtained through the Kronecker product[1] of the precision matrices for the space
and time effects interacting (Clayton, 1996; Knorr-Held, 2000).

7.1   Spatio-temporal disease mapping

Spatio-temporal disease mapping models are widely used in disease surveillance
studies (Abellan *et al.*, 2008; Lawson, 2009), when the interest is to identify the spatial and the temporal pattern of a disease. In practice, the standard disease mapping
model presented in Section 6.1.1 is extended to allow for a temporal component:

$$y_{it} \sim \text{Poisson}(\lambda_{it}); \qquad \lambda_{it} = E_{it}\rho_{it}$$

$$\log(\rho_{it}) = \eta_{it}$$

$$\eta_{it} = b_0 + u_i + v_i + \text{Temporal}_t \qquad (7.1)$$

with $t = 1, \ldots, T$. On Temporal$_t$ a parametric or nonparametric structure can be
specified.

---

[1] The Kronecker product (denoted by $\otimes$) consists in the multiplication of two matrices of arbitrary
size and results in a block matrix. For instance, if

$$A = \begin{pmatrix} a & b & c \\ d & e & f \\ g & h & i \end{pmatrix}$$

and B is another matrix of arbitrary size, then

$$A \otimes B = \begin{pmatrix} aB & bB & cB \\ dB & eB & fB \\ gB & hB & iB \end{pmatrix}.$$

In general, the Kronecker product is noncommutative, meaning that the order of the matrices influences
the results of the product.

Parametric trend

Bernardinelli *et al.* (1995) presented a parametric trend for the temporal component in Eq. (7.1) which assumes that the linear predictor can be written as

$$\eta_{it} = b_0 + u_i + v_i + (\beta + \delta_i) \times t. \tag{7.2}$$

This formulation includes the main spatial effect as presented in the previous chapter, the main linear trend β, which represents the global time effect, and a differential trend δ_i, which identifies the interaction between time and space.

Since for identifiability purposes a sum-to-zero constraint is imposed on $\delta = \{\delta_1, \ldots, \delta_n\}$ (recall that a similar constraint is also imposed on u), the terms δ_i represent the difference between the global trend β and the area-specific trend. If $\delta_i < 0$ then the area-specific trend is less steep than the mean trend, whilst $\delta_i > 0$ implies that the area-specific trend is steeper than the mean trend. We assume $\delta_i \sim$ Normal$(0, 1/\tau_\delta)$, but other specifications can be used, e.g., a conditional autoregressive structure, see Bernardinelli *et al.* (1995) and Schrödle and Held (2011) for a detailed description.

Lung cancer in Ohio

In this section, we build a parametric space–time disease mapping model using R-INLA for the Ohio lung cancer deaths example presented in Section 1.4.12. The number of deaths in each Ohio county ($i = 1, \ldots, 88$) and year ($t = 1, \ldots, 21$) follows a Poisson distribution as in Eq. (7.1) and the linear predictor η_{it} has a spatio-temporal specification as presented in Eq. (7.2). In R-INLA the model is specified as follows:

```
> formula.par<- y ~ 1 + f(county, model="bym",graph=Ohio.adj,
                      constr=TRUE),
               + f(county1, year, model="iid", constr=TRUE),
               + year
> model.par <- inla(formula.par,family="poisson",data=data,E=E,
                 control.predictor=list(compute=TRUE),
                 control.compute=list(dic=TRUE,cpo=TRUE))
```

Recall that county1 is a duplicate of county, but it is needed as in R-INLA each variable can be associated with an f() function only once. The first part of the formula specifies the BYM model as presented in Section 6.1.1, while year identifies the global time effect (estimated as a fixed effect) and f(county1,year,model="iid") is the differential trend, i.e., the interaction between space and time, modeled through an exchangeable prior.

Looking at model.par$summary.fixed shows the summary statistics for the fixed effects:

```
> round(model.par$summary.fixed[,1:5],3)
              mean    SD  0.025quant  0.5quant  0.975quant
(Intercept) -0.121 0.024    -0.169    -0.121      -0.073
year         0.001 0.001     0.000     0.001       0.003
```

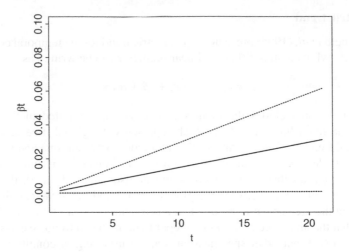

Figure 7.1   Global linear temporal trend for lung cancer mortality in Ohio. The solid line identifies the posterior mean for βt, while the dashed lines are the 95% credibility intervals.

Figure 7.1 plots the posterior mean of the main time effect together with its 95% credibility interval. A small but positive increment in the risk of respiratory cancer mortality for every subsequent year is visible.

Finally, the posterior mean of the spatial effect $\zeta_i = \exp(u_i + v_i)$ is obtained as usual through:

```
> m <- model.par$marginals.random[[1]][1:88]
> zeta.ST1 <- unlist(lapply(m,function(x)inla.emarginal(exp,x)))
```

and similarly we can get the differential time effect δ_i. Both the resulting maps are presented in Figure 7.2. The spatial effect is higher in the central-southern counties as well as in the far Western Counties. On the other hand, the differential temporal trend is below the average mostly in the north/northeast part of the state, while the southeast shows a differential trend higher than the average.

7.1.1   Nonparametric dynamic trend

In the model specified above, a linearity constraint is imposed on the differential temporal trend δ_i; nevertheless it is possible to release it using a dynamic nonparametric formulation for the linear predictor (Knorr-Held, 2000) as

$$\eta_{it} = b_0 + u_i + v_i + \gamma_t + \phi_t. \tag{7.3}$$

Here b_0, u_i, and v_i have the same parameterization as in Eq. (7.2); however, the term γ_t represents the temporally structured effect, modeled dynamically

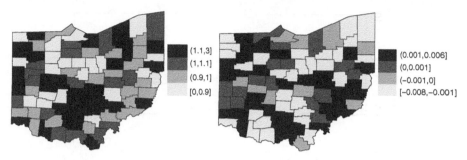

Figure 7.2   Posterior mean of the spatial main effect ζ_i (left) and of the differential time effect δ_i (right) for respiratory cancer mortality in Ohio.

(e.g., using a random walk of order 1 or 2) and defined as

RW of order 1

$$\gamma_t \mid \gamma_{t-1} \sim \text{Normal}(\gamma_{t-1}, \sigma^2) \tag{7.4}$$

RW of order 2

$$\gamma_t \mid \gamma_{t-1}, \gamma_{t-2} \sim \text{Normal}(2\gamma_{t-1} + \gamma_{t-2}, \sigma^2). \tag{7.5}$$

Finally, ϕ_t is specified by means of a Gaussian exchangeable prior: $\phi_t \sim \text{Normal}(0, 1/\tau_\phi)$.

Birth weight in Georgia

To show how to implement a nonparametric dynamic space–time model in R-INLA, we use the example of low birth weight in Georgia, presented in Section 1.4.13. The outcome consists of the counts of babies weighting less than 2500 g at birth, for the 159 counties in the US state of Georgia during 2000–2010 (Lawson, 2009).

The model presented in Eq. (7.3) is specified in R-INLA and run as

```
> formula.ST1 <- y ~
    f(ID.area,model="bym",graph=Georgia.adj) +
    f(ID.year,model="rw2") +
    f(ID.year1,model="iid")
> lcs <- inla.make.lincombs(ID.year = diag(11),  ID.year1 = diag(11))
> model.ST1 <- inla(formula.ST1,family="poisson",data=data,E=E,
                    control.predictor=list(compute=TRUE),
                    lincomb=lcs)
```

where ID.area is a vector going from 1 to n and identifies the counties (each county is repeated 11 times – one for each year), ID.year and ID.year1 are the rescaled years (1,...,11 – each year is repeated 159 times, once for each area).

Note that there are two parameters for the temporal trend (γ_t and ϕ_t) which we report on the natural scale using the code below and plot in Figure 7.3:

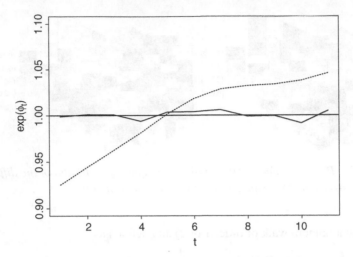

Figure 7.3   Posterior temporal trend for low birth weight in Georgia: unstructured effect exp(φ$_t$) (solid line) and temporally structured effect exp(γ$_t$) (dashed line).

```
> temporal.CAR <- lapply(model.ST1$marginals.random$ID.year,
                  function(X){
                      marg <- inla.tmarginal(function(x) exp(x), X)
                      inla.emarginal(mean, marg)
                  })
> temporal.IID <- lapply(model.ST1$marginals.random$ID.year1,
                  function(X){
                      marg <- inla.tmarginal(function(x) exp(x), X)
                      inla.emarginal(mean, marg)
                  })
```

An increasing trend is visible for the structured effect across the years, while the ustructured term shows some fluctuations around 1.

The two effects can also be combined through a linear combination using `inla.make.lincombs` before running the model. In the latter case when we run the model we need to add `lincomb=lcs`. For a detailed description of this function refer to Section 5.4.5. In this case, we need to create a linear combination $1 \times \gamma_t + 1 \times \phi_t$ for each year, obtained combining the tth element of two diagonal matrices, one for the unstructured and one for the structured temporal parameters.

7.1.2   Space–time interactions

It is easy to expand the model presented in Eq. (7.3) to allow for an interaction between space and time, which would explain differences in the time trend of low birth weight for different areas, e.g., using the following specification:

$$\eta_{it} = b_0 + v_i + v_i + \gamma_t + \phi_t + \delta_{it}. \tag{7.6}$$

Table 7.1   Interaction types: parameter interacting and rank of R_δ.

Interaction	Parameter interacting	Rank
I	v_i and ϕ_t	nT
II	v_i and γ_t	$n(T-1)$ for RW1 $\\$ $n(T-2)$ for RW2
III	ϕ_t and u_i	$(n-1)T$
IV	u_i and γ_t	$(n-1)(T-1)$ for RW1 $\\$ $(n-1)(T-2)$ for RW2

The parameter vector δ follows a Gaussian distribution with a precision matrix given by $\tau_\delta R_\delta$, where τ_δ is an unknown scalar, while R_δ is the structure matrix, identifying the type of temporal and/or spatial dependence between the elements of δ. Following Clayton (1996), R_δ can be factorized as the Kronecker product of the structure matrix of the corresponding main effects which interact. There are four ways to define the structure matrix, as presented in Knorr-Held (2000) and reported in Table 7.1. Note that given the noncommutative property of the Kronecker product, we stress that the order of the effects interacting is important.

Type I interaction

Type I assumes that the two unstructured effects v_i and ϕ_t interact. We write the structure matrix as

$$R_\delta = R_v \otimes R_\phi = I \otimes I = I,$$

because both v and ϕ do not have a spatial or temporal structure.[2] Consequently, we assume no spatial and/or temporal structure on the interaction either and therefore

$$\delta_{it} \sim \text{Normal}(0, 1/\tau_\delta).$$

---

[2] To better understand the Kronecker product, we introduce a simple example which we will use for the four types of interactions. Assuming these four matrices:

$$H = \begin{pmatrix} 1 & 0 & 1 & 1 \\ 0 & 1 & 0 & 0 \\ 1 & 0 & 1 & 0 \\ 1 & 0 & 0 & 1 \end{pmatrix}$$

is a typical (simplified) spatial adjacency matrix for $n = 4$ areas while

$$K = \begin{pmatrix} 1 & -1 & 0 \\ -1 & 2 & -1 \\ 0 & -1 & 1 \end{pmatrix}$$

The corresponding R-INLA coding for this model in the current example is

```
> formula.intI<- y ~ + f(ID.area,model="bym", graph=Georgia.adj) +
                      f(ID.year,model="rw2") +
                      f(ID.year1,model="iid") +
                      f(ID.area.year,model="iid")
```

where ID.area.year is the interaction index, going from 1 to 1749 (159 areas × 11 years) and the resulting model is saved in the object mod.intI:

```
> mod.intI <- inla(formula.intI,family="poisson",data=data,E=E,
                   control.predictor=list(compute=TRUE),
                   control.compute=list(dic=TRUE,cpo=TRUE))
```

Type II interaction

Type II combines the structured temporal main effect γ_t and the unstructured spatial effect v_i. We write the structure matrix as

$$R_\delta = R_v \otimes R_\gamma,$$

where $R_v = I$ and R_γ is the neighborhood structure specified for instance through a first- or second-order random walk. This leads to the assumption that for the ith area the parameter vector $\{\delta_{i1}, \ldots, \delta_{iT}\}$ has an autoregressive structure on the time component, which is independent from the ones of the other areas.[3] The matrix R_δ has a rank of $n(T - 1)$ for a first-order RW and $n(T - 2)$ for a second-order RW (see Table 7.1).

---

identifies the temporal structure using a first-order random walk for $T = 3$ time points,

$$J = \begin{pmatrix} 1 & 0 & 0 & 0 \\ 0 & 1 & 0 & 0 \\ 0 & 0 & 1 & 0 \\ 0 & 0 & 0 & 1 \end{pmatrix}$$

and

$$L = \begin{pmatrix} 1 & 0 & 0 \\ 0 & 1 & 0 \\ 0 & 0 & 1 \end{pmatrix}$$

are the identity matrices for unstructured effects on the areas and on the time points. In this case assuming an interaction of type I means imposing the Kronecker product of two unstructured effects, resulting in an identity matrix with dimensions 12 × 12.

[3] Going back to the simple example introduced above this means that we are calculating the Kronecker product of J and K, de facto replicating four times the structure of K as follows:

$$J \otimes K = \begin{pmatrix} 1 & -1 & 0 & 0 & 0 & 0 & 0 & 0 & 0 & 0 & 0 & 0 \\ -1 & 2 & -1 & 0 & 0 & 0 & 0 & 0 & 0 & 0 & 0 & 0 \\ 0 & -1 & 1 & 0 & 0 & 0 & 0 & 0 & 0 & 0 & 0 & 0 \\ \cdots & \cdots & \cdots & \cdots & \cdots & \cdots & \cdots & \cdots & \cdots & \cdots & \cdots & \cdots \\ 0 & 0 & 0 & 0 & 0 & 0 & 0 & 0 & 0 & 1 & -1 & 0 \\ 0 & 0 & 0 & 0 & 0 & 0 & 0 & 0 & 0 & -1 & 2 & 1 \\ 0 & 0 & 0 & 0 & 0 & 0 & 0 & 0 & 0 & 0 & -1 & 1 \end{pmatrix}$$

The corresponding R-INLA coding for this model in the current example is

```
> ID.area.int <- data$ID.area
> ID.year.int <- data$ID.year
> formula.intII<- y ~ f(ID.area,model="bym",graph=Georgia.adj) +
                     f(ID.year,model="rw2") +
                     f(ID.year1,model="iid") +
                     f(ID.area.int,model="iid", group=ID.year.int,
                     control.group=list(model="rw2"))
```

First, we create new area and year identifiers (ID.area.int and ID.year
.int, simply replicating the ones already available), which we will need
to specify the structure of the interaction. Then using f(ID.area.int,
model="iid", group=ID.year.int, control.group=list
(model="rw2")) we assume a random walk of order 2 (model="rw2")
across time (group=ID.year.int) for each area independently from all the
other areas as f(ID.area.int, model="iid"). The resulting model is
saved in the object mod.intII.

Type III interaction

Type III combines the unstructured temporal effect ϕ_t and the spatially structured
main effect u_i. We write the structure matrix as

$$R_\delta = R_\phi \otimes R_u,$$

where $R_\phi = I$ and R_u is a neighboring structure defined through the CAR specification. This leads to the assumption that the parameters of the tth time point
$\{\delta_1, \ldots, \delta_n\}$ have a spatial structure independent from the other time points.[4] The
matrix R_δ has a rank of $T(n-1)$. The corresponding R-INLA coding for this model
in the current example is

```
> formula.intIII<- y ~ f(ID.area,model="bym",graph=Georgia.adj) +
                     f(ID.year,model="rw2") +
                     f(ID.year1,model="iid") +
                     f(ID.year.int,model="iid", group=ID.area.int,
                     control.group=list(model="besag",
                                        graph=Georgia.adj))
```

---

[4] In the simple example introduced above this means that we are calculating the Kronecker product
of L and H, which means replicating three times the structure of H as follows:

$$L \otimes H = \begin{pmatrix}
1 & 0 & 1 & 1 & 0 & 0 & 0 & 0 & 0 & 0 & 0 & 0 \\
0 & 1 & 0 & 0 & 0 & 0 & 0 & 0 & 0 & 0 & 0 & 0 \\
1 & 0 & 1 & 0 & 0 & 0 & 0 & 0 & 0 & 0 & 0 & 0 \\
1 & 0 & 1 & 1 & 0 & 0 & 0 & 0 & 0 & 0 & 0 & 0 \\
\ldots & \ldots & \ldots & \ldots & \ldots & \ldots & \ldots & \ldots & \ldots & \ldots & \ldots & \ldots \\
0 & 0 & 0 & 0 & 0 & 0 & 0 & 0 & 1 & 0 & 1 & 1 \\
0 & 0 & 0 & 0 & 0 & 0 & 0 & 0 & 0 & 1 & 0 & 0 \\
0 & 0 & 0 & 0 & 0 & 0 & 0 & 0 & 1 & 0 & 0 & 0 \\
0 & 0 & 0 & 0 & 0 & 0 & 0 & 0 & 1 & 0 & 1 & 1
\end{pmatrix}$$

where f(ID.year.int,model="iid", group=ID.area.int, con-
trol.group=list(model="besag", graph=Georgia.adj)) means
that now we assume a conditional autoregressive structure on the area identifier
(group=ID.area.int, control.group=list(model="besag",
graph=Georgia.adj)) for each year independently from all the other years
as f(ID.year.int,model="iid"). The resulting model is saved in the
object mod.intIII.

Type IV interaction

Type IV is the most complex type of interaction, assuming that the spatially and
temporally structured effects u_i and γ_t interact.[5] The structure matrix can be written
as the Kronecker product of $R_\delta = R_u \otimes R_\gamma$ and has a rank of $(T - 1)(n - 1)$ for a
random walk of order 1, and of $(T - 2)(n - 1)$ for a random walk of order 2. The
corresponding R-INLA coding for this model in the current example is

```
> formula.intIV<- y ~ f(ID.area,model="bym",graph=Georgia.adj) +
                      f(ID.year,model="rw2") +
                      f(ID.year1,model="iid") +
                      f(ID.area.int,model="besag", graph=Georgia.adj,
                        group=ID.year.int,
                        control.group=list(model="rw2"))
```

which basically assumes that the temporal dependency structure for each area is
not independent from all the other areas anymore, but depends on the temporal
pattern of the neighboring areas as well. The resulting model is saved in the object
mod.intIV.

The spatio-temporal interactions are plotted in Figures 7.4–7.7. As expected
a spatial pattern is clear for mod.intIII and for mod.intIV which assumes
a spatial structure on the interaction. In addition, mod.intII and mod.intIV
show an increased number of areas becoming darker as the years passed, which is
in line with the main temporal trend observed in Figure 7.3.

---

[5] Note that due to the noncommutative property of the Kronecker product, the order of the matrices
changes the results. For this type of interaction going back to the simple example this means that we
are calculating the Kronecker product of H and K, de facto combining the H spatial structure on the K
temporal pattern as follows:

$$H \otimes K = \begin{pmatrix} 1 & -1 & 0 & 0 & 0 & 0 & 1 & -1 & 0 & 1 & -1 & 0 \\ -1 & 2 & -1 & 0 & 0 & 0 & -1 & 2 & 1 & -1 & 2 & -1 \\ 0 & -1 & 1 & 0 & 0 & 0 & 0 & -1 & 1 & 0 & -1 & 1 \\ \cdots & \cdots & \cdots & \cdots & \cdots & \cdots & \cdots & \cdots & \cdots & \cdots & \cdots & \cdots \\ 1 & -1 & 0 & 0 & 0 & 0 & 0 & 0 & 0 & 1 & -1 & 0 \\ -1 & 2 & -1 & 0 & 0 & 0 & 0 & 0 & 0 & -1 & 2 & -1 \\ 0 & -1 & 1 & 0 & 0 & 0 & 0 & 0 & 0 & 0 & -1 & 1 \end{pmatrix}.$$

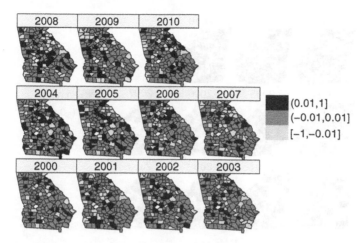

Figure 7.4   Posterior mean of the spatio-temporal interaction δ_{it} for low birth weight in Georgia under mod.intI *(nonspatially or temporally structured interaction).*

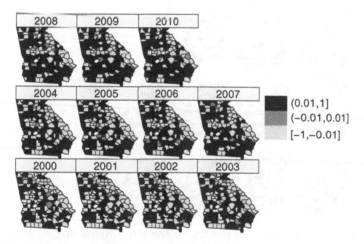

Figure 7.5   Posterior mean of the spatio-temporal interaction δ_{it} for low birth weight in Georgia under mod.intII *(temporally structured interaction).*

Equivalently to what we have presented in the previous chapter, if covariates (e.g., risk factors, exposures, confounders) are available, the spatio-temporal models described above can easily incorporate these in the formula environment and be transformed in spatio-temporal ecological regressions. Then the interpretation of the spatial, temporal, and spatio-temporal effects would be "residual," after accounting for the covariates included in the model.

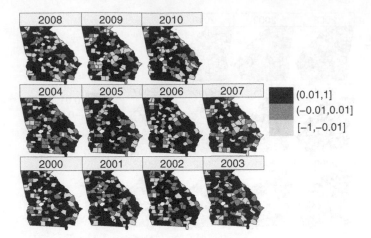

Figure 7.6   Posterior mean of the spatio-temporal interaction δ_{it} for low birth weight in Georgia under mod.intIII *(spatially structured interaction).*

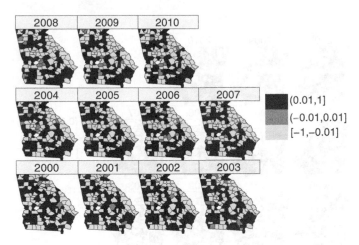

Figure 7.7   Posterior mean of the spatio-temporal interaction δ_{it} for low birth weight in Georgia under mod.intIV *(spatially and temporally structured interaction).*

7.2   Spatio-temporal modeling particulate matter concentration

In this section, we present a spatio-temporal model for the particulate matter (PM_{10} in µg/m^3) data described in Section 1.4.14. In particular, the focus is on the prediction of particulate matter concentration in the considered continuous spatial domain, where no monitoring stations are displaced. In addition, we describe how to get a map for the probability of exceeding a specific threshold (e.g 50 µg/m^3 fixed by the European Community for health protection).

We denote by y_{it} the logarithm of the PM$_{10}$ concentration measured at site s_i ($i = 1, \ldots, n$) and day $t = 1, \ldots, T$. The following distribution is assumed for the observations:

$$y_{it} \sim \text{Normal}(\eta_{it}, \sigma_e^2),$$

with σ_e^2 being the variance of the measurement error defined by a Gaussian white-noise process, both serially and spatially uncorrelated, and

$$\eta_{it} = b_0 + \sum_{m=1}^{M} \beta_m x_{mi} + \omega_{it},$$

where b_0 is the intercept and $\beta_1, \ldots, \beta_M$ are the fixed effects related to mete-orological and orographical covariates $x_1, \ldots, x_M$. The term ω_{it} refers to the latent spatio-temporal process (i.e., the true unobserved level of pollution) which changes in time with first-order autoregressive dynamics and spatially correlated innovations:

$$\omega_{it} = a\omega_{i(t-1)} + \xi_{it}, \tag{7.7}$$

with $t = 2, \ldots, T$, $|a| < 1$ and $\omega_{i1} \sim \text{Normal}(0, \sigma^2/(1 - a^2))$. Moreover, ξ_{it} is a zero-mean Gaussian field, assumed to be temporally independent and characterized by the following spatio-temporal covariance function:

$$\text{Cov}\left(\xi_{it}, \xi_{ju}\right) = \begin{cases} 0 & \text{if} \quad t \neq u \\ \text{Cov}(\xi_i, \xi_j) & \text{if} \quad t = u \end{cases} \tag{7.8}$$

for $i \neq j$, where $\text{Cov}(\xi_i, \xi_j)$ is given by the Matèrn spatial covariance func-tion defined in Eq. (6.15). As demonstrated by Cameletti *et al.* (2011), the spatio-temporal covariance function in Eq. (7.8) is separable as it can be rewritten as the product of a purely spatial and a purely temporal covariance function.

To run this model in R-INLA, we first load the PM$_{10}$ data, the monitoring station coordinates, and the Piemonte region borders, all available as csv files. Hence, in the workspace three dataframes named Piemonte_data, coordinates, and borders are created. To check how the data are structured, we print the first part of the Piemonte_data dataframe

```
> head(Piemonte_data)
```

ID	Date	A	UTMX	UTMY	WS	TEMP	HMIX	PREC	EMI	PM10
1	01/10/05	95.2	469.45	4972.85	0.90	288.81	1294.6	0	26.05	28
2	01/10/05	164.1	423.48	4950.69	0.82	288.67	1139.8	0	18.74	22
3	01/10/05	242.9	490.71	4948.86	0.96	287.44	1404.0	0	6.28	17
4	01/10/05	149.9	437.36	4973.34	1.17	288.63	1042.4	0	29.35	25
5	01/10/05	405.0	426.44	5045.66	0.60	287.63	1038.7	0	32.19	20
6	01/10/05	257.5	394.60	5001.18	1.02	288.59	1048.3	0	34.24	41

and notice that the data are stacked by day (in the first rows we have the data for the first day in all the stations, then the values for the second day and so on); the variable Station.ID identifies the station. For computational convenience we store the number of stations, data, and days in three separate objects

```
> n_stations <- length(coordinates$Station.ID) #24 stations
> n_data <- length(Piemonte_data$Station.ID) #4368 space-time data
> n_days <- n_data/n_stations #182 time points
```

Moreover, we add to the Piemonte_data dataframe a new variable for time indexing, defined as the sequence of integer from 1 to 182, each of them repeated 24 times:

```
> Piemonte_data$time <- rep(1:n_days, each=n_stations)
```

In addition, we create a matrix – which will be used later – containing the station coordinates repeated for all the days of the year (they are extracted from the coordinates object according to the Piemonte_data$Station.ID indexes):

```
> coordinates.allyear <- as.matrix(
                    coordinates[Piemonte_data$Station.ID,
                    c("UTMX","UTMY")])
> dim(coordinates.allyear)
[1] 4368    2
```

Finally, we compute the logarithmic transformation of PM_{10} data

```
> Piemonte_data$logPM10 <- log(Piemonte_data$PM10)
```

and standardize the covariates (contained in columns from 3 to 10; see Section 1.4.14 for their description) using the scale function

```
> mean_covariates <- apply(Piemonte_data[,3:10],2,mean)
> sd_covariates <- apply(Piemonte_data[,3:10],2,sd)
> Piemonte_data[,3:10] <- scale(Piemonte_data[,3:10],
                    center=mean_covariates, scale=sd_covariates)
```

As we are interested in the prediction of particulate matter concentration on a regular grid of 4032 points for a particular day (e.g., i_day=122 corresponding to 30/01/2006), we upload all the covariate data at the grid level, standardize them, and extract the values for the selected day (the code is not shown here). The final object is a dataframe named covariate_matrix_std with 4032 rows (given by the number of grid points) and 8 columns (as the number of covariates). The regular grid of 4032 points is plotted in Figure 7.8. It is now possible to create the mesh for the Piemonte spatial domain, following the approach described in Section 6.7.1:

```
> Piemonte_mesh <- inla.mesh.2d(
    loc=cbind(coordinates$UTMX,coordinates$UTMY),
    loc.domain=borders,
    offset=c(10, 140),
    max.edge=c(50, 1000))
```

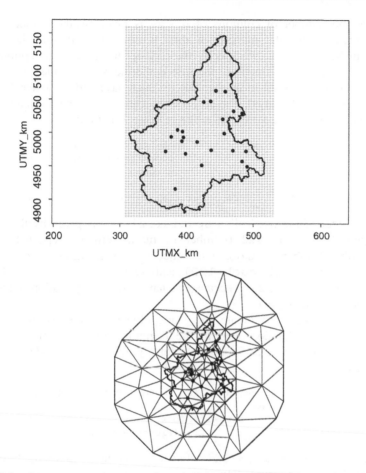

Figure 7.8   Piemonte grid (top) and mesh (bottom). Black dots denote the 24 monitoring stations.

The resulting mesh, which is formed by $G = 122$ vertices, is plotted in Figure 7.8. Given the mesh, it is possible to create the Matérn SPDE object through the following code:

```
> Piemonte_spde <- inla.spde2.matern(mesh=Piemonte_mesh, alpha=2)
```

and the projector matrix A

```
> A_est <- inla.spde.make.A(mesh=Piemonte_mesh,
                            loc=coordinates.allyear,
                            group=Piemonte_data$time,
                            n.group=n_days)
> dim(A_est)
[1]   4368 22204
```

Note that the number of columns of A_est is given by the number of mesh vertices (122) times the number of time points (182). In fact, here, differently from Section 6.7.2, we specify the group and n.group options in the inla.spde.make.A function: the first is the index which identifies the time grouping (i.e.,we have 24 measurements for each day) and the latter defines the number of groups (182 days). The group specification has to be taken into account also when using the inla.spde.make.index function:

```
> s_index <- inla.spde.make.index(name="spatial.field",
                               n.spde=Piemonte_spde$n.spde,
                               n.group=n_days)
> names(s_index)
[1] "spatial.field"      "spatial.field.group" "spatial.field.repl"
```

The first object of the list (called spatial.field) is given by the sequence of integers from 1 to 122 (number of mesh vertices) repeated as many times as the number of days. The sequence spatial.field.group is defined as rep(1:182,each=122) and spatial.field.repl is just rep(1,times=182*122) (because we have a single replication of the spatial process at each time point).

We are now ready to create the stack object for the estimation of the spatio-temporal model described at the beginning of the section. Similar to what has been described in Section 6.8 for a purely spatial model, we run the following code:

```
> stack_est <- inla.stack(data=list(logPM10=Piemonte_data$logPM10),
                       A=list(A_est, 1),
                       effects=list(c(s_index,list(Intercept=1)),
                               list(Piemonte_data[,3:10])), tag="est")
```

where Piemonte_data[,3:10] refers to the columns containing the covariate values for the 24 monitoring stations.

We create the same objects also for the prediction step performed on the regular grid

```
> A_pred <- inla.spde.make.A(mesh=Piemonte_mesh,
                         loc=as.matrix(Piemonte_grid),
                         group=i_day,   #selected day for prediction
                         n.group=n_days)
> stack_pred <- inla.stack(data=list(logPM10=NA),
                       A=list(A_pred,1),
                       effects=list(c(s_index,list(Intercept=1)),
                               list(covariate_matrix_std)),
                       tag="pred")
```

and combine all in the full stack object:

```
> stack <- inla.stack(stack_est, stack_pred)
```

Note that, differently from Section 1.4.11 and Cameletti *et al.* (2013), we include at this stage the grid information for spatial prediction (and not after having performed the estimation step). This means that the output of the inla function will provide directly the estimates of the linear predictor at the grid level for the selected day.

The formula

```
> formula <- logPM10 ~ -1 + Intercept +
    A + UTMX + UTMY + WS + TEMP + HMIX + PREC + EMI +
    f(spatial.field, model=Piemonte_spde,
      group=spatial.field.group, control.group=list(model="ar1"))
```

includes an explicit intercept and all the meteorological and geographical covariates. Moreover, using the options group and control.group in the f($\cdot$) term, we specify that at each time point the spatial locations are linked by the spde model object (named spatial.field.group), while across time, the process evolves according to an AR(1) process (see Eq. (7.7)).

In the final step we run the inla function:

```
> #Attention: the run is computationally intensive!
> output <- inla(formula,
           data=inla.stack.data(stack, spde=Piemonte_spde),
           family="gaussian",
           control.predictor=list(A=inla.stack.A(stack), compute=TRUE))
```

We can retrieve the posterior summary statistics for the fixed effects β with output\$summary.fixed and for $1/\sigma_e^2$ and the AR(1) coefficient a through output\$summary.hyperpar. The posterior estimates for the spatial variance σ^2 and the range r can be obtained applying the inla.spde2.result function, as described in Section 6.7.3. All the posterior summaries are reported in Table 7.2.

To obtain the prediction of the smooth (i.e., without the measurement error) air pollution field for the selected day, we just need to extract the posterior marginals of the linear predictor – which are available for all the grid locations – from output\$summary.linear.predictor

```
> index_pred <- inla.stack.index(stack,"pred")$data
> lp_marginals <- output$marginals.linear.predictor[index_pred]
```

and then compute the posterior mean of the exponentiated distribution to go back to the natural PM_{10} scale (recall that we log transformed the data at the beginning)

```
> lp_mean <- unlist(lapply(lp_marginals,
                    function(x) inla.emarginal(exp, x)))
```

and reshape it properly in accordance with the grid size

```
> lp_grid_mean <- matrix(lp_mean, 56, 72, byrow=T)
```

The map of the posterior mean is reported in Figure 7.9. Note that in the map, only the results for elevation below 1000 m are shown in order to exclude inappropriate linear extrapolation of the effect of elevation (since the monitoring stations cover only a limited range of altitude).

It may also be of interest to compute for each grid point the probability of exceeding a specific threshold. For instance, we might consider the 50 μg/m^3 limit value

Table 7.2   Posterior estimates (mean, standard deviation (SD), and quantiles) for the Piemonte air pollution model.

Parameter	Mean	SD	2.5%	50%	97.5%
b_0	3.696	0.457	2.784	3.698	4.596
β_1 (A)	−0.209	0.052	−0.313	−0.209	−0.107
β_2 (UTMX)	−0.173	0.170	−0.512	−0.172	0.161
β_3 (UTMY)	−0.179	0.155	−0.487	−0.179	0.125
β_4 (WS)	−0.058	0.008	−0.075	−0.058	−0.042
β_5 (TEMP)	−0.121	0.035	−0.190	−0.120	−0.051
β_6 (HMIX)	−0.025	0.013	−0.051	−0.025	0.001
β_7 (PREC)	−0.054	0.009	−0.071	−0.054	−0.037
β_8 (EMI)	0.035	0.015	0.005	0.035	0.064
σ_e^2	0.032	0.001	0.030	0.032	0.035
σ^2	1.309	0.211	0.956	1.286	1.783
r	269.909	17.034	238.500	269.079	305.408
a	0.960	0.007	0.946	0.960	0.972

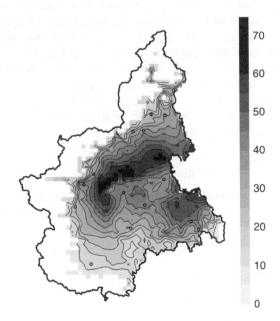

Figure 7.9   Posterior mean of particulate matter concentration for the selected day 30/01/2006. Only locations with an altitude below 1000 m are shown.

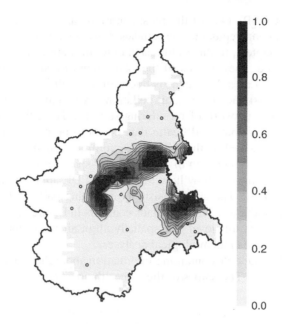

Figure 7.10   Posterior probability of exceeding the 50 µg/m³ *limit value for 30/01/2006. Only locations with an altitude below 1000* m *are shown.*

imposed by EU. The probability can easily be computed by using the built-in function `inla.pmarginal`:

```
> threshold <- log(50)
> prob   <- lapply(X=lp_marginals,
                FUN=function(x) inla.pmarginal(marginal=x,threshold))
> tailprob_grid <- matrix(1-unlist(prob),56,72, byrow=T)
```

The resulting map with the posterior exceedance probabilities is reported in Figure 7.10 and can be used to detect the areas where it is more likely to observe air pollution levels higher than the threshold; thus, they do not meet the national and European air quality regulations. The concept of exceedance probability can be extended to find regions – and not single grid points as shown here – where the process exceeds a certain level. The method for calculating probabilistic excursion sets, contour credible regions, and simultaneous confidence bands for latent Gaussian stochastic processes and fields is described by Bolin and Lindgren (2015) and is implemented in a R package named `excursions`.

7.2.1   Change of support

This section focuses on the change of support problem (COSP, Gotway and Young, 2002; Gelfand *et al.*, 2010) which concerns the spatial misalignment between the prediction of the process of interest and the observed data (see Cameletti, 2013, for a review on COSP). One of the most common cases of spatial misalignment occurs in environmental epidemiology studies (Lawson, 2009). As seen extensively in the previous chapters, in this field health outcomes are usually available at the aggregated level, i.e., they consist of the total count of deaths or hospitalizations registered in a given area (e.g., census tracts, municipalities). On the other hand, the environmental risk factors (e.g., air pollution) are usually measured at the point level by means of a network of monitoring stations. Thus, the spatial misalignment of exposure variables and health data needs to be managed in a modeling framework. The drawback is that COSP is a computationally demanding task as it involves stochastic integration of the continuos spatial process over the area of interest; in this section we show how to use the SPDE approach in order to deal effectively with COSP. The aim consists in predicting daily PM_{10} concentration for the Piemonte health districts (see black contours in Figure 7.11). By predicting PM_{10} concentration at this level, we spatially align air pollution exposure to the health outcome for the epidemiological analyses.

We first load the shapefile containing information about Piemonte health districts (named *asl* in Italian). The names of the 12 health areas are

```
> asl@data$COD
 [1] TO4 BI  NO  VC  VCO TO5 TO3 CN1 CN2 AT  AL  TO
Levels: AL AT BI CN1 CN2 NO TO TO3 TO4 TO5 VC VCO
```

In order to detect in which health district the PM_{10} monitoring stations lie, the function `over` (available in the sp library) is used

```
> library(sp)
> #coords of the stations
  coords <- SpatialPoints(coordinates[,2:3]*1000)
> match_coords_asl <- over(coords,asl)
> table(match_coords_asl$COD)
 AL  AT  BI CN1 CN2  NO  TO TO3 TO4 TO5  VC VCO
  5   1   2   1   1   3   2   2   2   2   2   1
```

The contingency table reported above shows that, for example, in the area named AL there are five monitoring stations. We repeat the same procedure for the 4032 points of the regular grid displayed in Figure 7.11:

```
> grid <- SpatialPoints(Piemonte_grid*1000) #change km -> m
> match_grid_asl <- over(grid,asl)
> table(match_grid_asl$COD)
 AL  AT  BI CN1 CN2  NO  TO TO3 TO4 TO5  VC VCO
229  86  52 366  69  74   8 177 202  49 127 150
```

It is worth noting that there are some NA in the `match_grid_asl` object since some grid points are located outside the health districts. We remove them through the following command:

```
> sum(is.na(match_grid_asl$ID)) #number of NAs
[1] 2443
> match_grid_asl <- match_grid_asl[!is.na(match_grid_asl$ID),]
```

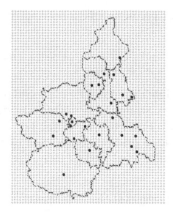

Figure 7.11   Map of the 12 health districts in Piemonte. Black points denote the PM$_{10}$ monitoring stations, while gray diamonds show the 4032 points of the regular grid.

The upscaling (i.e., the prediction of PM$_{10}$ concentration at the health district level) is performed in INLA by computing linear combinations of the linear predictor. Basically, for a given time point t and area B_i we compute a linear combination of the values from the linear predictor (η_{jt}^{pred}) in all the s_j grid locations belonging to area B_i:

$$\text{PM}_{B_i t}^{\text{Area}} = \sum_{j \in B_i} \eta_{jt}^{\text{pred}} K_{ij},$$

where K_{ij} is the weight for the prediction. Here we choose equal weights for each grid point in the same area so that $K_{ij} = 1/\#(s_j \in B_i)$.

As described by Martins *et al.* (2013), linear combinations of the latent field nodes can be obtained in INLA through `inla.make.lincomb`. In Section 5.4.5, we introduced a way of dealing with multiple linear combinations (through `inla.make.lincombs` – note the plural), while here we build a linear combination once at a time; thus, we use `inla.make.lincomb`, but the approach for obtaining these is the same. For each health district, we define the indexes of the grid points (selected from the `match_grid_asl`) which lie in the considered area. For example for the health district named AL we run the following code

```
> AL_ind <- as.numeric(
    rownames(match_grid_asl[match_grid_asl$COD=="AL",]))
> length(AL_ind)
[1] 229
```

The resulting object `AL_ind` is a vector of indexes for the grid points falling into the AL area. We repeat the procedure for the remaining 11 areas (code not shown here). We now define for each health district the vector containing the linear combination weights. We start creating an empty vector whose length is given by the dimension of the linear predictor (the following code refers to the AL health district):

```
> dim_lp <- nrow(inla.stack.A(stack)) + ncol(inla.stack.A(stack))
> lc_AL_vec <- rep(NA,times=dim_lp)
```

As specified above the weights are equal for each grid point in the AL area (given by 1/length(AL_ind)), while for the points outside the considered area, the weights are set equal to NA. From the full vector lc_AL_vec we first select the elements referring to the 4032 grid points (indexed by the index_pred vector defined in the previous section), and then the elements in the AL area (through the AL_ind indexes):

```
> lc_AL_vec[index_pred][AL_ind] <- 1/length(AL_ind)
```

Finally, we make use of the inla.make.lincomb function to create the linear combinations of the linear predictor components (it is important to note that the linear predictor has a predefined name given by Predictor):

```
> lc_AL <- inla.make.lincomb(Predictor = lc_AL_vec)
```

and specify a unique name for the linear combination

```
> names(lc_AL) <- "lc_AL"
```

We repeat the procedure for the remaining health districts (code not included) and then combine the 12 linear combination objects:

```
> lc_all_ASL <- c(lc_AL, lc_AT, lc_BI, lc_CN1, lc_CN2,
                  lc_NO, lc_TO, lc_TO3, lc_TO4, lc_TO5,
                  lc_VC, lc_VCO)
> length(lc_all_ASL)
[1] 12
```

We run the inla formula as usual except for the specification of the lincomb option:

```
> #Attention: the run is computationally intensive!
> output_asl <-
    inla(formula,
         data=inla.stack.data(stack, spde=Piemonte_spde),
         family="gaussian",
         lincomb = lc_all_ASL,
         control.predictor=list(A=inla.stack.A(stack), compute=TRUE))
```

The summary statistics of the linear combinations (on the logarithmic scale) can be obtained through

```
> output_asl$summary.lincomb.derived
```

Since we are interested in producing a map of PM_{10} concentration on the original scale, we back-transform the linear combination distributions and compute the posterior mean:

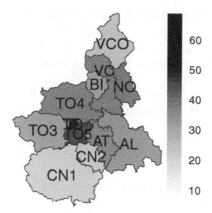

Figure 7.12   Map of the PM$_{10}$ posterior mean at the health district level for 30/01/2006.

```
> asl_lp_marginals <- output_asl$marginals.lincomb.derived
> asl_lp_mean_exp <- lapply(asl_lp_marginals,
                            function(x) inla.emarginal(exp,x))
```

Finally, as usual, we merge the obtained posterior means with the original shapefile

```
> asl_lp <- data.frame(exp.mean = unlist(asl_lp_mean_exp))
> asl_lp$COD <- substr(rownames(asl_lp),4,6)
> attr(asl, "data") <- merge(attr(asl, "data"),asl_lp,by="COD",sort=F)
```

and the resulting map is reported in Figure 7.12.

In this example each grid point contributes equally to the linear combination, but in practice it is also possible to include different weights based for example on the population in each area. Moreover, if the dimension of the area is not so wide as in this case (for instance, when municipalities are used), it would make sense to compute the probability – at the area level – of exceeding a given threshold, as shown in the previous section.

References

Abellan, J., Richardson, S., and Best, N. (2008). Use of space-time models to investigate the stability of patterns of disease. *Environ Health Perspective*, **116**(8), 1111–1119.

Bernardinelli, L., Clayton, D., Pascutto, C., Montomoli, C., Ghislandi, M., and Songini, M. (1995). Bayesian analysis of space-time variation in disease risk. *Statistics in Medicine*, **14**(21–22), 2433–2443.

Bolin, D. and Lindgren, F. (2015). Excursion and contour uncertainty regions for latent Gaussian models. *Journal of the Royal Statistical Society, Series B (Statistical Methodology)*, **77**(1), 85–106.

Cameletti, M. (2013). The change of support problem through the INLA approach. *Statistica & Applicazioni*, **1**, 29–43. 2013 Special Issue.

Cameletti, M., Ignaccolo, R., and Bande, S. (2011). Comparing spatio-temporal models for particulate matter in Piemonte. *Environmetrics*, **22**, 985–996.

Cameletti, M., Lindgren, F., Simpson, D., and Rue, H. (2013). Spatio-temporal modeling of particulate matter concentration through the SPDE approach. *Advances in Statistical Analysis*, **97**(2), 109–131.

Clayton, D. (1996). Generalised linear mixed models. In W. Gilks, S. Richardson, and D. Spiegelhalter, editors, *Markov Chain Monte Carlo in Practice*, pp. 275–301. Chapman & Hall.

Cressie, N. and Huang, H. (1999). Classes of nonseparable, spatio-temporal stationary covariance functions. *Journal of the American Statistical Association*, **94**(448), 1330–1340.

Gelfand, A., Diggle, P., Fuentes, M., and Guttorp, P., editors (2010). *Handbook of Spatial Statistics*. Chapman & Hall.

Gneiting, T. (2002). Nonseparable, stationary covariance functions for space-time data. *Journal of the American Statistical Association*, **97**(458), 590–600.

Gneiting, T., Genton, M., and Guttorp, P. (2006). Statistical methods for spatio-temporal systems. In B. Finkenstädt, L. Held, and V. Isham, editors, *Statistical Methods for Spatio-temporal Systems*, pp. 151–175. CRC Press, Chapmann and Hall.

Gotway, C. and Young, L. (2002). Combining incompatible spatial data. *Journal of the American Statistical Association*, **97**(458), 632–648.

Harvill, J. (2010). Spatio-temporal processes. *Wiley Interdisciplinary Reviews: Computational Statistics*, **2**(3), 375–382.

Knorr-Held, L. (2000). Bayesian modelling of inseparable space-time variation in disease risk. *Statistics in Medicine*, **19**(17–18), 2555–2567.

Lawson, A. (2009). *Bayesian Disease Mapping. Hierarchical Modeling in Spatial Epidemiology*. CRC Press.

Martins, T. G., Simpson, D., Lindgren, F., and Rue, H. (2013). Bayesian computing with INLA: New features. *Computational Statistics & Data Analysis*, **67**, 68–83.

Schrödle, B. and Held, L. (2011). A primer on disease mapping and ecological regression using INLA. *Computational Statistics*, **26**, 241–258.

8

Advanced modeling

Elias T. Krainski

This chapter aims at presenting advanced spatio-temporal models which can be specified and run through R-INLA. In particular, we will focus on four applications: the first considers spatially misaligned data, e.g., response and a covariate observed at different spatial locations; the second deals with a joint model of data coming from two different distributions; the third presents a spatio-temporal dynamic model and the last deals with data where the resolution is too high and needs to be reduced for computational reasons. Throughout the chapter, we will use simulated or real data and introduce some R and R-INLA functions which we have not previously used in the book.

8.1 Bivariate model for spatially misaligned data

In this section, we implement a spatial model for geostatistical data involving a response variable and a covariate which are spatially misaligned, i.e., they are observed at different spatial locations. This is a particular case of the change of support problem and represents a new feature with respect to the spatial and spatio-temporal models implemented in Chapters 6 and 7 where we assume that the response variable and covariate values refer to the same spatial locations. To illustrate this misalignment case, we simulate $n_y = 15$ and $n_x = 20$ locations for the response variable and the covariate, respectively, for a square spatial domain between 0 and 1 (we use the runif function for generating values from a Uniform distribution between 0 and 1, see Section 4.3):

```
> n_y <- 15
> n_x <- 20
> set.seed(2)
> loc_y <- cbind(runif(n_y), runif(n_y))
```

Spatial and Spatio-temporal Bayesian Models with R-INLA, First Edition.
Marta Blangiardo and Michela Cameletti.
© 2015 John Wiley & Sons, Ltd. Published 2015 by John Wiley & Sons, Ltd.

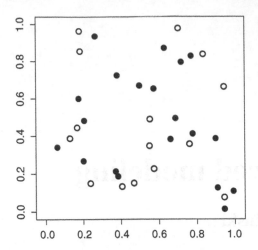

Figure 8.1   Simulated locations for the response variable (white dots) and for the covariate (black dots).

```
> set.seed(1)
> loc_x <- cbind(runif(n_x), runif(n_x))
```

The two simulated set of locations are plotted in Figure 8.1. Note that it may happen that some of the locations provide data for the response as well as for the covariate.

To deal with the misalignment, a distribution for the covariate has to be assumed, in addition to the one for the response variable. Given this, the easiest solution would consist in predicting the value of the covariate at the n_y locations where the response variable is observed. Then, by means of a plug-in approach, the predicted values of the covariate would be used as *fixed* while modeling the response (as done in the examples presented in Chapters 6 and 7). The drawback of this approach is that the uncertainty on the covariate prediction is not fed forward into the model for the response. The alternative approach consists in implementing a joint bivariate model for both covariate and response, in order to take into account all sources of uncertainty.

In R-INLA, a joint bivariate model can be easily implemented using the new features described in Martins *et al.* (2013) for dealing with multiple likelihoods (in this case given by the two distributions for the response and the covariate). Moreover, as the same spatial process is used in more than one linear predictor, we will make use of the copy feature.

Note that assuming a distribution for the covariate means that we can have missing data in it, which will be predicted using the model, while in the previous chapters covariates were considered as fixed quantities and no missing values were allowed.

In the following sections we present two examples with simulated data: in Section 8.1.1, we assume that both covariate and response follow a Normal distribution, while in Section 8.1.2, we consider the case of a Poisson distribution combined with a Binomial distribution.

8.1.1   Joint model with Gaussian distributions

We assume the following distribution for the covariate x_j at the generic location s_j:

$$x_j \sim \text{Normal}(\xi_j, \sigma_x^2), \tag{8.1}$$

where the spatial random effect ξ_j is the realization of a zero-mean Matérn GF $\xi(s)$ (see Sections 6.4 and 6.5), and σ_x^2 is the measurement error variance.

The response y_i at location s_i is assumed to be distributed like

$$y_i \sim \text{Normal}(\eta_i, \sigma_e^2) \tag{8.2}$$

$$\eta_i = b_0 + \beta_1 \xi_i + u_i, \tag{8.3}$$

where b_0 is the intercept, β_1 is the coefficient for the covariate mean ξ_i, and u_i is the realization of an additional spatial effect (i.e., a zero-mean Matérn GF). Finally the parameter σ_e^2 represents the residual variance. Note that it would be possible to include additional nonmisaligned covariates in Eqs. (8.1) and (8.3).

It is worth noting that the model defined in Eq. (8.3) introduces a link between the covariate and the response through the mean ξ_i. It would also be possible to assume that y_i depends directly on x_i including also the measurement error variance σ_x^2. This can be implemented in R-INLA using a measurement error approach, as described by Muff _et al._ (2013).

Data simulation

In order to simulate the covariate and observation values using Eqs. (8.1) and (8.3), we need to fix the parameters for both the random fields $\xi(s)$ and $u(s)$, i.e., the values of the spatial variance and of the scale parameter κ of the Matérn covariance function (see Eq. (6.15)):

```
> kappa_xi <- 5
> sigma2_xi <- 0.5
> kappa_u <- 7
> sigma2_u <- 0.3
```

In practice, to simulate values from a multivariate Normal distribution with covariance matrix defined by the Matérn covariance function, we use a standard algorithm based on the Cholesky factorization.[1] In particular, in the case study we are considering that the mean vector is equal to zero and the covariance matrix is obtained from the $n \times n$ distance matrix computed considering all pairs of locations.

---

[1] To simulate values from a Gaussian multivariate distribution $X \sim \text{MVNormal}(\mu, \Sigma)$, the linear transformation $X = \mu + LZ$ is used, where L is the Cholesky factorization of Σ (the Cholesky decomposition or factorization takes a positive definite matrix and transforms it in the product of a lower triangular matrix and its conjugate transpose, i.e., $\Sigma = LL'$) and Z is a collection of iid standard Normal random variables Normal(0, 1). Basically, to obtain a sample z from the n-dimensional Z, we compute the Cholesky factorization for Σ, we create x with n values drawn independently from a standard Normal distribution and compute $x = \mu + Lz$.

We define a new function named `simulate_GF` to sample data from a Matérn Gaussian field (see Section 2.5 for details about how a new function is defined in R):

```
> simulate_GF <- function(coords, kappa, variance, lambda=1) {
+    #Compute the number of locations
+    n <- nrow(coords)
+    #Compute the distance matrix
+    dist.m <- as.matrix(dist(coords))
+    #Compute the Matern correlation matrix
+    cor.m <- 2^(1-lambda)/gamma(lambda)*(kappa*dist.m)^lambda*
+            besselK(x=dist.m*kappa, nu=lambda)
+    diag(cor.m) <- 1
+    #Compute the covariance matrix
+    Sigma <- variance * cor.m
+    #Simulate date using standard algorithm based on Cholesky fact.
+    c(chol(Sigma) %*% rnorm(n=n,mean=0,sd=1))
+ }
```

The arguments of the function are the coordinate matrix (`coords`) and the parameters of the Matérn covariance function (the scale parameter `kappa` and the variance `variance`; note that, as reported in Section 6.5 λ is fixed and equal to 1). The Cholesky decomposition is computed by means of the `chol` function which returns L'; the `besselK` function provides the Bessel function of second kind (see Eq. (6.15)).

By using the `simulate_GF` function and the values chosen for the Matérn parameters, we simulate the values for the spatial process $u(s)$ at the n_y locations with

```
> set.seed(223)
> u <- simulate_GF(coords=loc_y,
+                   kappa=kappa_u, variance=sigma2_u)
> length(u)
[1] 15
```

and the realizations of the process $\xi(s)$ at both set of spatial sites (first for the n_x covariate locations) with

```
> set.seed(233)
> xi <- simulate_GF(coords=rbind(loc_x, loc_y),
+                   kappa=kappa_xi, variance=sigma2_xi)
> length(xi)
[1] 35
```

It is worth noting that we need the values ξ_i also in the n_y response locations in order to be able to simulate the observations using Eq. (8.3). However, when we fit the model we will consider only the covariate values available at the n_x locations.

Before simulating the values for x_i and y_i according to Eqs. (8.1) and (8.3), we set the values for b_0 (intercept), β_1 and the variances σ_e^2 and σ_x^2:

```
> b0 <- 10
> beta1 <- -0.5
> sigma2_e <- 0.16
> sigma2_x <- 0.25
```

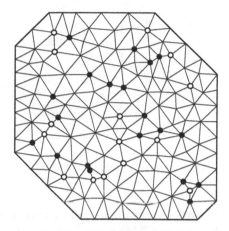

Figure 8.2   Mesh for the misaligned data example. White and black dots denote the response and covariate locations, respectively.

Finally, the simulated values for the covariate and the response are obtained through

```
> set.seed(4455)
> x <- xi[1:n_x] + rnorm(n=n_x, mean=0, sd=sqrt(sigma2_x))
> set.seed(5544)
> y <- b0 + beta1*xi[n_x + 1:n_y] + u +
+        rnorm(n=n_y, mean=0, sd=sqrt(sigma2_e))
```

Model fitting

The SPDE approach is used to estimate the spatial model. As usual the first step consists in creating the mesh. Here we create a simple mesh with only one outer extension by passing just one value for the max.edge argument:

```
> mesh <- inla.mesh.2d(loc=rbind(loc_x, loc_y), max.edge=0.15,
+                      cutoff=0.03, offset=0.1)
```

It includes 147 nodes and can be visualized in Figure 8.2.

We now define one SPDE model which will be used for both spatial effects $\xi(s)$ and $u(s)$:

```
> spde <- inla.spde2.matern(mesh=mesh, alpha=2)
```

Due to the misalignment, in order to link the locations with the mesh we have to define two projection matrices:

```
> A_x <- inla.spde.make.A(mesh=mesh, loc=loc_x)
> dim(A_x)
[1]   20 147
> A_y <- inla.spde.make.A(mesh=mesh, loc=loc_y)
> dim(A_y)
[1]   15 147
```

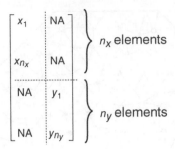

Figure 8.3   Schematic representation of the data matrix for the case with two likelihoods.

The model we are implementing is characterized by two likelihoods, one for the covariate and one for the response. This setting can be implemented in R-INLA using the approach described in Martins *et al.* (2013) and rewriting the response data as a matrix where the number of columns is given by the number of likelihoods. Thus, for the present case study a two-column response matrix has to be defined, with the first column containing the covariate values x_i and the second one the response values y_i. Note that, since the linear predictor for each component is different, the matrix values should be misaligned. This means that the lines containing the x_i values will have NAs in the second column and vice versa. Figure 8.3 displays a representation of the data matrix structure for the considered case with two likelihoods.

This particular data structure, with multiple columns according to the number of likelihoods, has to be taken into account when using the inla.stack function. The following code, for example, which defines the stack object for the covariate, specifies in the data argument a two-column matrix created using the cbind function (the first column contains the x_i values in the n_x locations while the second one is filled with NAs):

```
> stk_x <- inla.stack(data=list(y=cbind(x, NA)),
+                       effects=list(xi.field=1:spde$n.spde),
+                       A=list(A_x),
+                       tag="est.x")
```

As we do not have replicates or any grouping, the index set for the spatial effect (xi.field) is just a sequence of integers from 1 to the number of nodes on the mesh. Moreover, since there are no other components in the linear predictor, the effects list is just the index set for the spatial random effect (so in this simple case we do not use the inla.spde.make.index function).

The stack object for the response is slightly more complicated (it includes also the intercept and the spatial field $u(s)$) and is defined as

```
> stk_y <- inla.stack(data=list(y=cbind(NA, y)),
+                 effects=list(
+                   list(u.field=1:spde$n.spde, x.field=1:spde$n.spde),
+                   list(intercept=rep(1,n_y))),
```

```
+                A=list(A_y, 1),
+                tag="est.y")
```

with the observed response values y_i in the second column of the `data` matrix. The `effect` argument is a list with two elements: the first includes two index sets for the two spatial random effects (with same projector matrix), while the second is the intercept vector. It is now possible to define the full stack object through

```
> stk <- inla.stack(stk_x, stk_y)
```

The estimation procedure is carried out using the R-INLA `copy` feature described in Martins *et al.* (2013), which is adopted when a latent field is needed more than once in the model formulation. In fact, in the example under study, the spatial field $\xi(s)$ is used both in the specification of the covariate and response linear predictor. The `copy` feature has to be defined when specifying the `formula`

```
> formula <- y ~ -1 + f(xi.field, model=spde) +
+                intercept + f(u.field, model=spde) +
+                f(x.field, copy="xi.field", fixed=FALSE,
+                  hyper=list(theta=list(param=c(-1, 10)))))
```

In this case, the random effect $\xi(s)$ is copied as it enters both in the linear predictor of x_i and of y_i (see Eqs. (8.1) and (8.3)). But it can be seen in Eq. (8.3) that the relationship between ξ_i and y_i involves β_1 which is treated as hyperparameter in the estimation step.[2] In our example, we estimate the hyperparameter β_1 (`fixed=FALSE`) and, in the prior specification, we center the distribution on -1 and assign a variance equal to 10 (this is sufficient to include zero). The β_1 hyperparameter is called `theta` in R-INLA and the default prior distribution is Gaussian. So, we just change the `param` argument to specify our prior. Some other details can be seen typing `?inla.models`.

We also change the prior for σ_x^2 and σ_e^2, choosing an informative logGamma with parameters 1 and 0.1 for both precisions.

```
> precprior <- list(theta=list(param=c(1, 0.1)))
```

The final step is the run of the `inla` function:

```
> output <- inla(formula, family=c("gaussian","gaussian"),
+                data=inla.stack.data(stk),
+                control.predictor=list(compute=TRUE,
+                                       A=inla.stack.A(stk)),
+                control.family=list(list(hyper=precprior),
+                                    list(hyper=precprior)))
```

where it is important to point out that the `family` argument specifies a vector of two likelihoods, both Gaussian in this case. Moreover, the same prior values for

---

[2] Note that the `copy` feature in R-INLA defines a copy of a generic effect θ as $\theta^\star = \beta\theta + \epsilon$, where $\epsilon \sim \text{Normal}(0, b)$, with b being a large and fixed value, and β is a hyperparameter. By fixing $\beta = 1$, it means that $\theta^\star$ is an exact copy of θ. According to the specification of the `fixed` option (as FALSE or TRUE), the hyperparameter β is estimated or kept fixed.

both the variances σ_x^2 and σ_e^2 are specified entering twice the precprior list in control.family.

Getting the results

The true values and the posterior summaries of the intercept b_0 and of the precisions ($1/\sigma_x^2$ and $1/\sigma_e^2$) are extracted from the output through the following code:

```
> round(cbind(True=b0,output$summary.fixed[1,1:5,drop=FALSE]), 4)
              True     mean      SD 0.025quant 0.5quant 0.975quant
intercept      10 10.4898  0.8615     9.0744    10.486    11.8772
> round(cbind(True=1/c(Prec.x=sigma2_x, Prec.e=sigma2_e),
+                output$summary.hyperpar[1:2,1:5]), 4)
          True     mean      SD 0.025quant 0.5quant 0.975quant
Prec.x    4.00   3.7891  1.5322     1.5741   3.5375     7.4915
Prec.e    6.25  14.9023 10.8982     2.7281  12.1824    43.2504
```

where drop=FALSE inside [ ] is used to avoid the result to be coerced to a vector (when the result has just one line or row). By using drop=FALSE, we obtain a matrix object. For the precision, due to the asymmetry, it is better to look at the posterior marginal distribution, as reported in Figure 8.4. The same quantities can be retrieved for β_1 through

```
> round(cbind(True=beta1,
              output$summary.hyperpar[7,1:5, drop=FALSE]), 4)
                     True     mean      SD 0.025quant 0.5quant 0.975quant
Beta for x.field     -0.5  -1.0304  0.282    -1.5971  -1.0246      -0.49
```

The posterior marginal distributions of the parameters b_0, β_1, σ_x^2, and σ_e^2 are reported in Figure 8.4: all the posterior marginal distributions contain the true parameter values used for data simulation.

The posterior summaries of the spatial parameters (for the process $\xi(s)$ and $u(s)$) can be extracted from the output using the inla.spde2.result function:

```
> xi_field <- inla.spde2.result(output, name="xi.field", spde)
> u_field <- inla.spde2.result(output, name="u.field", spde)
```

In particular, the true values and posterior summaries (mean and 95% highest posterior density interval) for the spatial variances σ_ξ^2 and σ_u^2 can be obtain through

```
> round(cbind(True=c(sigma2.xi=sigma2_xi, sigma2.u=sigma2_u),
+    mean=c(inla.emarginal(function(x) x, xi_field$marginals.var[[1]]),
+           inla.emarginal(function(x) x, u_field$marginals.var[[1]])),
+    rbind(inla.hpdmarginal(.95, xi_field$marginals.var[[1]]),
+          inla.hpdmarginal(.95, u_field$marginals.var[[1]]))), 4)
             True    mean     low    high
sigma2.xi     0.5  0.2865  0.0330  0.6862
sigma2.u      0.3  0.2116  0.0026  0.6864
```

The true values for the range parameters r_ξ and r_u (computed as $\sqrt{8}/\kappa$) and the summary of the corresponding posterior marginal distributions are reported here:

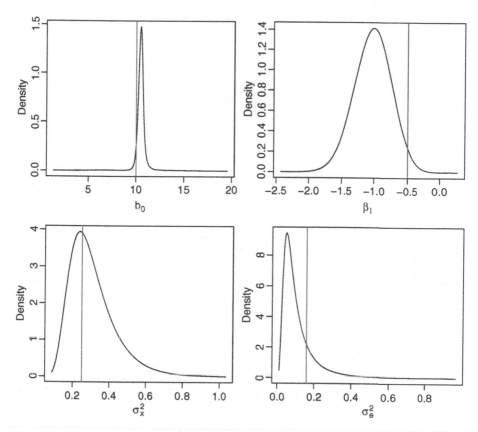

Figure 8.4   Posterior marginal distributions of the parameters b_0, β_1, σ_x^2, and σ_e^2. The vertical lines denote the true values used to simulate the data.

```
> round(cbind(True=c(range.xi=sqrt(8)/kappa_xi, range.u=sqrt(8)/kappa_u),
+       mean=c(inla.emarginal(function(x) x, xi_field$marginals.range[[1]]),
+              inla.emarginal(function(x) x, u_field$marginals.range[[1]])),
+       rbind(inla.hpdmarginal(.95, xi_field$marginals.range[[1]]),
+             inla.hpdmarginal(.95, u_field$marginals.range[[1]]))), 4)
             True    mean    low    high
range.xi  0.5657  0.8114  0.1872  1.6998
range.u   0.4041  0.6832  0.0051  2.4119
```

The posterior marginal distributions of the spatial parameters for both random fields are included in Figure 8.5.

8.1.2   Joint model with non-Gaussian distributions

In this section, we consider the case when both the covariate and the response assume discrete values: in particular, the covariate is modeled as a Poisson distribution while the response is modeled as a Binomial. This means that for the covariate

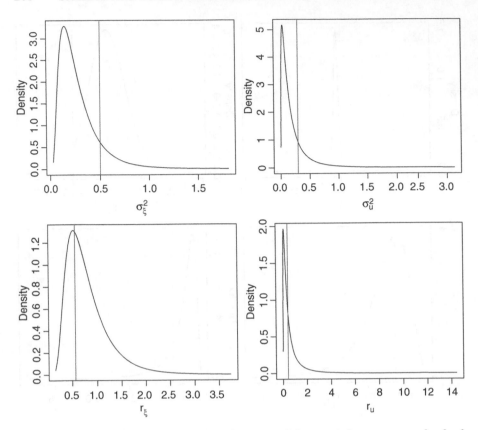

Figure 8.5   Posterior marginal distributions of the spatial parameters for both random fields. The vertical lines denote the true values used to simulate the data.

x_i we assume the following likelihood:

$$x_j \sim \text{Poisson}(\lambda_j),$$

where $\lambda_j = E_j \rho_j$, with E_j being the expected number of cases at location s_j. The rate ρ_j is modeled as

$$\log(\rho_j) = \eta_j = \xi_j,$$

with ξ_j coming from a Matérn Gaussian field as in the example in Section 8.1.1 (see Eq. (8.1)). The following Binomial distribution is assumed for y_i

$$y_i \sim \text{Binomial}(\pi_i, n_i),$$

where n_i is the number of trials at location s_i and the probability π_i is defined as

$$\text{logit}(\pi_i) = b_0 + \beta_1 \xi_i + u_i \tag{8.4}$$

and b_0, β_1, and u_i are defined as in Section 8.1.1 (see Eq. (8.3)). The difference here is that the linear predictors are specified at different scales through the logarithmic and logit link functions.

Data simulation

To simplify the example, for the spatial random fields we use the values ξ_i and u_i simulated in Section 8.1.1. Given this, we only need to simulate data for the covariate and the response. For the simulation of the covariate values x_i (through the rpois function) the expected values E_i are required, which are here generated using the Gamma distribution:

```
> set.seed(134)
> E <- rgamma(n=n_x, shape=10, rate=10)
> rho <- exp(xi[1:n_x])
> set.seed(14)
> x <- rpois(n=n_x, lambda=E*rho)
```

To simulate the response data, the intercept value has to be fixed (equal to 1)

```
> b0 <- 1
```

and the number of trials is randomly generated

```
> set.seed(19)
> ntrials <- 5 + rpois(n=n_y, lambda=10)
```

Finally, using Eq. (8.4) and the antilogit transformation (see Section 5.3), we get the response values:

```
> eta_y <- b0 + beta1 * xi[n_x + 1:n_y] + u
> set.seed(553)
> y <- rbinom(n=n_y, size=ntrials, prob=exp(eta_y)/(1 + exp(eta_y)) )
```

Fitting the model

To fit the model, we use the same mesh, SPDE model object, and projector matrices defined in Section 8.1.1. We only need to create new data stack objects, since we have now new values for the covariate and the response. Note that the data list specified inside the inla.stack function may contain anything associated with the "left-hand side" of the model, such as for example the type of link function, the expected number of cases (E) for the Poisson likelihood or the number of trials for the Binomial case. As in Section 8.1.1, we have two likelihoods and adopt the two columns structure for the data matrix:

```
> stk_x <- inla.stack(data=list(y=cbind(x, NA), E=E, link="log"),
+              effects=list(xi.field=1:spde$n.spde),
+              A=list(A_x),
+              tag="est.x")
> stk_y <- inla.stack(data=list(y=cbind(NA, y),
+                          Ntrials=ntrials, link="logit"),
```

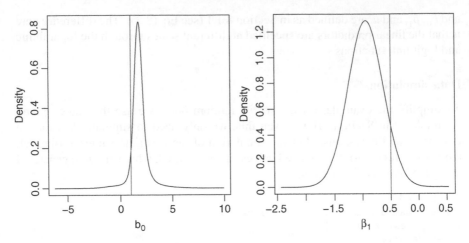

Figure 8.6   Posterior distributions of b_0 and β_1. The vertical lines denote the true values used to simulate the data.

```
+        effects=list(list(x.field=1:spde$n.spde, u.field=1:spde$n.spde),
+                          list(intercept=rep(1,length(y)))),
+             A=list(A_y, 1),
+             tag="est.y")
> stk <- inla.stack(stk_x, stk_y)
```

The formula is the same as in Section 8.1.1. To fit the model with the `inla` function, we specify the Poisson and Binomial families as well as the expected number of cases and of trials (extracted from the object `stk` by means of the `inla.stack.data` function):

```
> output2 <- inla(formula,
+                data=inla.stack.data(stk),
+                family=c("poisson", "binomial"),
+                E=inla.stack.data(stk)$E,
+                Ntrials=inla.stack.data(stk)$Ntrials,
+           control.predictor=list(compute=TRUE, A=inla.stack.A(stk)))
```

The posterior marginal distributions for the intercept b_0 and for the regression parameter β_1 are reported in Figure 8.6, while the posterior distributions of the spatial parameters (variances and ranges) are displayed in Figure 8.7 (the complete code is not reported here as is similar to the one used in Section 8.1.1).

8.2   Semicontinuous model to daily rainfall

For some applications it is difficult to fit the data using a single distribution. This is the case, for example, of daily rainfall data for which it is common to specify a distribution for the rain occurence (because there are days with no rain) and one for

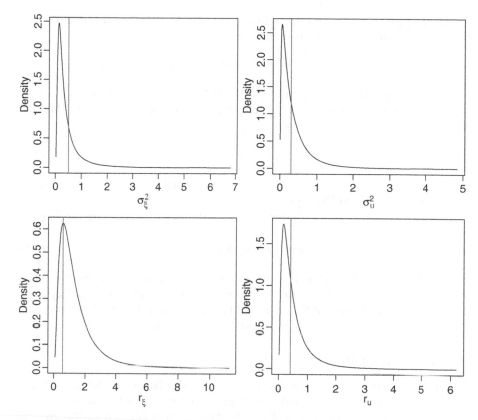

Figure 8.7 Posterior marginal distributions of the spatial parameters (variances and ranges). The vertical lines denote the true values used to simulate the data.

the rain amount. In particular, the distribution for the precipitation amount is chosen to be asymmetric because usually there are more days with small precipitation quantities. In this section, we show how to combine in a joint model the Gamma distribution, used for modeling rain amount, with the Bernoulli distribution for rain occurence. We refer to it as semicontinuous model because it takes into account at the same time zeros and positive continuous values.

The rainfall amount at location s_i can be zero or a positive number. We first define the rain occurrence at location s_i as

$$z_i = \begin{cases} 1, & \text{if it rains at location} s_i \\ 0, & \text{otherwise} \end{cases}$$

and the rainfall amount as

$$y_i = \begin{cases} \text{NA}, & \text{if it does not rain at location } s_i \\ \text{rainfall amount at location } s_i, & \text{otherwise} \end{cases}.$$

This setting gives rise to a model with two likelihoods given by a Bernoulli distribution for z_i and a Gamma distribution for y_i:

$$z_i \sim \text{Binomial}(\pi_i, n_i = 1) \quad \text{and} \quad y_i \sim \text{Gamma}(a_i, b_i).$$

Regarding the Gamma distribution, in R-INLA, we consider that $E(y_i) = \mu_i = a_i/b_i$ and $Var(y_i) = a_i/b_i^2 = \mu_i^2/\tau$, where τ is the precision parameter. Then the linear predictor is defined on $\log(\mu_i)$ and is given by

$$\log(\mu_i) = b_0^y + \xi_i, \tag{8.5}$$

where b_0^y is the intercept and ξ_i comes from a spatial random effect, i.e., a GF modeled through the SPDE approach.

As usual the linear predictor for the Bernoulli is specified using the logistic transformation

$$\text{logit}(\pi_i) = b_0^z + \beta_1 \xi_i + u_i, \tag{8.6}$$

with b_0^z being the intercept and β_1 the scaling parameter for ξ_i, which is a shared spatial random effect with the first component of the model defined in Eq. (8.5). The term u_i is an additional Gaussian field modeled through the SPDE approach, similar to what we have on the joint modeling example in Section 8.1.

Paraná state rainfall data

The rainfall data, we consider are provided by the Brasillian National Water Agency. The data were collected at 616 gauge stations – in Paraná State in the South of Brasil – for each day in 2011. The data are available in R-INLA and can be loaded by

```
> data(PRprec)
> dim(PRprec)
[1] 616 368
```

Note that the first three columns of the PRprec data frame contains longitude, latitude, and altitude for each gauge station. The following code extracts a portion of the data frame with the rainfall data for the first seven days (in January) at three different stations:

```
> PRprec[1:3, 1:10]
  Longitude Latitude Altitude d0101 d0102 d0103 d0104 d0105 d0106 d0107
1  -50.8744 -22.8511      365     0     0     0   0.0     0     0   2.5
3  -50.7711 -22.9597      344     0     1     0   0.0     0     0   6.0
4  -50.6497 -22.9500      904     0     0     0   3.3     0     0   5.1
```

For the same selection of days, it is possible to obtain a summary over stations of the rain amount through the apply function:

```
> apply(X=PRprec[,4:10], MARGIN=2, FUN=summary)
         d0101  d0102  d0103  d0104  d0105  d0106  d0107
Min.    0.0000  0.00  0.000  0.000  0.000  0.000  0.000
```

1st Qu.	0.0000	0.00	0.000	0.000	0.000	0.000	0.000
Median	0.0000	0.00	0.300	0.000	0.000	0.000	0.000
Mean	0.8074	2.87	5.928	3.567	2.793	4.059	5.999
3rd Qu.	0.0000	2.10	7.000	3.475	0.600	3.850	6.700
Max.	43.8000	55.60	78.500	62.900	64.100	81.400	75.700
NA's	6.0000	7.00	7.000	6.000	6.000	8.000	8.000

and the number of stations with rain

```
> colSums(PRprec[,4:10]>0, na.rm=TRUE)
d0101 d0102 d0103 d0104 d0105 d0106 d0107
   72   210   315   237   181   240   239
```

It can be noted, for example, that the third quartile for the first day ($d0101$) is zero and we have rain only in 72 out of 616 stations. Also for each day there are some missing data due to operational problems in collecting the measurements at the sites.

In this section, we consider only the data observed during the third day ($d0103$) in order to fit a semicontinuous model. The two response variables z_i and y_i are defined as follows:

```
> jday <- 6 #column in which data are stored
> z <- as.numeric(PRprec[,jday] > 0)
> sum(z==0,na.rm=T) #stations with no rain
[1] 294
> y <- ifelse(PRprec[,jday] > 0, PRprec[,jday], NA)
```

The function ifelse returns the amount of rain (when it rains, PRprec[,jday] > 0) or NA (otherwise), as defined in Eq. (8.5). Figure 8.8 displays the map with the rain data for the selected day together with the histogram for the rain amount y_i.

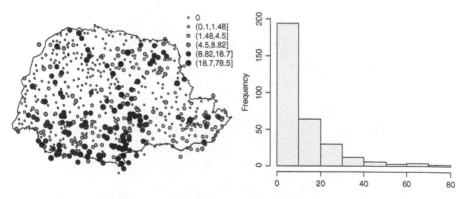

Figure 8.8   *The map on the left side shows the station locations together with the rain amount. The histogram on the right side refers to the distribution of the positive rain amount y_i.*

Fitting the model

Before fitting the two likelihoods model, the first step consists in defining the mesh considering all the gauges (also where rain amount is zero). Since the study region is not convex, we can avoid having too many triangles by using the `inla.nonconvex.hull` function in the mesh construction, as shown in Section 6.7.1:

```
> prec.coords <- cbind(PRprec$Longitude, PRprec$Latitude)
> boundary <- inla.nonconvex.hull(points=prec.coords,
+                                 convex=0.2, concave=0.2)
> mesh <- inla.mesh.2d(loc=prec.coords, boundary=boundary,
+                      max.edge=c(0.3, 0.8), cutoff=0.1)
```

By providing the boundary in the `inla.mesh.2d` function, we do not have small triangles in the northeast side of the Paraná region when an outer extension is used. Here, we create a mesh with few nodes by using a relative small outer extension and a quite high `cutoff` parameter; moreover, we set the maximum length of the inner edges by means of the `max.edge` option. The final mesh, with 865 vertices, is displayed in Figure 8.9.

The SPDE model is defined through

```
> spde <- inla.spde2.matern(mesh=mesh, alpha=2)
```

and the corresponding predictor matrix is given by

```
> A <- inla.spde.make.A(mesh=mesh, loc=prec.coords)
> dim(A)
[1] 616 865
```

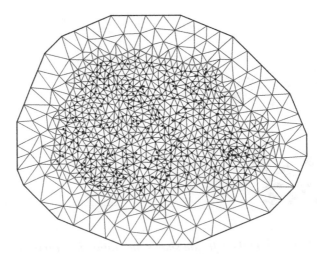

Figure 8.9   Mesh for the Paraná state with 865 nodes; black points denote the 616 rain gauges.

The procedure now requires the definition of the stack objects for the joint model (rain occurrence and amount), using the two columns structure for the response as described in Sections 8.1.1 and 8.1.2. In addition, for comparison purpose, we fit two separate (or single) models, one with rainfall occurrence only and the other with the rainfall amount. Using the flexibility of the `inla.stack` function, it is possible to define the single and joint models in a single stack object by specifying a multiple list in the `data` argument. Thus, the stack object for the precipitation amount is defined as

```
> stk.y <- inla.stack(data=list(amount=y, #for the single model
+                     alldata=cbind(y, NA)), #for the joint model
+                 A=list(A, 1),
+                 effects=list(
+                     list(y.field=1:spde$n.spde),
+                     list(y.intercept=rep(1,length(y)))),
+                 tag="est.y")
```

In the same way, it is possible to create the stack object for the occurrence data:

```
> stk.z <- inla.stack(data=list(occurence=z, #for the single model
+                     alldata=cbind(NA, z)), #for the joint model
+             A=list(A, 1),
+             effects=list(
+                 list(z.field=1:spde$n.spde, zc.field=1:spde$n.spde),
+                 list(z.intercept=rep(1,length(z)))),
+             tag="est.z")
```

The single model with Gamma likelihood for the rain amount is fitted using the following code:

```
> formula.y <- amount ~ -1 + y.intercept + f(y.field, model=spde)
> out.y <- inla(formula.y, family="gamma", data=inla.stack.data(stk.y),
+               control.predictor=list(A=inla.stack.A(stk.y)),
+               control.compute=list(dic=TRUE),
+               control.inla=list(strategy="laplace"))
```

The single model with Bernoulli likelihood for the occurence data is

```
> formula.z <- occurence ~ -1 + z.intercept + f(z.field, model=spde)
> out.z <- inla(formula.z, family="binomial", data=inla.stack.
                                          data(stk.z),
+               control.predictor=list(A=inla.stack.A(stk.z)),
+               control.compute=list(dic=TRUE),
+               control.inla=list(strategy="laplace"))
```

where we do not specify the number of trials for the Binomial distribution as `Ntrials=1` is the default value in the `inla` function. Finally, the joint model is fitted as follows:

```
> stk.yz <- inla.stack(stk.y, stk.z)
> formula.yz <- alldata ~ -1 + y.intercept + z.intercept +
+     f(y.field, model=spde) + f(z.field, model=spde) +
+     f(zc.field, copy="y.field", fixed=FALSE)
```

```
> out.yz <- inla(formula.yz, family=c("gamma", "binomial"),
+               data=inla.stack.data(stk.yz),
+               control.predictor=list(A=inla.stack.A(stk.yz)),
+               control.compute=list(dic=TRUE, config=TRUE),
+               control.inla=list(strategy="laplace"))
```

We choose to use the `strategy="laplace"` because we have asymmetric non-Gaussian data and we need a more accurate approximation than the one provided by R-INLA as default (see Section 4.7.2 for a description of the different types of approximations). In `control.compute` the argument `config` is set to TRUE for later use.

Note that we use the `copy` feature as the same spatial GF $\xi(s)$ is used in two linear predictors (see Eqs. (8.5) and (8.6)). In particular, the GF in the rain amount model of Eq. (8.6) is a copy – through the hyperparameter β_1 – of the GF defined in the occurrence model of Eq. (8.5). Here we use the default prior Normal(1, 10) for β_1 because we believe that when there is a high probability of raining, the actual amount of precipitation is supposed to be larger than for a low probability of raining. It is also possible to define and copy the spatial GF in the Bernoulli linear predictor (z) and copy it on the Gamma linear predictor for y.

We can compare the results obtained for the two separate models with the one for the joint model looking at the DIC values. However, we have to be careful when computing the DIC for the joint model. In R-INLA, the local DIC is returned, i.e., the DIC value for each observation. So when we deal with multiple likelihoods, a correct DIC value for each response (y_i and z_i) has to be computed by summing the local DIC values corresponding to each likelihood. This can be done using the following commands:

```
> rbind(separate=c(y=out.y$dic$dic, z=out.z$dic$dic),
+       joint=tapply(out.yz$dic$local.dic, out.yz$dic$family, sum))
                   y         z
separate 2078.905 695.6875
joint    2075.880 689.4337
```

and we can see that the joint model is characterized by a slightly lower DIC, hence by a marginally better fit for the data.

The posterior mean of the linear predictor expressed in the original response scale can be computed through the corresponding inverse link function (exponential for y and antilogit for z). To compute the expected value of the posterior marginal distributions on the response scale we use the `inla.emarginal` function:

```
> idy <- which(PRprec[,jday]>0)
> exp.y <- sapply(out.yz$marginals.linear.pred[idy], function(m)
+                 inla.emarginal(exp, m))
> idz <- which(!is.na(z))
> exp.z <- sapply(out.yz$marginals.linear.pred[nrow(PRprec) + idz],
+                 function(m) inla.emarginal(inla.link.invlogit, m))
```

These values can be compared to the observed mean for the rain occurence and amount:

```
> c(yPositive.obs=mean(PRprec[which(PRprec[,jday]>0),jday],
                                       na.rm=TRUE),
+   yPositive.pred=mean(exp.y))
 yPositive.obs yPositive.pred
      11.46063       11.56729
> c(z.obs=mean(z, na.rm=TRUE), z.pred=mean(exp.z))
    z.obs    z.pred
0.5172414 0.5170477
```

The posterior marginal distributions of b_0^z, b_0^y, τ, and β_1 are represented in Figure 8.10. It can be appreciated that β_1 is significantly different from zero, meaning that the rainfall occurrence and amount share the same spatial pattern.

Significance of the spatial effects

To assess if the occurrence and amount of rain are spatially dependent, we test the significance of the spatial random effect $\xi(s)$ and $u(s)$. One approach consists in looking at the 2.5% and 97.5% quantiles of each element of the random effect.

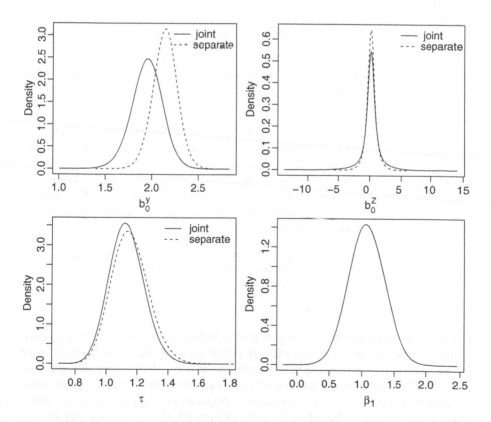

Figure 8.10   Posterior marginal distributions of b_0^y (top left), b_0^z (top right), τ (bottom left), for both separate and joint models, and β_1 (bottom right).

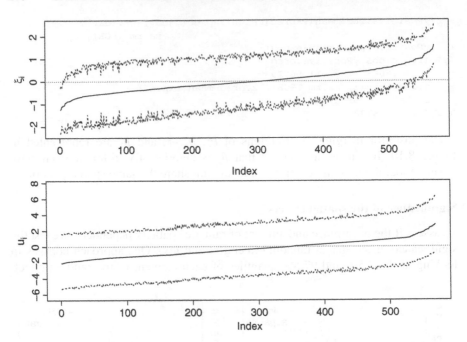

Figure 8.11   Posterior mean (continuous line) of each ξ_i (top) and u_i (bottom) and 2.5% and 97.5% quantiles of the posterior marginal distributions (dashed lines).

If for some of these both quantiles have the same sign, then the corresponding $\xi(s)$ are significantly different from zero. As we have modeled $\xi(s)$ at mesh nodes, we can plot only the ones inside the Paraná state domain. We see in Figure 8.11 the mean and quantiles for each ξ_i and u_i ordered by their posterior mean. For ξ_i, we have 38 of those completely above or below zero. As it is more than 5% of those (expected by using a 95% credibility intervals), we can conclude that this spatial component is significantly different from 0.

```
> c(n.nodes.in.pr=length(in.pr), expected.out=0.05*length(in.pr),
+     observed.out=sum(out.yz$summary.random$y.field[in.pr,4]>0 |
+         out.yz$summary.random$y.field[in.pr,6]<0))
n.nodes.in.pr  expected.out  observed.out
        569.00        28.45        38.00
```

Using the same approach, we can also conclude that $u(s)$ is not significant (as each u_i includes zero). However, this strategy considers individual tests for each entry of the random effect vector ignoring their correlation. Also, for the specific case of the SPDE approach, the number of effects far from zero depends on the mesh nodes design. For example, we can put more nodes around regions where the spatial effect is far from zero. Based on the plots in Figure 8.11, one can see that there is in fact a trend in the values of ξ_i and u_i. So, instead of testing each ξ_i or each u_i independently we should consider these jointly.

A typical approach to test significance of effects on a model consists in comparing the DIC values between different models. The models with smaller DIC can be chosen as the best fit for the data in hand. We already have two models for each response (rainfall amount and occurrence). The joint model has a smaller DIC indicating that it is preferrable to treat these together. To complete the range of possible models, we can fit one for each response without any spatial component.

```
> form.nospatial <- alldata ~ -1 + z.intercept + y.intercept
> out.nospatial <- inla(form.nospatial, family=c("gamma", "binomial"),
+                         data=inla.stack.data(stk.yz),
+                         control.predictor=list(A=inla.stack.A(stk.yz)),
+                         control.compute=list(dic=TRUE),
+                         control.inla=list(strategy="laplace"))
```

Also, we can fit a model with only one spatial component which is shared by both responses, i.e., we take out the u_i term in Eq. (8.6):

```
> form.oneshared <- alldata ~ -1 + y.intercept + z.intercept +
+        f(y.field, model=spde) + f(z.field, model=spde)
> out.oneshared <- inla(form.oneshared, family=c("gamma", "binomial"),
+                         data=inla.stack.data(stk.yz),
+                         control.predictor=list(A=inla.stack.A(stk.yz)),
+                         control.compute=list(dic=TRUE),
+                         control.inla=list(strategy="laplace"))
```

From the summary table with the DIC values for the model with and without spatial effect

```
> rbind(nospatial=tapply(out.nospatial$dic$local.dic,
+                         out.nospatial$dic$family, sum),
+        one.shared=tapply(out.oneshared$dic$local.dic,
+                         out.oneshared$dic$family, sum),
+        separated=c(out.y$dic$dic, out.z$dic$dic),
+        joint=tapply(out.yz$dic$local.dic, out.yz$dic$family, sum))
                  1         2
nospatial  2157.415  857.7367
one.shared 2079.681  700.9380
separated  2078.905  695.6875
joint      2075.880  689.4337
```

we can conclude that the joint model is to be preferred (column=1 is the Gamma likelihood, column=2 is the Binomial likelihood). Note that there is a big reduction in the DIC when any spatial effect is included (separated, shared or both). The model with only the shared spatial effect does perform similarly to the one which includes also the extra spatial effect (u_i) for the rain occurrence.

The spatial random effects

The results for the spatial random field can be extracted as usual with the `inla.spde2.result` function:

```
> y.field <- inla.spde2.result(out.yz, "y.field", spde)
> z.field <- inla.spde2.result(out.yz, "z.field", spde)
```

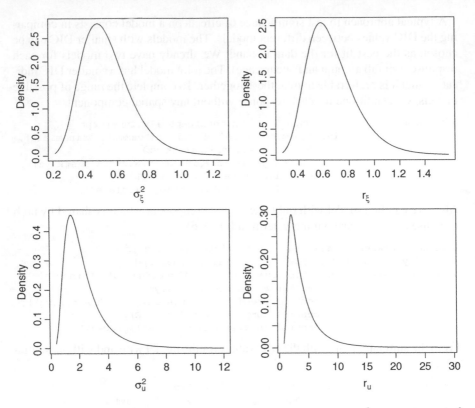

Figure 8.12   Posterior marginal distribution of the variances σ_ξ^2 (top left) and σ_u^2 (bottom left) and of the practical ranges r_ξ (top right) and r_u (bottom right).

The corresponding posterior marginals are reported in Figure 8.12 (the range is defined on degree units).

Another interesting result is the map of the spatial random field. As described in Section 6.10, the easiest approach is the spatial interpolation of the posterior marginal mean of the spatial field on a regular grid. In the following, we define a link between the mesh and a grid with square pixels that covers the Paraná state:

```
> data(PRborder) #state boundary
> nxy <- round(c(diff(range(PRborder[,1]))),
+                   diff(range(PRborder[,2]))) /.02)
> nxy #grid size
[1] 330 210
> projgrid <- inla.mesh.projector(mesh,
+                                 xlim=range(PRborder[,1]),
+                                 ylim=range(PRborder[,2]),
+                                 dims=nxy)
```

Then the posterior mean and standard deviation of the spatial random field are interpolated on the regular grid through the `inla.mesh.project` function

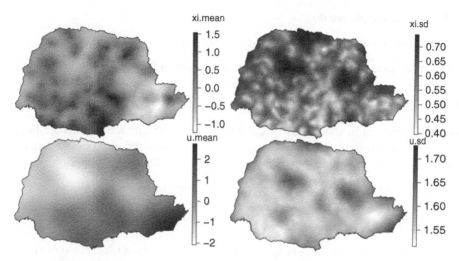

Figure 8.13   Posterior mean (left) and standard deviation (right) of the spatial random fields $\xi(s)$ *(top) and* $u(s)$ *(bottom).*

```
> rf.grid <- list(xi.mean = inla.mesh.project(projgrid,
+                         out.yz$summary.random$y.field$mean))
> rf.grid$xi.sd <- inla.mesh.project(projgrid,
+                             out.yz$summary.random$y.field$sd)
> rf.grid$u.mean <- inla.mesh.project(projgrid,
+                             out.yz$summary.random$z.field$mean)
> rf.grid$u.sd <- inla.mesh.project(projgrid,
+                             out.yz$summary.random$z.field$sd)
```

The resulting maps are reported in Figure 8.13.

Because we only have the intercept and the spatial effect for the rainfall amount, it is possible to associate the map of $\xi(s)$ with the rainfall amount.

Prediction of the responses

It is easy to carry out predictions from our model anywhere in the domain as we do not have any other covariate (which we would need at the target locations). The predicted values are computed at the data locations when we use `compute=TRUE` in the `control.predictor`, but to map these on a fine grid it would be expensive having too many points on it. A common approach would consist in building a new stack of data considering prediction over the grid and assigning NA to the observations.

However, a computational cheaper option consists in computing the linear predictor at the mesh nodes and project it onto the grid taking into account the uncertainty by sampling from its posterior distribution. In R-INLA this can be done using the `inla.posterior.sample` function which needs the output from the `inla` function by setting `config=TRUE` in the `control.compute` option.

To get one sample we do

```
> s1 <- inla.posterior.sample(n=1,result=out.yz)
```

The `inla.posterior.sample` function returns a list with several objects

```
> names(s1[[1]])
[1] "hyperpar" "latent"   "logdens"
```

We are interested in the values of the latent field (`latent`). Since all the latent field components are stacked, we need to query the index for each component. For example, to find the index for the intercept b_0^y, we use the grep[3] function:

```
> grep("y.intercept", rownames(s1[[1]]$latent), fixed=TRUE)
[1] 4892
```

We repeat it for each component with

```
> ids <- lapply(c('y.intercept', 'z.intercept', 'y.field', 'z.field',
                                                  'zc.field'),
+           function(x) grep(x, rownames(s1[[1]]$latent), fixed=TRUE))
```

and then we define a function to return the predicted values for each response:

```
> pred.y.f <- function(s)
+     exp(s$latent[ids[[1]], 1] + s$latent[ids[[3]], 1])
> pred.z.f <- function(s)
+     1/(1 + exp(-(s$latent[ids[[2]], 1] + s$latent[ids[[4]], 1] +
+                   s$latent[ids[[5]], 1])))
```

We draw 1000 samples from the posterior joint distribution in `out.yz`

```
> s1000 <- inla.posterior.sample(1000, out.yz)
```

compute the predicted values at the mesh nodes for each response

```
> prd.y <- sapply(s1000, pred.y.f)
> prd.z <- sapply(s1000, pred.z.f)
```

and finally project the average of the predicted values

```
> prd <- list(y.mean=inla.mesh.project(projgrid,
                                       field=rowMeans(prd.y)))
> prd$y.sd <- inla.mesh.project(projgrid, field=apply(prd.y, 1, sd))
> prd$z.mean <- inla.mesh.project(projgrid, field=rowMeans(prd.z))
> prd$z.sd <- inla.mesh.project(projgrid, field=apply(prd.z, 1, sd))
> for (j in 1:4) prd[[j]][!xy.in] <- NA
```

Figure 8.14 shows the prediction for both responses together with their standard deviations: large amount of rain is predicted for the southern and southeastern side of the region, while more uncertainty is present on the northeastern side and on the Western borders.

---

[3] grep(a,b) returns the position on the character vector b which matches the character a.

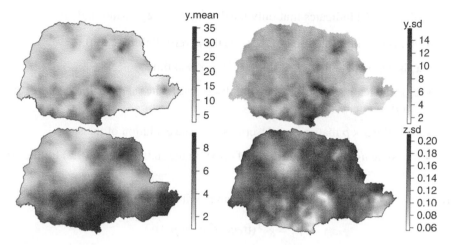

Figure 8.14   Posterior mean (left) and standard deviation (right) of both responses y and z.

8.3   Spatio-temporal dynamic models

Dynamic models are extensively used in the time series framework (see, for instance, West and Harrison, 1997 or Petris *et al.*, 2009). One particular version of these models is a hierarchical version of a time series with the regression coefficients varying smoothly over time. In this framework, it is also possible to assume that the regression coefficients change only in space, obtaining the so-called spatially varying coefficient models (see Assunção *et al.*, 1999, Assunção *et al.*, 2002; Gamerman *et al.*, 2003). Finally, if we combine the spatial and temporal dimension we get spatio-temporal dynamic models which were proposed by Gelfand *et al.* (2003).

Several univariate and multivariate time-series structures can be specified in a dynamic model. We focus on the class where each time series has a degree of spatial dependence and in particular at each time point we define a convolution of proper Gaussian Markov random fields over space. This class of spatio-temporal models has also been proposed by Vivar and Ferreira (2009) using the MCMC algorithm, but is rather computationally expensive; an alternative approach using INLA is proposed by Ruiz-Cárdenas *et al.* (2012), which is what we describe in this section.

We define a parametric family for the vector of observations at time t for a set of n areas, given by y_t $(t = 1, \ldots, T)$. A dynamic model is specified on the mean $E(y_t) = \mu_t$ as follows:

$$\mu_t = g^{-1}(\text{trace}(x_t' \xi_t^*))$$
$$(\xi_t^* - \mu_\xi^*) = G_t(\xi_{t-1}^* - \mu_\xi^*) + \omega_t, \tag{8.7}$$

where the trace($\cdot$) indicates that only the diagonal of $x'_t \xi^*_t$ counts and

- $g(\cdot)$ is the link function (so $g^{-1}(\cdot)$ is the inverse link function),

- x_t is a covariate matrix of dimension $p \times n$ at time t,

- ξ^*_t is the realization of p latent (unobservable) states at n areas and time t (this is a $p \times n$ matrix),

- G_t is the $p \times p$ matrix that describes the time evolution of the states,

- ω_{tk} is the n-dimensional vector of errors in the state equation (8.7) for the kth state ($k = 1, \dots, p$) at time t.

To simplify the estimation process, we can rewrite Eq. (8.7) as

$$\mu_t = g^{-1}(\text{trace}(x'_t(\xi_t + \mu^*_\xi)))$$

$$\xi_t = G_t \xi_{t-1} + \omega_t, \tag{8.8}$$

where $\xi = \xi^* - \mu^*_\xi$ and $E(\xi) = 0$.

It is assumed that ω_{tk} are independent realizations (over time) of each state k and that $\omega_{tk} \sim \text{MVNormal}(0, \Sigma_k)$, with $k = 1, \dots, p$ and Σ_k as the variance–covariance matrix over space for each state k.

The matrix G_t is considered fixed over time (and denoted by G) and defines the correlation structure of ξ_t. If G is assumed to be a diagonal matrix, it means that there is no correlation between states (or covariates) for the ξ_t matrix.

Going back to the observations, we need to specify a distribution for each entry of y_t. Here we assume that y_t are counts (e.g., of diseases) observed in a set of n areas at time t so, as shown in the previous chapters, we choose a Poisson distribution and an inverse link function $g^{-1}(\cdot) = \exp(\cdot)$.

To define the spatial component, we assume that Σ_k (recall that this is different for each state) is a covariance matrix defined by any of the spatial models presented in Chapters 6 and 7.

In the following sections, we consider data on a discrete spatial domain and describe two examples based on the neighborhood structure: one using the besag-proper model in Section 8.3.1 and one using the generic1 model in Section 8.3.2.

8.3.1   Dynamic model with Besag proper specification

The proper Besag prior for spatial dependence has been introduced in Chapter 6.1.1 and is a (less used) alternative to the intrinsic conditional autoregressive structure that we used extensively in the previous two chapters. In R-INLA the specification for the proper Besag model is as follows:

$$u_i | u_{-i} \sim \text{Normal}\left(\frac{1}{(d + \mathcal{N}_i)} \sum_{j=1}^{n} a_{ij} u_j, 1/\tau(d + \mathcal{N}_i) \right),$$

which is slightly different from the one presented in Chapter 6.1.1 as it uses the d parameter (instead of ϕ) to ensure properness. The precision matrix for this model is

$$Q = \tau(dI + \text{diag}(\mathcal{N}_i) - R), \tag{8.9}$$

where $\mathcal{N}_i$ is the number of neighbors of area i and R is a structure matrix given by

$$R_{ij} = \begin{cases} 0 & \text{if } i = j \\ 1 & \text{if } i \sim j \\ 0 & \text{otherwise} \end{cases}$$

where $i \sim j$ means that the areas i and j are neighbors. This setting can be specified with model=besagproper in the f() environment of the R-INLA formula.

Data simulation

As an example, we will use simulated data of time series from $n = 26$ counties from the Republic of Ireland available as a shapefile through the spdep package (Bivand *et al.*, 2012).

```
> file <- system.file("etc/shapes/eire.shp", package="spdep")[1]
> require(maptools)
> pol <- readShapePoly(file)
```

We define the precision matrix $Q = \tau(dI + \text{diag}(\mathcal{N}_i) - R)$ using the neighborhood list returned by the poly2nb function and transforming it in an adjacency matrix using the nb2mat function (poly2nb and nb2mat are from the spdep package):

```
> require(spdep)
> nbl <- poly2nb(pol)
> n <- length(nbl)
> R <- Matrix(nb2mat(nbl, style="B"))
```

Considering the simple case of one intercept and one covariate ($p = 2$), we have that G is a 2×2 matrix which is assumed to be diagonal with temporal parameters γ_1 and γ_2 (so no correlation between the intercept and the covariate is specified). Moreover, we set a Poisson distribution for the observations y_t. We have to perform inference for the bidimensional state ξ_t, for the precision parameters τ_1 and τ_2, for the diagonal parameters d_1, and d_2 of the precision matrix and for the temporal correlation parameters (γ_1 and γ_2).
We set the parameter values as follows:

```
> mu.xi <- c(-10, 0.5);        tau <- c(0.5, 0.3)
> ddiag <- c(0.3, 0.5);        gamma <- c(.8, .6)
```

where mu.xi represents the vector $\boldsymbol{\mu}_\xi$. The state variance–covariance matrix $\Sigma_{k=1}$ and $\Sigma_{k=2}$ are defined according to the besagproper specification in R-INLA and the inverse precision matrix defined in Eq. (8.9):

```
> n <- 26
> nnb <- colSums(R) #number of neighbors
> n <- length(nnb)
> Q1bp <- tau[1]*(diag(ddiag[1],n)+diag(nnb)-R)
> Q2bp <- tau[2]*(diag(ddiag[2],n)+diag(nnb)-R)
```

We can generate samples from a Normal distribution given a known precision matrix using the `inla.qsample` function already presented in Chapter 6. In our case, we need to simulate samples from a spatio-temporal dynamic model as specified in Eq. (8.8). This can be done by simulating T (time length) samples from ω_t and then computing ξ_t as follows:

```
> T <- 30
> xi1 <- omega1 <- inla.qsample(n=T, Q=Q1bp, seed=1)
> xi2 <- omega2 <- inla.qsample(n=T, Q=Q2bp, seed=2)
> xi1[,1] <- sqrt(1-gamma[1]^2)*omega1[,1]
> xi2[,1] <- sqrt(1-gamma[2]^2)*omega2[,1]
> for (j in 2:T) {
+     xi1[, j] <- gamma[1]*xi1[, j-1] + sqrt(1-gamma[1]^2)*omega1[, j]
+     xi2[, j] <- gamma[2]*xi2[, j-1] + sqrt(1-gamma[2]^2)*omega2[, j]
+ }
```

The term $\sqrt{1 - \gamma^2}$ is multiplied by the innovation error (ω_t) as the `ar1` latent model in R-INLA is defined in this way (see the description of `ar1` on the INLA website).

Additionally, we simulate a covariate matrix and an offset (the expected number of cases for the Poisson distribution) and finally the response:

```
> #Covariate matrix
> set.seed(3)
> x2 <- matrix(runif(T*n), nrow=n)
> #Expected values
> set.seed(4)
> ee <- outer(rgamma(n, 5000000, scale=0.1),
              rgamma(T, 100, scale=0.01)) *
+             rgamma(n*T, 100, scale=0.01)
> #Observations
> set.seed(5)
> yy <- rpois(n=n*T,
+             lambda=ee*exp((xi1+mu.xi[1]) + (xi2+mu.xi[2])*x2))
```

We use the `outer` product between n Gamma(5000000,0.1) and T Gamma(100,0.01) samples to have more variation on `ee` between different areas at the same time and less between different times in the same area.

Estimation through the `group` feature

After simulating the data, we estimate the parameters of the space–time dynamic model by specifying a Kronecker product between the spatial and temporal structure (see Chapter 7), i.e., by defining the `besagproper` GMRF and group it by the `ar1` on time (note that this would be the equivalent proper version of a type IV interaction as described in Chapter 7).

We prepare the data and set the R-INLA formula environment as follows:

```
> dat.bp <- data.frame(y=yy, x=as.vector(x2),  e=as.vector(ee),
+                      xi1=rep(1:n, T), index.t=rep(1:T, each=n))
> dat.bp$xi2 <- dat.bp$xi1
> dat.bp$index.t2 <- dat.bp$index.t
> form.bp <- y ~ x +
+     f(xi1, model="besagproper", graph=R,
+       group=index.t, control.group=list(model="ar1")) +
+     f(xi2, x, model="besagproper", graph=R,
+       group=index.t2, control.group=list(model="ar1"))
```

Then we run the `inla` function

```
> res.bp <- inla(form.bp, family="poisson", data=dat.bp, E=dat.bp$e,
+                control.predictor=list(compute=TRUE))
```

The posterior distributions for μ_ξ and for the model hyperparameters $\{\tau_1, \tau_2, \gamma_1, \gamma_2, d_1, d_2\}$ are reported in Figure 8.15.

Moreover, we can investigate the latent fields (or states) ξ_1 and ξ_2. First, it is possible to analyze the temporal pattern for some given areas as done in Figure 8.16: Note that the estimated line is able to reproduce the true one generally well in all the areas. We can also create maps of the latent fields for specific time points. In Figure 8.17, we present the maps for the first, middle and last time point for the true and estimated values of ξ_1 and ξ_2. From the maps, it is clear that the spatial pattern is well reconstructed using the `inla` model, as the pairs of maps (true and estimated) are very close to each others.

Finally, it is possible to summarize the results by computing the correlation between the simulated and estimated values for ξ_1 and ξ_2:

```
> c(xi1=cor(as.vector(xi1), res.bp$summary.random$xi1$mean),
+   xi2=cor(as.vector(xi2), res.bp$summary.random$xi2$mean))
      xi1       xi2
0.9235725 0.7306488
```

which is above 0.7 for both states suggesting a good ability of the inferential process to reproduce the spatial and temporal pattern specified in the simulation.

8.3.2 Dynamic model with `generic1` specification

In this section, we present another example of dynamic model. In particular, we show how to fit a spatio-temporal dynamic model without using the `group` feature described in the previous section but by means of the data augmentation strategy used in Ruiz-Cárdenas *et al.* (2012). This strategy can be applied to any multivariate distribution already implemented in R-INLA as well as to dynamic models of different order (e.g., second-order dynamic model presented by Ruiz-Cárdenas *et al.* (2012)).

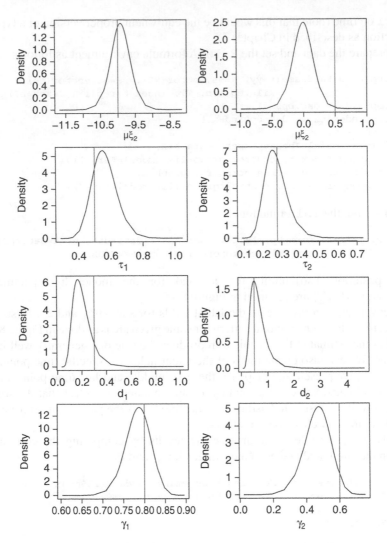

Figure 8.15   Posterior marginal distributions for the dynamic spatial model with besagproper *spatial distribution. The vertical line represents the true values used for simulating the data.*

We now specify the spatial correlation structure using the generic1 latent specification in R-INLA. This assumes that the precision matrix is $Q = \tau(I - \frac{\phi}{\lambda_{\max}}R)$, where τ is the precision parameter, ϕ is the spatial correlation parameter (correlation between neighbor areas), R is a structure matrix and $\lambda_{\max}$ is the maximum eigenvalue of R so that $\phi \in [0, 1)$. In this example, we set R equal to the adjacency matrix (or neighborhood matrix) defined earlier.

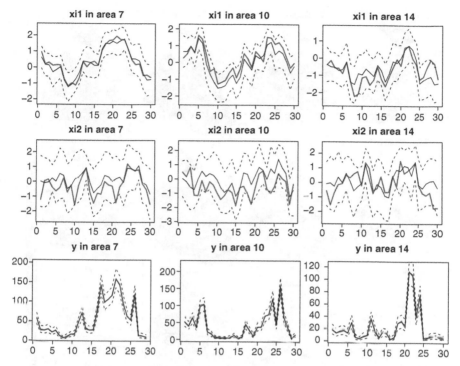

Figure 8.16   Simulated time series (gray solid line) of $\boldsymbol{\xi}_1$, $\boldsymbol{\xi}_2$ and $\mathbf{y}$ in three given areas, posterior mean (black solid line), 2.5 and 97.5 quantiles for fitted values (dashed lines).

This specification is equivalent to the following set of conditional distributions:

$$u_i \mid \boldsymbol{u}_{-i} \sim \text{Normal}\left(\frac{1}{\lambda_{\max}}\sum_{j=1}^{n}a_{ij}u_j, 1/(\tau\lambda_{\max})\right),$$

which does not depend on the number of neighbors. However, $\lambda_{\max}$ is related to the average number of neighbors of all areas and it increases as the number of neighbors increases (Assunção and Krainski, 2009).

Assuming the `generic1` model definition, the precision matrix for the kth state is given by

$$\boldsymbol{Q}_k = \boldsymbol{\Sigma}_k^{-1} = \tau\left(\boldsymbol{I} - \frac{\phi_k}{\lambda_{\max}}\boldsymbol{R}\right),$$

where τ is the scale parameter and $0 \leq \phi_k < 1$ controls the degree of spatial correlation (ϕ_k is different for each state).

If we consider the simple case of an intercept varying over time and space, it follows that $\boldsymbol{G} = \gamma_1$ and $\phi_k = \phi$. This defines a spatio-temporal interaction model similar to those proposed by Knorr-Held (2000) and introduced in Chapter 7. Note

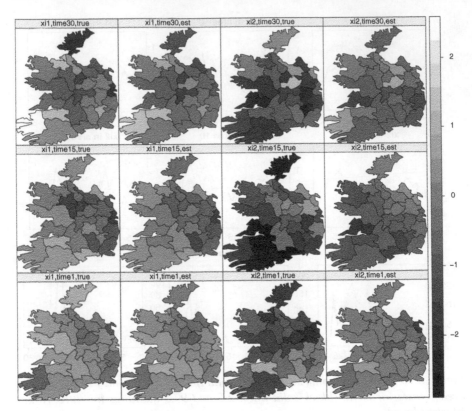

Figure 8.17 *Maps of the latent fields (ξ_1 and ξ_2) for the true (simulated) and estimated posterior mean. Each line corresponds to a different time point (1, 15, and 30, from bottom to top).*

that the case $\gamma = \phi = 0$ defines type I interaction (i.e., iid) and $\gamma = \phi = 1$ defines type IV interaction (i.e., a spatial structure product with a temporal structure); when $\gamma = 0$ and $\phi = 1$ we have type III interaction (spatial structure independent of each time point) and when $\gamma = 1$, $\phi = 0$ type II interaction (temporal structure independent for each area). This model is also similar to the one proposed by Cameletti *et al.* (2012), which is also of type IV class interaction. In the example, we are considering in this section, we show how the dynamic spatio-temporal model works when both intercept and the covariate coefficients vary over space and time. Similarly to what we did in the previous section, we simulate time series for each area using the same parameters as before, with the exception of the spatial correlation parameters ϕ_1 and ϕ_2 and precisions τ_1 and τ_2:

```
> phi <- c(0.95, 0.85)
> tau <- c(3, 5)
```

The precision matrices are computed as follows:

```
> lamb.max <- max(eigen(R, only.values=TRUE)$values)
```

```
> Q1g1 <- tau[1]*(diag(n)-phi[1]/lamb.max*R)
> Q2g1 <- tau[2]*(diag(n)-phi[2]/lamb.max*R)
```

and finally it is possible to draw samples for ξ_1, ξ_2 and y

```
> xi1 <- omega1 <- inla.qsample(n=T, Q=Q1g1, seed=1)
> xi2 <- omega2 <- inla.qsample(n=T, Q=Q2g1, seed=2)
> for (j in 2:T) {
+     xi1[, j] <- gamma[1]*xi1[, j-1] + omega1[, j]
+     xi2[, j] <- gamma[2]*xi2[, j-1] + omega2[, j]
+ }
> set.seed(5)
> yy <- rpois(n=n*T,
+                 lambda=ee*exp((mu.xi[1]+xi1) + (mu.xi[2]+xi2)*x2))
```

The data augmentation strategy

The data augmentation strategy is used here to estimate the parameters of the temporal correlation structure in the model (γ_1 and γ_2). To understand it, it is convenient to rewrite the state formula in Eq. (8.8) as

$$0 = \xi_i - G\xi_{i-1} - \omega_i, \tag{8.10}$$

where we create a vector of faked zeros on the left-hand side assuming to be distributed like a zero-mean Gaussian with fixed large precision. On the right-hand side, we have p independent components for ξ_i (in our example $p = 2$: intercept and one regression coefficient). Moreover, we define three latent models: one for ω_i, one for ξ_i and another one for ξ_{i-1}.

In the augmentation strategy, we have to model directly the $n \times T$ errors ω_i in the state equation (8.10). The model for ω_i includes the spatial structure which is assumed to be independent across time (type III interaction). On the other hand, ξ is characterized by a spatio-temporal interaction of type IV. The spatial part defined through the generic1 model needs a structure matrix R. So we define it as the Kronecker product between a diagonal matrix with dimension T and the spatial structure matrix. As said before the order of the Kronecker product matters, and here we put first the temporal matrix because we are going to stack our data into a vector ordered by time (e.g., observations for all areas at the first time point enter as the first n elements, then the observations for the second time and so on):

```
> stc.mat <- kronecker(diag(T), R)
```

The model for ξ_i is chosen to be a multivariate Gaussian distribution with independent components and fixed high precision. Then, a model is defined for ξ_{i-1} (the same effect but lagged) using the copy feature as described in Martins et al. (2013) and Ruiz-Cárdenas et al. (2012). In this case, the copy parameter defines the diagonal of G.

As seen in the previous section, we deal with the response, the spatio-temporal random intercept and the spatio-temporal varying regression coefficient for one

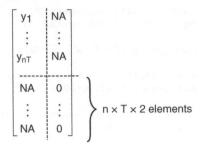

Figure 8.18   Schematic representation of the data structure for the augmented model.

covariate (everything stacked in a vector). By using the data augmentation strategy and the faked zero-observation vector, we have to define a two-column matrix similar to the one in Figure 8.18. Note that the number of rows in this matrix is three times the number of observations $n \times T$.

We now define a list containing vectors for the offset (ee), the intercept (x1), the covariate (x2) and the response (Y). Each vector has the same length as the number of rows of the response matrix, i.e., $n \times T \times 3$.

```
> dat.aug <- list(e=c(as.vector(ee), rep(NA, n*T*2)),
+                 x1=rep(1:0, c(n*T, n*T*2)),
+                 x2=c(as.vector(x2), rep(0, n*T*2)))
> dat.aug$Y <- cbind(c(yy, rep(NA, n*T*2)),
+                    rep(c(NA, 0), c(n*T, n*T*2)))
```

To implement the data augmentation approach, we need to take care of the index sets. We have to define one index for each error term and one for each latent spatio-temporal random effect. Let $m = n \times T$, then the index for the first error is from row $m + 1$ to row $2m$ and the index for the second error is from row $2m + 1$ to row $3m$.

```
> dat.aug$o1 <- c(rep(NA, n*T), 1:(n*T), rep(NA, n*T))
> dat.aug$o2 <- c(rep(NA, n*T*2), 1:(n*T))
```

When $t = 1$, we have $\xi_1 = \omega_1$ so that the index set for the errors starts at $t = 2$, going from $n + 1$ to $n \times T$.

We have to define an index set for each state on the observation equation and also a lagged index for the faked zero observations:

```
> dat.aug$xi1 <- c(1:(n*T), 1:(n*T), rep(NA, n*T))
> dat.aug$xi1d <- c(rep(NA, n*T+n), 1:(n*(T-1)), rep(NA, n*T))
> dat.aug$xi2 <- c(1:(n*T), rep(NA, n*T), 1:(n*T))
> dat.aug$xi2d <- c(rep(NA, n*T*2+n), 1:(n*(T-1)))
```

Also, we need to define the weights, because ξ_{t-1} and ω_t have negative signs on the faked zero-observation equation:

```
> dat.aug$wo1 <- dat.aug$wxi1d <- rep(c(0,-1,0), c(n*T, n*T, n*T))
> dat.aug$wo2 <- dat.aug$wxi2d <- rep(c(0,0,-1), c(n*T, n*T, n*T))
```

The dynamic intercept is on the observation equation and in the first m elements of the stacked state observations, the rows from $m + 1$ to $2m$ of the second column of the Y matrix. We assign the weights for this effect as

```
> dat.aug$wxi1 <- rep(1:0, c(n*T*2, n*T))
```

As the covariate x_t in Eq. (8.8) multiplies μ_ξ^* and ξ_t, we need to include it twice in the formula to fit the model properly using the inla function. First, we consider it as an usual covariate (to estimate μ_ξ^*) and then we include it as a weight for the latent field ξ_t.[4] Since ξ_{2t} appears in the observation equation and in the faked zeros equation, we need to define the proper weight. On the observation equation, the weights are exactly given by the covariate values, while in the second equation they are equal to zero for the first $n \times T$ elements (the faked zero observations for the dynamic intercept) and equal to 1 for the last $n \times T$ elements:

```
> dat.aug$wxi2 <- c(as.vector(x2), rep(0:1, c(n*T, n*T)))
```

The formula definition needs to take everything into account, as follows:

```
> form.aug <- Y ~ -1 + x1 + x2 +
+     f(o1, wo1, model="generic1", Cmatrix=stc.mat) +
+     f(o2, wo2, model="generic1", Cmatrix=stc.mat) +
+     f(xi1, wxi1, model="iid",
+        hyper=list(theta=list(initial=-10, fixed=TRUE))) +
+     f(xi1d, wxi1d, copy="xi1", range=c(0,1),
+        hyper=list(beta=list(fixed=FALSE, param=c(0, 1.5)))) +
+     f(xi2, wxi2, model="iid",
+        hyper=list(theta=list(initial=-10, fixed=TRUE))) +
+     f(xi2d, wxi2d, copy="xi2", range=c(0,1),
+        hyper=list(beta=list(fixed=FALSE, param=c(0, 1.5))))
```

where initial=-10 is used as the fixed (fixed=TRUE) low log precision for the two effects to allow it to be flexible here as it can be any value. We make it varying smoothly on time (the value for time t is (almost) a copy of the value for time $t - 1$). It is almost a copy because we put the copy parameter not fixed to one but varying in the (0, 1) interval. We have $0 = \xi_t - \gamma\xi_{t-1} - \omega_t$ by fixing the precision of the faked zero observations on a large enough value.

The γ parameters, estimated through the copy feature, can be outside the stationary range (0, 1). So, we include a restriction on the copy by considering a range interval. When we specify a range interval, the actual copy parameter, named β, is transformed and treated internally as $\theta = \log(-(a - \beta)/(b - \beta))$, where a and b define the range (a, b). So, with $a = 0$ and $b = 1$ we have $\theta = \log(\beta/(1 - \beta))$. In this case, we have to take care of the prior specification on θ which is by default Normal(0, 10). To understand what this prior means on the β scale we have to transform θ back into β. An easy way to do this consists in simulating a sample from the density of θ, applying the transformation $\beta = 1/(1 + \exp(-\theta))$ on the simulated values of θ and looking at the histogram of the values on the β scale. We decide to

---

[4] A weight for a random effect is provided as the second argument of f() function.

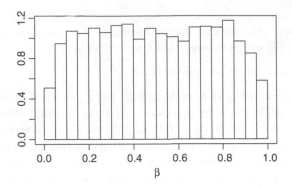

Figure 8.19   Histogram from the simulated prior distribution for the temporal correlation parameter estimated using the copy *feature.*

use a Normal(0, 1) prior for θ, which corresponds to a prior on the β scale whose (simulated) distribution is plotted through an histogram in Figure 8.19.

Finally, we can use the `inla` function. Having specified each term of the likelihood for the zero observations, we have to fix the precision for the Gaussian likelihood equal to a high value; thus, we set `inital=10` for the log precision:

```
> res.aug <- inla(form.aug, c("poisson", "gaussian"),
+            data=dat.aug, E=dat.aug$e,
+            control.family=list(list(), list(
+                hyper=list(theta=list(initial=10, fixed=TRUE)))),
+            control.predictor=list(compute=TRUE, link=1))
```

The option `link=1` is used to specify that the fitted values are computed with the link function from the first likelihood.

Results

We can see the posterior marginal distributions for μ_x and for the model hyperparameters in Figure 8.20; they always cover the true values (vertical lines).

Also, we can see how this works for the latent field. First, we take a look over time in some areas. Figure 8.21 shows the time series for some specific areas.

We can also draw maps for the latent fields on some specific time points. As in the previous example, we use the first, median, and the last time points. To compare true and estimated values, we show the two maps next to each others in Figure 8.22.

We can summarize the results by looking at the correlation between the simulated values for the states and the posterior mean

```
> c(xi1=cor(as.vector(xi1), res.aug$summary.random$xi1$mean),
+    xi2=cor(as.vector(xi2), res.aug$summary.random$xi2$mean))
      xi1        xi2
0.9691602 0.4826942
```

and as before we can conclude that the correlations between observed and estimated values are reasonably large to suggest that the inferential process works well in reproducing the simulated spatio-temporal dependencies.

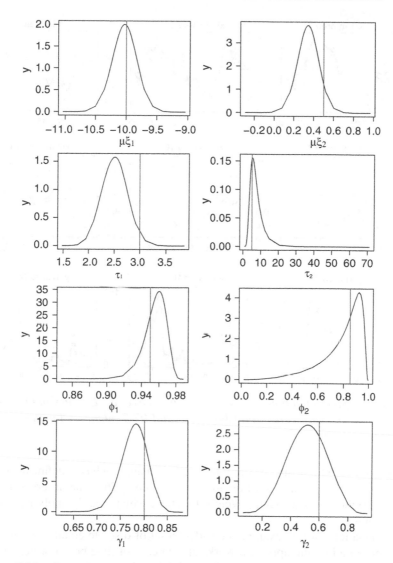

Figure 8.20   Posterior marginal distributions for the dynamic spatio-temporal model with generic1 *used to specify the spatial distribution. Vertical lines represent the true values.*

8.4   Space–time model lowering the time resolution

In this section, we present a type of spatio-temporal model characterized by a high-resolution time series (e.g., hourly data) at different locations. As seen extensively, it is natural and realistic to include some dependency structure in space and time and this makes the model very computational expensive.

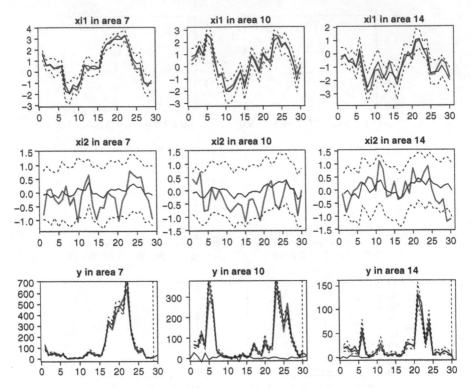

Figure 8.21   Simulated time series (black solid line) of ξ_1, ξ_2 and y in three given areas, posterior mean (gray solid line), 2.5 and 97.5 quantiles for fitted values (dashed lines).

To deal with the high-time resolution, an efficient approach is to define the model on a set of time knots instead of on all the time points. The time observations can be linked to the knots through a weight function, which could simply be a linear interpolation.

The simulation for this example considers a set of discrete equally spaced time points (nevertheless the approach works also in case of time points which are not equally spaced as our approach avoids any kind of data aggregation over time by using a map from the discretized time domain. Let us assume that we have daily data but we specify a model on the months: specifically we suppose to have four observations and consider them as two pairs. The observations for the first pair refer to the end of January and at the beginning of February, while those of the second pair are observed at the beginning of January and at the end of February. It is clear that for the second pair the time difference is bigger. However, if we just use the month as an index, then we assume that the observations on both pairs are equally spaced over time. The approach discussed in this section preserves the distance between observations, so it takes into account that the first pair is closer in time than the second pair.

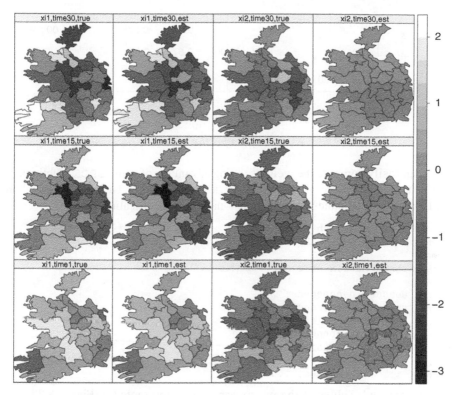

Figure 8.22   Maps of the latent fields, ξ_1 and ξ_2, for the true (simulated) and estimated posterior mean. Each line corresponds to a different time point (1, 15 and 30, from bottom to top).

We start defining the following model for one time series:

$$y_t = \sum_{j=1}^{J} w_{tj} x_j + e_t,$$ (8.11)

where e_t is an independent Gaussian error term with zero mean and precision τ_e. The term x_j is the latent value for the jth knot ($j = 1, \ldots, J$) and can be modeled as previously seen through a first-order autoregressive model; finally w_{ij} is the weight of the linear interpolator for time t on knot j.

Let the set of irregularly observed time points and equally spaced knots be the following:

```
> obst <- c(1:2,4:7,10)
> n <- length(obst)
> knots <- c(2, 5, 8)
> k <- length(knots)
```

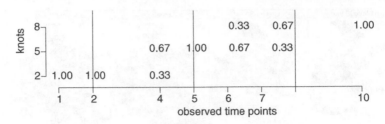

Figure 8.23   Knot weights for the observed time points.

We can easily compute the weights taking advantage of some SPDE functions. In particular, we make use of inla.spde.make.A and inla.mesh.1d, where the latter function creates a one-dimensional mesh specification.

```
> mesh1d <- inla.mesh.1d(loc=knots)
> wmat <- inla.spde.make.A(mesh=mesh1d, loc=obst)
> wmat
7 x 3 sparse Matrix of class "dgCMatrix"

[1,] 1.0000000 0.0000000 .
[2,] 1.0000000 0.0000000 .
[3,] 0.3333333 0.6666667 .
[4,] .         1.0000000 0.0000000
[5,] .         0.6666667 0.3333333
[6,] .         0.3333333 0.6666667
[7,] .         0.0000000 1.0000000
```

The (transposed) values of the matrix wmat are represented in Figure 8.23. The weight matrix is sparse, with at least two nonzero values on each row (column in Figure 8.23). When an observed time point is between two knots, the weight is inversely proportional to the distance from each knot. For example, the observed time point 7 is between knots 5 and 8 and the corresponding weights are $1/3$ and $2/3$. When an observed time point corresponds to a knot or is outer the knots domain, its weight is set equal to 1 and is associated to the nearest knot (see, e.g., the time points 1, 2, 5, and 10 in Figure 8.23).

We now draw samples from the model in Eq. (8.11). First, we need to define the time points for the observations:

```
> n <- 1000
> obst <- 1:n
```

the knots set:

```
> k <- 200
> knots <- seq(n/k, n, n/k) - 0.5*n/k
```

and the weight matrix:

```
> mesh1d <- inla.mesh.1d(loc=knots)
> wmat <- inla.spde.make.A(mesh=mesh1d, loc=obst)
> dim(wmat)
[1] 1000  200
```

We draw the time-series observations at knots from a first-order autoregressive model with the autoregressive parameter γ and variance $1/\tau_x$. Then, the observed time series y is computed as the product of the weight matrix and the simulated values from the AR(1) model (obtained through the `arima.sim` function) plus an error (e) simulated from a zero-mean Normal distribution with variance $1/\tau_e$:

```
> taue <- 5;      taux <- 3;      gamma <- 0.7
> set.seed(1)
> x <- as.vector(arima.sim(n=k,
+                  model=list(ar=gamma), sd=sqrt(1/taux)))
> e <- rnorm(n=n, mean=0, sd=sqrt(1/taue))
> y <- drop(wmat%*%x) + e
```

We can fit two models: one on the set of knots (with and without weights) and another one on the observed time points and then compare them using the DIC. To fit the model on the observed time points we write

```
> formula <- y ~ -1 + f(i, model="ar1")
> ar1 <- inla(formula, data=list(y=y, i=1:n),
+              control.predictor=list(compute=TRUE),
+              control.compute=list(dic=TRUE))
```

while to fit the same model on the reduced set of time points (knots) without weights, we use the following code:

```
> id.mid.knots <- findInterval(obst, c(0.5, knots+n/k))
> ar1k <- inla(formula, data=list(y=y, i=id.mid.knots),
+              control.predictor=list(compute=TRUE),
+              control.compute=list(dic=TRUE))
```

where `findInterval` is used to define the knots associated with each observed time points. Finally, to fit the model on the knots with the weights, we need to provide the weight matrix wmat as projector matrix in `control.predictor`:

```
> ar1w <- inla(formula, data=list(y=y, i=1:k),
+              control.predictor=list(A=wmat, compute=TRUE),
+              control.compute=list(dic=TRUE))
```

Computing the DIC values for all the three models returns:

```
> c(ar1$dic$dic, ar1k$dic$dic, ar1w$dic$dic)
[1] 1488.253 1623.827 1495.867
```

The autoregressive model estimated on the observed time points has the smallest DIC value. However, we can see that the model built on the knots and taking into account the weights has a slightly bigger DIC, while not considering the weights makes the DIC much larger.

We can look at the predicted values and 2.5% and 97.5% quantiles for all the three models in Figure 8.24 (just for the first 50 time points).

We can conclude that the model with the knots is a good simplification in terms of model fit. In our example, the model with the knots provides a reduction of

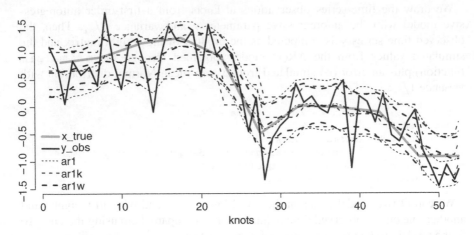

Figure 8.24   Predictions for the first 50 time points from the three models.

the random effect size only by a factor of 5 (we have 200 knots instead of 1000 observed time points), but for more complex models such reduction could be greater and would mean a reduced computational burden, for example, for spatio-temporal models. Of course, there is a tradeoff between accuracy and computer effort, but when it is unfeasible to build a model over all the entire time series this strategy provides a good alternative.

8.4.1   Spatio-temporal model

Here, we present a space–time extension of the previous model, specified as

$$y_t = \sum_{j=1}^{k} w_{tj}\xi_j + e_t,$$

where e_t are Gaussian errors with zero-mean and diagonal-precision matrix (independent over space) and assumed to be independent in time, while ξ_j can be modeled by defining a multivariate structure over time, for example, a dynamic model. As seen in the previous section, the term w_{ij} is the weight of the linear interpolation for time t and knot j. In this example, we assume a simplified version of the space–time dynamic model considered in Section 8.3 (we do not specify any covariate). First, we draw a sample for ξ:

```
> file <- system.file("etc/shapes/eire.shp", package="spdep")[1]
> pol <- readShapePoly(file)
> nbl <- poly2nb(pol)
> nbmat <- Matrix(nb2mat(nbl, style="B"))
> n <- nrow(nbmat)
> T <- 20
```

```
> nnb <- colSums(nbmat)
> tau <- c(1, 5)
> gamma <- 0.7
> Qbp <- tau[1]*(diag(nnb+1e-5) - nbmat)
> xi <- omega <- inla.qsample(n=T, Q=Qbp, seed=1,
+                            constr=list(A=matrix(1,1,n), e=0))
> xi[,1] <- sqrt(1-gamma^2)*omega[,1]
> for (j in 2:T)
+    xi[, j] <- gamma*xi[, j-1] + sqrt(1-gamma^2)*omega[, j]
```

The small value 1×10^{-5} added on the diagonal ensures that the precision matrix is proper. As it is very close to zero, we can assume it zero in the inference step when using the besag model.

Also, to have the simulated values centered around zero we add a linear constraint through the constr argument. This argument lists two elements A and e. A is a matrix $1 \times n$ with 1 and e is zero in our case and it means that $Ax = e$, where x is the random sample.

Then, we define the knots and the observed time points. We have $T = 20$ knots and choose the number of observations equal to four times the number of knots.

```
> knots <- seq(from=2, to=T*4-2, by=4)
> length(knots)
[1] 20
> obst <- 1:(T*4)
> k <- length(obst)
> mesh1d <- inla.mesh.1d(loc=knots)
> wmat <- inla.spde.make.A(mesh=mesh1d, loc=obst)
> dim(wmat)
[1] 80 20
```

Now, we complete the data simulation taking into account that we have the same number of areas, but with different time dimension

```
> yy <- matrix(NA, nrow=nrow(xi), ncol=length(obst))
> set.seed(2)
> for (i in 1:n)
+     yy[i, ] <- drop(wmat %*% xi[i,]) +
+                 rnorm(n=k, mean=0, sd=sqrt(1/tau[2]))
```

To fit the model, we proceed in a similar way as for the first example in Section 8.3. The difference here is that we define a random effects model on a set of knots over time and consider the weight matrix for the interpolation of the effects in the observed time points.

The dataset needs to be organized into a list, as there is a difference in the length of the response and of the index set

```
> ldat <- list(y.resp=as.vector(t(yy)),
+              xi.idx=rep(1:n, each=T), time=rep(1:T, n))
> length(ldat$y.resp)
[1] 2080
> length(ldat$xi.idx)
[1] 520
```

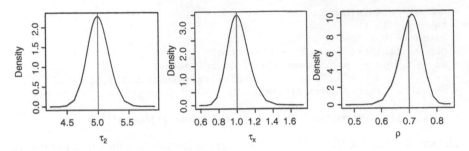

Figure 8.25   *Posterior marginal distributions for the model hyperparameters.*

```
> length(ldat$time)
[1] 520
```

The formula remains the same as before

```
> formula <- y.resp ~ -1 +
+      f(xi.idx, model="besag", graph=nbmat, scale.model=FALSE,
+        group=time, control.group=list(model="ar1"))
```

but now we have to define the projection matrix for the linear predictor, starting from the weight matrix wmat and taking into account that at each time point we have a set of observations over the areas. So, the projection matrix is the Kronecker product of an *n*-dimensional diagonal matrix and of the weight matrix

```
> A <- kronecker(Diagonal(n), wmat)
```

which enters in the control.predictor argument of the inla function

```
> out.st.low <- inla(formula, data=ldat,
+                     control.predictor=list(A=A, compute=TRUE))
```

The posterior distributions of the three hyperparameters (τ_e, τ_x and ρ) are displayed in Figure 8.25.

It is also possible to plot the temporal trend of the latent field ξ for some given areas (see Figure 8.26). Moreover, in Figure 8.27, we provide the maps for the latent fields at some specific time points. The posterior mean maps are similar to the maps of the simulated values.

Finally, it is possible to compute the correlation between the simulated values and the posterior mean, which is above 0.9:

```
> cor(as.vector(xi), out.st.low$summary.random$xi$mean)
[1] 0.9432829
```

and suggests once again that the inferential process works well in reproducing the simulated values.

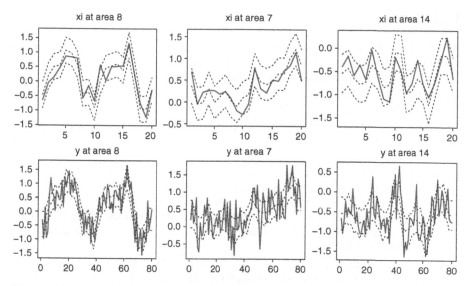

Figure 8.26 Simulated time series of ξ_t and y_t at some given areas (solid gray line), posterior mean and 2.5 and 97.5 quantiles for fitted values (dashed black lines).

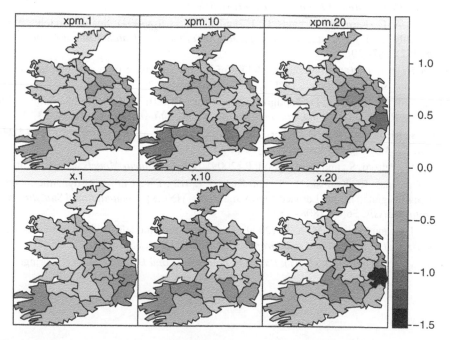

Figure 8.27 Maps of the latent field ξ for the simulated (second line) and posterior mean (first line). Each column corresponds to a different time point (1, 15, and 30, from left to right).

References

Assunção, J. J., Gamerman, D., and Assunção, R. M. (1999). Regional differences in factor productivities of Brazilian agriculture: A space-varying parameter approach. Technical Report, Universidade Federal do Rio de Janeiro, Statistical Laboratory.

Assunção, R. M. and Krainski, E. T. (2009). Neighborhood dependence in Bayesian spatial models. *Biometrical Journal*, **51**(5), 851–869.

Assunção, R. M., Potter, J. E., and Cavenaghi, S. M. (2002). A bayesian space varying parameter model applied to estimating fertility schedules. *Statistics in Medicine*, **21**, 2057–2075.

Bivand, R., with contributions by Micah Altman, Anselin, L., ao, R. A., Berke, O., Bernat, A., Blanchet, G., Blankmeyer, E., Carvalho, M., Christensen, B., Chun, Y., Dormann, C., Dray, S., Halbersma, R., Krainski, E., Legendre, P., Lewin-Koh, N., Li, H., Ma, J., Millo, G., Mueller, W., Ono, H., Peres-Neto, P., Piras, G., Reder, M., Tiefelsdorf, M., and Yu., D. (2012). *SPDEP: Spatial Dependence: Weighting Schemes, Statistics and Models*. R package version 0.5-55.

Cameletti, M., Lindgren, F., Simpson, D., and Rue, H. (2012). Spatio-temporal modeling of particulate matter concentration through the SPDE approach. *Advances in Statistical Analysis*, **97**(2), 109–131.

Gamerman, D., Moreira, A. R. B., and Rue, H. (2003). Space-varying regression models: Specifications and simulation. *Computational Statistics and Data Analysis – Special Issue: Computational Econometrics*, **42**(3), 513–533.

Gelfand, A. E., Kim, H., Sirmans, C. F., and Banerjee, S. (2003). Spatial modeling with spatially varying coefficient processes. *Journal of the American Statistical Association*, **98**(462), 387–396.

Knorr-Held, L. (2000). Bayesian modeling of inseparable space-time variation in disease risk. *Statistics in Medicine*, **19**(17–18), 2555–2567.

Martins, T. G., Simpson, D., Lindgren, F., and Rue, H. (2013). Bayesian computing with INLA: New features. *Computational Statistics and Data Analysis*, **67**(0), 68–83.

Muff, S., Riebler, A., Rue, H., Saner, P., and Held, L. (2013). *Measurement error in GLMMs with INLA*. http://arxiv.org/abs/1302.3065

Petris, G., Petroni, S., and Campagnoli, P. (2009). *Dynamic Linear Models with R*. Springer.

Ruiz-Cárdenas, R., Krainski, E. T., and Rue, H. (2012). Direct fitting of dynamic models using integrated nested Laplace approximations – {INLA}. *Computational Statistics and Data Analysis*, **56**(6), 1808–1828.

Vivar, J. C. and Ferreira, M. A. R. (2009). Spatio-temporal models for Gaussian areal data. *Journal of Computational and Graphical Statistics*, **18**(3), 658–674.

West, M. and Harrison, J. (1997). *Bayesian Forecasting and Dynamic Models*. Springer.

Index